THE A–Z OF WOMEN'S

Also in this series:
ALTERNATIVE HEALTH CARE FOR WOMEN — Patsy Westcott
BRITTLE BONES AND THE CALCIUM CRISIS — Kathleen Mayes
COMING LATE TO MOTHERHOOD — Joan Michelson and Sue Gee
CREDIBILITY GAP — Kathryn Stechert
CYSTITIS: THE NEW APPROACH — Dr Caroline Shreeve
FERTILITY AWARENESS WORKBOOK — Barbara Kass-Annese and Hal Danzer
MENOPAUSE: THE WOMAN'S VIEW — Nikki Henriques and Anne Dickson
NOW OR NEVER? — Yvonne Bostock and Maggie Jones
PRE-MENSTRUAL SYNDROME — Dr Caroline Shreeve
SECOND NINE MONTHS — Judith Gansberg and Dr A Mostel
SINGLE WOMAN'S SURVIVAL GUIDE — Lee Rodwell
WOMAN: HER CHANGING IMAGE — Ann Shearer
WOMEN ON HYSTERECTOMY — Nikki Henriques and Anne Dickson
WOMEN ON RAPE — Jane Dowdeswell
WORKING THROUGH YOUR PREGNANCY — Lee Rodwell
WORKING WOMEN'S GUIDE — Liz Hodgkinson
YOUR BODY — in association with the Maries Stopes Clinic

THE A–Z OF
WOMEN'S HEALTH

by

Christine Ammer

GRAPEVINE

First published in 1983 by Everest House, 79 Madison Avenue, New York, N.Y. 10016, simultaneously with McClelland and Stewart Limited, Toronto, Canada.
This edition first published in 1988

For
My mother,
Dr. Helene Reitmann Parker

Ammer, Christine
    The A–Z of women's health.
    1. Women. Health
    I. Title
    613.04244

ISBN — 0 7225 1611 8

Grapevine is part of the Thorsons Publishing Group, Wellingborough, Northamptonshire, NN8 2RQ, England

Printed in Great Britain by Woolnough Bookbinding Limited, Irthlingborough, Northamptonshire

10 9 8 7 6 5 4 3 2 1

Foreword

The colonel's lady and Judy O'Grady
Are sisters under their skins.

Although Kipling was talking about something quite different, that statement is both true and appropriate when discussing our anatomy and physiology; our reproductive diseases and their outcomes.

Christine Ammer, a layperson with a long experience in women's health and the issues affecting it, has created a compendium of facts and explanations which will be of great value to the laywoman and medical people in training — student doctors or nurses.

Although the A–Z was written by an American, users in the UK, be they men or women, patients, doctors or nurses will find their way about this 'vade–mecum' with ease. After all, women are the same the world over.

Medicine is a dynamic discipline and there are inevitable changes and alterations in its practice and many different opinions. Not every person in health care will agree with everything in this book, nor will the advice given be appropriate to *every* patient, but it gives every patient adequate information so that she may discuss her treatment intelligently with her medical advisers.

For far too long, women have had operations, in particular D and Cs and hysterectomies without really understanding the reasons why it's being done and what the expected outcome will be. In the USA more than 650,000 hysterectomies are performed annually. In the UK D and Cs and hysterectomies are two of the most commonly performed operations. Although the number of women having a hysterectomy by the age of fifty in the UK nowhere near reaches that of the US, there is some cause for concern regarding unnecessary and inappropriate procedures.

Whatever you wish to know, whatever words you find incomprehensible, you will find your answers in this encyclopaedia.

DR PAT LAST
DIRECTOR OF WOMEN'S SCREENING
BUPA MEDICAL CENTRE
1988

Author's note

The underlying assumption of this book is that every woman wants to take responsibility for her own health, and the only way she can act intelligently and safely in her own best interest is to understand the workings of her body and to know what kinds of care and treatment are available. Medicine is not yet a 'hard' science; indeed, it may never be one, and certainly not for many years to come. An enormous number of things about our bodies still are not known or are at best imperfectly understood. Therefore it is especially important to know the various options and to choose among them with the fullest possible information. There is more than one way to deal with breast cancer, more than one way to treat a vaginal infection, more than one way to practice birth control. We women are the major consumers of health care. We live longer than men and see doctors more often. We are entitled to the best care, but we must learn to recognize it and know how to obtain it.

The body of medical knowledge is growing constantly. While great care has been taken to make sure that the information in this book is accurate, new facts are constantly coming to light and new treatments and procedures are being developed. For any serious health problem, therefore, the reader is urged to consult her doctor and, if there is still doubt in her mind, to follow the practice

recommended throughout this book, and by all reputable professionals, and *get a second opinion*. No book can be a substitute for clinical examination, diagnosis, or treatment. If something seems to be wrong, check it out.

The entries in this concise encyclopaedia cover a broad range, from the anatomy of the female and male reproductive systems to the basic workings of the endocrine system, from the events of puberty through those of the childbearing years to menopause and old age. They cover the functioning and malfunctioning of the sexually active woman, the decisions involved in whether or not to bear children, how to prevent pregnancy, and how to overcome infertility. They cover all aspects of pregnancy and birth, as well as some of the common problems that occasionally arise for either mother or baby after birth. Included also are articles pertaining to the maintenance of good health, to diet and exercise, to weight control, drinking, smoking, drug use. They describe what a woman should expect (and demand) during a thorough medical check-up, what tests and procedures are necessary, and when. And finally, they include the principal diseases and disorders that affect women's bodies and minds, their diagnosis, their treatment (including home and herbal remedies as well as prescription drugs and surgery), their outlook, and, in the case of chronic diseases, their effect on a woman's sexuality and childbearing.

Despite the technical nature of some of the material, every effort has been made to present subjects simply and clearly, in everyday language. For this reason comparatively complex subjects, such as the menstrual cycle or the different kinds of mastectomy, are treated at greater length than other, equally important subjects; the space allotted reflects only the practical considerations of adequate explanation. With controversial questions or issues, every attempt has been made to present all sides, including all the known alternatives, and the advantages and disadvantages of each.

I am deeply grateful to the many experts and friends who have answered questions and made valuable suggestions, criticisms, and corrections. Special warm thanks go to Belita Cowan of the National Women's Health Network; Joan Caly of the erstwhile Cambridge Women's Community Health Center; and the many women who have shared their personal experiences concerning health, disease, and medical care with me, expecially Helen Citron Boodman, Sigrid Harrison, Anne Novak, and Maia Sherman. Thanks also is due to the women who expressed and explored their concerns in special workshops, consciousness-raising groups, and other discussion groups. The common ground of our experiences gave the original impetus to this book.

Finally, gratitude and appreciation must go to the practitioners in many fields who have critically read relevant portions of this encyclopedia. They include Cynthia P. Anderson, ACSW, American Association of Sex Education Counselors and Therapists, sex and family therapist; Elisabeth Bing, co-founder American Society for Psychoprophylaxis in Childbirth, author and childbirth educator; Katherine Gulick Fricker, Ed.M., science teacher and naturalist; Peter T. Bruce, M.D., F.R.C.S., Senior Lecturer in Urology, Melbourne University; Stephen Fricker, M.D., Massachusetts Eye and Ear Infirmary; A. Gordon Gauld, M.D., formerly obstetrics-gynaecology staff, Boston Hospital for Women; Nancy Greenleaf, R.N., Ph.D., Professor, University of Southern Maine School of Nursing; Cheryl E. Kraley, M.S., R.N., R.N.C., certified nurse-practitioner in obstetrics-gynaecology, Harvard Community Health Plan; James Gavin Manson, M.D., Chief Orthopaedic Surgeon, Mt. Auburn Hospital; Esther Rome, Boston Women's Health Collective and Ananda Health Collective, author, nutritionist, and masseuse; David Satcher, M.D., Ph.D., Chairman, Department of Community Medicine and Family Practice, Morehouse College School of Medicine; Nathan T. Sidley, M.D., Fellow, American Psychiatric Association and President, American Academy of Psychiatry and the Law; David Singer, M.D., American Diabetes Association, private practice; Vincent R. Sites, M.D., Teaching Associate in Radiology, Massachusetts General Hospital, and private practice; Louis R. Slattery, M.D., Acting Director of Surgery, Bellevue Hospital; Samuel Stein, M.D., Assistant Director, M.I.T. Health Service; and Alan Ziskind, M.D., M.P.H., Fellow, American Academy of Pediatrics, private practice. Thanks are also due to Clare Glassman at Women Against Rape, for her work on the 'Rape' entry. This book has been vastly improved through their expertise. Its errors and shortcomings remain my own responsibility.

CHRISTINE AMMER

How to use this book

The terms in this encyclopaedia, whether they consist of one word or several words, are listed in alphabetic order, letter by letter, up to the comma in case of inversion. Identical or related terms with different meanings are defined under a single heading in a series of number definitions.

Terms that are mentioned in one entry but are further explained in another, where the reader is advised to seek them out, are printed in small capital letters, for example, PAGET'S DISEASE or LABOUR or CANCER, BREAST.

For terms that have several common names, or both common and scientific names, all the important versions of the term are included. In the case of herbs, common usage varies considerably, the same name sometimes being used for several different herbs, so to avoid confusion every herb mentioned is identified by its botanical name.

The reader who wants to look up all the articles pertaining to a larger subject such as birth control or diagnostic tests and procedures, is advised to look in the subject index, beginning on page 329, which lists all the articles pertaining to various large topics.

A

Abnormal presentation In childbirth, any position in which a part of the baby other than the crown of its head will emerge first (see under CEPHALIC PRESENTATION). The principal kinds of abnormal presentation are breech, brow, face, posterior, and shoulder; there is a separate entry for each of them.

Abortifacient A drug, herb, or other chemical agent that dilates the cervix and/or causes the uterus to contract, resulting in the ending of a pregnancy before the foetus can survive on its own. Plants of various kinds have been used for this purpose since ancient times. Among the most effective for cervical dilatation is LAMINARIA, a marine plant whose stem gradually expands when it is moist. Dried laminaria, when inserted in the cervix, causes it to open and, over a period of hours, gradually stretches the cervical canal. It does not, however, induce uterine contractions.

A number of herbs are said to be EMMENAGOGUES, that is, they allegedly induce menstruation delayed by illness or emotional stress, and sometimes also by pregnancy. As abortifacients they allegedly work best when taken very early after conception, even before the next menstrual period is due, and generally they must be brewed to a fairly concentrated strength. When effective, they then induce abdonimal cramps and uterine contractions, ending in abortion. This procedure also tends to be accompanied by pain, vomiting, and diarrhoea; indeed, some herbalists warn that an herb-induced abortion is more traumatic than an early medical procedure such as VACUUM ASPIRATION. In addition, some vegetable compounds so used are toxic in large doses, and the oil of at least two plants, pennyroyal (or squawmint; *Mentha pulegium*) and Eastern red cedar (*Juniperus virginiana*), has caused a number of deaths. Among the herbs said to be effective abortifacients are blue cohosh or squaw root (*Caulophyllum thalictroides*), common rue (*Ruta graveolens*), pennyroyal, black cohosh or black snakeroot (*Cimicifuga racemosa*), and tansy (*Chrysanthemum* or *Tanacetum vulgare*). The last three are toxic in large doses, and black cohosh should be avoided if a woman has low blood pressure. An abortifacient long used in the American Deep South is cotton bark (*Gossypium herbaceum*), which brings on uterine contractions when chewed. The cotton tree is often a host to ERGOT, a parasitic fungus whose derivatives have long been used in childbirth under medical supervision to strengthen uterine contractions.

A more recent discovery that stimulates uterine contractions and may effectively terminate pregnancies of four to eight weeks – that is, before the second missed menstrual period – are PROSTAGLANDINS, compounds naturally occurring in various animal tissues, including human, that have been synthesized in the laboratory. They are used in a vaginal suppository, which causes uterine contractions to begin a few hours after insertion. For pregnancies of longer duration, prostaglandin suppositories tend to be ineffective or to result in incomplete abortion, with part of the products of conception being retained; then bleeding continues for more than two weeks, and a curettage, either vacuum or surgical, must be performed to eliminate the remaining tissue.

In pregnancies of sixteen weeks or longer, the replacement of some of the amniotic fluid with a strong solution of salt, urea, or prostaglandins brings on labour (see AMNIOINFUSION).

Where therapeutic abortion has not been available, women have used a variety of ineffective but often life-endangering agents to try to end a pregnancy. Among them are concentrated soap solution used as a douche, the insertion of suppositories of potassium permanganate, and the ingestion of quinine pills, or of castor oil or other strong laxatives. None of these is an effective abortifacient.

Some authorities point out that both intrauterine devices and some oral contraceptives are actually abortifacients, since they do not prevent the fertilization of an egg by a sperm but rather prevent the implantation of the egg in the uterine wall, with the result that it is expelled during the next menstrual period. See also ABORTION.

Abortion The interruption or loss of any pregnancy before the foetus is viable (capable of living). In common usage, however, a *spontaneous* or *natural abortion* is usually called a MISCARRIAGE, and the term 'abortion' is reserved for *induced* or *elective abortion*, that is, the intentional termination of a pregnancy. A *therapeutic abortion* is an elective abortion that is legal; a *criminal abortion* is an illegal abortion. The procedures used for elective abortion depend on the length of the pregnancy. For pregnancies of twelve weeks or less, Menstrual extraction or VACUUM ASPIRATION (definition 1) have largely replaced surgical dilatation and curettage (D AND C). For pregnancies of thirteen to eighteen weeks, DILATATION AND EVACUATION are used, and for sixteen to twenty-four weeks, AMNIOINFUSION or HYSTEROTOMY.

Unlike most medical procedures, abortion has long been the subject of moral and legal controversy, owing to disagreement as to what constitutes a living human being and when life actually begins. Those who believe that a life is created at the moment of conception regard abortion as equivalent to murder. Many other views have prevailed, ranging from the idea that life begins when a foetus's movements first are felt (St Thomas Aquinas) to a particular time period after conception (Aristotle said forty days for boys and ninety days for girls) to after delivery (the ancient Hebrews). In the late 19th century Pope Leo XIII declared that all abortion is a sin, even if it is performed to save the mother's life, and the present-day Roman Catholic Church has retained this view. During the course of the 19th century most countries of the Western world made abortion illegal. This did not prevent women from seeking abortions, often from unskilled persons who performed the procedure for money alone and frequently botched the job. These criminal abortions were often *septic abortions*, that is, serious complications (usually infection and/or haemorrhage) resulted from them. The women who survived them often could not bear subsequent children, either because of scar tissue blocking their tubes or because the only way their lives had been saved was by hysterectomy (removal of the UTERUS).

In Britain the 1967 abortion act allows abortions to be carried out legally when there is a greater risk to the life or physical and mental health of the woman and her existing children than if the pregnancy were allowed to continue. It also allows for abortion when there is a substantial risk of the child being born with a serious mental or physical handicap. Two doctors have to certify that these conditions have been satisfied.

Women who are considering abortion should remember that the earlier it is performed, the safer it is.

In Britain abortions are either carried out in an NHS hospital, at a clinic run by one of the charitable organizations such as the British Pregnancy Advisory Service, or privately by a gynaecologist. Referral to a hospital is carried out by the woman's family doctor or alternatively she can approach one of the charitable organizations directly.

Prior to performing an abortion a doctor should review the woman's medical and menstrual history, with special attention to disorders contraindicating abortion in a clinic (such as a cardiac condition or bleeding disorders); administer a pregnancy test and blood tests for anaemia and blood type, as well as Rh factor and venereal disease; check blood pressure, temperature, pulse, and respiration; perform breast and pelvic examinations; and take a Pap smear and gonorrhaea culture. Rh-negative women can have serious difficulties with a later pregnancy if they are not given anti-D immune globulin within seventy-two hours following an abortion (or delivery or miscarriage; see RH FACTOR). Many hospitals and clinics provide a trained counsellor to discuss the woman's decision with her, as well as to explain the procedure in detail and advise her on birth control methods. When there is no such counsellor, it is up to the doctor to explain the procedure and discuss subsequent birth control. See also ABORTIFACIENT, HABITUAL MISCARRIAGE.

Abruptio placentae also *placental abruption, premature separation of the placenta*. The separation of all or part of the PLACENTA from the uterine wall after the twentieth week of pregnancy but before the baby is delivered. Such detachment can also occur before the twentieth week and is a frequent cause of MISCARRIAGE. However, the clinical features of early and later detachment differ, the latter having far more serious consequences. Along with PLACENTA PRAEVIA, abruptio placentae is one of the two most common causes of haemorrhage in late pregnancy, but it is still relatively rare, occuring mostly in women who have borne six or more children. The cause is unknown, and the symptoms vary, depending on the degree of placenta separation and how much blood loss is involved. Bleeding tends to begin just under the placenta, which by the seventh month of pregnancy is generally attached to the fundus, front, or rear wall of the uterus. Blood accumulates and the placenta begins to break loose from its delicate fastening. In some cases, the blood passes through the cervix and out of the vagina (external haemorrhage), in others it is retained inside the uterus (concealed haemorrhage), and in still others some blood is retained and some is expelled. Concealed haemorrhage is the most dangerous because it hides the severity of the condition more than profuse vaginal bleeding does. During this process the uterus becomes tightly contracted, point tenderness develops, the patient begins to show signs of shock, and there are signs of foetal distress, including absence of a foetal heartbeat.

Aburptio placentae calls for immediate emergency treatment, with transfusions to replace lost blood and fight shock, antibiotics to protect against infection, and delivery of the foetus, either vaginally, with labour induced through rupture of the membranes and/or administering OXYTOCIN, or surgically, by CAESAREAN SECTION. Most authorities believe the foetus should be delivered within six hours, the method chosen depending on the degree of abruption. Although prompt treatment will nearly always save the mother, the foetus, which depends on the placenta for its oxygen, has much less chance for survival – practically none in severe cases and only forty to seventy per cent in moderate to mild cases. Many obstetricians believe an immediate Caesarean section yeilds the best results for mother and baby.

Abscess 1 An accumulation of pus in a well-circumscribed area, resulting from acute bacterial infection. Abscesses can occur in many parts of the body, both internally and externally.

2 **Pelvic abscess** An abscess inside the genital tract, usually following childbirth, abortion, or surgery or, more rarely, in the ovaries or Fallopian tubes as a result of PELVIC INFLAMMATORY DISEASE. Such abscesses are usually caused by bacterial infection. The bacteria may already be present in the vagina or, more often, are introduced from the outside (by nonsterile instruments, for example). Early symptoms are pain in the pelvic region and the development of a fever. With severe infection, high temperature, chills, vomiting, and an abnormally fast heartbeat may also occur, singly or in combination. The white blood count will rise markedly, and a softened area becomes discernible in the pelvic mass. Treatment is usually with antibiotics, often a combination of two drugs administered intravenously, the kind depending on what organisms are found to cause the infection. As soon as the abscess has ripened and begun to drain, a soft rubber tube may be inserted into the pelvic area through the abdomen and left in place for several weeks, until drainage is complete. See also PUERPERAL FEVER

3 **Breast abscess** Also *submammary abscess*. An abscess that develops most often during breast-feeding when the nipples become dry and cracked. These cracks, or fissures, give access to bacteria, often staphylococci, present on the skin or in the baby's mouth. The area around the fissure becomes red, swollen, and tender. Fever and chills may occur, and soon a large hard lump is palpable. Treatment consists of antibiotics, and when the abscess ripens surgical drainage may be performed. Breast abscess was once a very common occurrence after childbirth, especially with a first baby, but today early antibiotic treatment frequently cures such infections before an abscess can form. See also MASTITIS.

Absolute contraindication See under CONTRAINDICATION.

Abstinence, periodic See under NATURAL FAMILY PLANNING.

Acini (*Sing. acinus.*) The milk-producing glands in the breast. Each lobe inside the female BREAST is made up of many smaller lobules, which in turn contain anywhere from ten to one hundred acini. Each acinus is made up of glandular cells spherically arranged around a central space, or lumen. The cells secrete milk into the lumen, which is connected to a collecting duct. The acini and ducts are surrounded by a layer of cells with the ability to contract. When they contract, they produce a milking action, that is, they express milk from the lumen into the collecting duct; from there it is in turn forced through other ducts into the terminal duct for each lobe, which exits on the surface of the nipple. See also LACTATION.

Acne A common inflammatory skin disease, most often affecting the face, neck, chest, and upper back. It is characterized by lesions called comedones (pimples), pustules (pus-filled lesions), and sometimes cysts. Contrary to older thought, acne is not the result of eating certain foods like chocolate and fats, nor of overindulging in sexual fantasies or masturbation. Rather, it is caused by a complex interaction among hormones, sebum (produced by the sebaceous or oil glands of the skin), and bacteria. It usually begins at PUBERTY, when the increase in androgens – male hormones produced in girls by the adrenal gland and in boys by both the testes and adrenals – causes an increase in the size and activity of the sebaceous glands. The glands secrete more oil, some of the tiny follicles on the skin become blocked, and comedones form. A simple blockage, called a *blackhead* or *open comedo*, is an oil-blocked pore, part of which is exposed to air and turns dark, or black. A *closed comedo*, or *whitehead*, forms in the same way except that the pore has no opening to the air, the oil cannot drain, and a small cyst forms under the skin. Bacterial action causes pus to form, seen on the outside as a small white area; often the area around the whitehead is painful. Occasionally acne will erupt later in life, in women particularly premenstrually (sometimes flaring up before each menstrual period), or while taking oral contraceptives, or after discontinuing oral contraceptives. In these instances, too, the triggering mechanism seems to be changed hormone levels, though the culprit then is thought to be progesterone, which apparently is somewhat similar to the androgens. With post-Pill acne the condition usually clears up within six months of stopping oral contraceptives.

Treatment for acne, basically palliative, depends on the severity of the case. With superficial acne, washing the face thoroughly two or three times a day with either a mild toilet soap or one containing special drying agents (resorcinol, salicylic acid, or benzoyl peroxide) is recommended. Greasy lotions and cosmetics should be avoided. The hair should also be kept clean – washed two or three times a week – since oily hair can aggravate the eruptions. Sunlight (in moderate doses) and topical irritating agents, which cause dryness and scaling, may dry up superficial lesions. Tretinoin (vitamin A acid) in liquid or gel form may be effective but must be used with caution; it is applied nightly, or less often, for several weeks – during which time exposure to sunlight and other medications must be avoided – and usually requires several weeks to take effect. Other topical irritants include benzoyl peroxide and various sulphur resorcinol combinations, applied twice a day. Squeezing and other manipulation of the comedones and pustules, except with a special extractor, are to be avoided, because they can produce permanent scars. For severe acne, a course of antibiotic therapy for several months, usually tetracycline, may be helpful, but it should be noted that this drug makes women more prone to vaginal infection, especially YEAST INFECTION, and long-term use can lead to further complications. Cryotherapy (freezing skin to make it peel) sometimes helps. X-ray therapy, topical application of corticosteroids, and the use of hormones in general are not recommended. No matter how severe the case, acne nearly always clears up by itself after puberty when hormone levels subside, which is the only real cure.

Acromegaly Overproduction of the pituitary growth hormone, which is marked by excessive body growth, especially of the hands, feet, nose, and lower jaw. Laboratory tests will reveal the presence of an increase in the pituitary hormones and usually a decrease in sex hormones, resulting in amenorrhoea (no menstruation) in young women. Acromegaly may be caused by a pituitary tumour, which is usually treated with radiation therapy or surgery.

Acute Developing suddenly, having severe symptoms, and usually (but not always) brief in duration. The opposite of acute is CHRONIC.

Adenocarcinoma 1 A cancer involving gland tissue (see CANCER), or one whose cells take the form of gland tissue. Most breast cancers are adenocarcinomas.
2 **Clear-cell adenocarcinoma** A cancer of the vagina and cervix first noted in the 1960s in daughters of women who had received diethylstilboestrol (DES) while pregnant. In normal women the vaginal lining has no gland tissue, so adenocarcinomas cannot develop there, but many daughters of women who took DES while pregnant have been found to have many tiny glands in their vagina (see ADENOSIS, definition 1), presumably caused by DES in the developing foetus. Since that discovery and the realization that DES daughters, as they are called, have a much higher risk of developing vaginal and cervical cancer, there has been a widespread effort to locate and warn all such women to undergo frequent examination. See also DIETHYLSTILBOESTROL.
3 **Of the uterus** The most common kind of uterine cancer, arising in the endometrium (uterine lining). See CANCER, ENDOMETRIAL.

Adenofibroma Another name for FIBROADENOMA.

Adenomyosis A condition in which fragments of endometrial tissue (from the lining of the uterus) become embedded in the muscular wall of the uterus. Like ENDOMETRIOSIS, it represents a displacement of endometrial tissue. It tends to occur somewhat later, between the ages of thirty-five and fifty. The symptoms of adenomyosis include menorrhagia (longer, more profuse menstrual periods) and dysmenorrhoea (painful periods), which range from mild pressure and discomfort to severe, colicky pain (caused when the endometrial tissue becomes swollen). Pelvic examination shows the uterus to be enlarged, soft, and boggy. For minor symptoms no treatment is required. More severe symptoms may be treated with hormones to interrupt the menstrual cycle, as in endometriosis, or a D AND C to scrape out some of the endometrial tissue. If neither treatment is effective and severe pain persists, hysterectomy (surgical removal of the uterus) may be recommended. Adenomyosis tends to disappear after menopause, when oestrogen production is greatly reduced.

Adenosis 1 The presence of abnormal, mucus-secreting gland tissue in the cervix or vagina. It is an extremely rare condition except in daughters of women who took DIETHYLSTILBOESTROL (DES) during the first trimester of pregnancy, about 90 per cent of whom have been found to have adenosis. Since it is believed to be a precancerous lesion, which may develop into ADENOCARCINOMA (see definition 2), careful diagnosis and regular follow-up care are urged. Diagnosis involves a SCHILLER TEST and a biopsy on any tissue that does not absorb the iodine stain; COLPOSCOPY is even more accurate. If adenosis is found, a PAP SMEAR and pelvic examination should be performed every six months, and colposcopy at least yearly. Some doctors treat the condition with more aggressive methods, ranging from electric cautery (burning) and cryosurgery (freezing) to surgical excision of the abnormal tissue, but most prefer a more conservative approach. Some doctors recommend avoiding the use of oral contraceptives lest they encourage the growth of the lesions, but others see no connection between the two.
   2 See SCLEROSING ADENOSIS.

Adhesion Also *synechia, scar tissue.* A dense layer of connective tissue that forms over a healing abrasion, cut, or other lesion. In the pelvic area, especially in the Fallopian tubes, uterus, and cervix, adhesions can cause infertility (see ASHERMAN'S SYNDROME).

Adjuvant treatment Any treatment used in addition to some other treatment in order to enhance its effects. The term is used particularly for additional treatment following surgery for CANCER, such as radiation therapy, hormone therapy, and/or chemotherapy.

Adnexae Neighbouring organs. This term is frequently used by gynaecologists and obstetricians for the organs adjacent to the uterus, that is, the Fallopian tubes and ovaries.

Adolescence See PUBERTY.

Adolescent nodule A smooth, round enlargement directly under the nipple of the breast, seen most often in girls of nine to eleven and in boys aged twelve to fourteen. The nipple is usually tender to the touch. The nodule results from hormone stimulation of gland tissue during puberty, a condition that generally subsides after some months. No treatment of any kind is advisable.

Adrenalectomy Surgical removal of the ADRENAL GLANDS, a treatment sometimes used for advanced breast cancers whose growth is stimulated by oestrogen (see OESTROGEN-RECEPTOR ASSAY). Since the adrenal glands produce some oestrogen, their removal reduces the levels of that hormone. After such surgery the patient must receive replacement of the vital adrenal hormones, usually in the form of hydrocortisone, for the rest of her life. Adrenalectomy may be performed at the same time as oophorectomy (removal of the ovaries) or, if the cancer is progressing despite oophorectomy, as an additional procedure. In postmenopausal women with an oestrogen-dependent malignancy, adrenalectomy is sometimes performed before oophorectomy. However as yet not enough cases have been studied to predict the effectiveness of adrenalectomy combined with radical mastectomy. See also CANCER, BREAST. Adrenalectomy may also be performed in aldosteronism (see ALDOSTERONE).

Adrenal glands a pair of ENDOCRINE glands that are located on top of each kidney (*ad-* means 'on', *renal* means 'pertaining to the kidney'). Each gland consists of a *cortex*, a firm outer portion that constitutes most of the gland, and a *medulla*, a soft inner part. The medulla produces the hormone *adrenalin* while the cortex produces more than thirty different hormones, some of which are indispensable to life. The adrenals also produce other steriods such as oestrogen, which can in some cases aggravate a disease process. Thus they are sometimes removed in treating an advanced oestrogen-dependent breast cancer (see ADRENALECTOMY).

The adrenal glands are subject to a number of diseases, two of which in particular affect women, causing menstrual irregularities and other problems. They are ADRENOGENITAL SYNDROME and CUSHING'S SYNDROME.

Adrenal hyperplasia See ADRENO-GENITAL SYNDROME.

Adrenal steroid A steroid hormone produced by the adrenal glands. See also HORMONE.

Adrenogenital syndrome Also *adrenal virilism, adrenal hyperplasia*. A disorder, usually present from birth, that is characterized by overproduction of androgens by the adrenal glands, resulting in the development of male secondary sex characteristics in girls and precocious sexual development in boys. The effects depend on the age of the patient and are more marked in females. The underlying cause is usually either a tumour of the adrenal glands or hyperplasia (overgrowth of gland tissue), which in turn may be caused by an inherited enzyme deficiency that prevents the adrenal glands from synthesizing cortisol. The principal symptom is hirsutism (excess body hair), which appears even in mild cases. Other symptoms include baldness, acne, deepening of the voice, cessation of menstruation, atrophy of the uterus, deformed genitals (especially growth of the clitoris so that it resembles a small penis), decreased breast size, and increased muscularity. Treatment with cortisone usually eliminates the condition; in the congenital form of the disease it must be continued for life.

Afterbirth Another name for PLACENTA.

Afterpains Uterine contractions following the delivery of a baby. See under CONTRACTION, UTERINE

Agalactia The inability to lactate (secrete milk) after childbirth. True total agalactia is a rare condition. When the quantity of milk secreted is smaller than desired, the condition can usually be corrected by more frequent stimulation of the breasts by suckling. See also BREAST-FEEDING; LACTATION.

Age, childbearing In theory, the years from the first ovulation following MENARCHE (average age, 12.8) through MENOPAUSE (average age, 50). Physically, the ideal years for childbearing are from the late teens through the twenties. Indeed, any woman who becomes pregnant when she is under the age of sixteen or over thirty-four is considered at risk (see HIGH-RISK PREGNANCY). The risk is to both mother and child. Pregnant women over thirty-four run a greater risk of developing complications such as pre-eclampsia and placenta praevia. Chronic conditions that are more common in older women, such as diabetes, kidney disease, hypertension, and heart disease, add to possible complications. Labour and delivery are likely to be more difficult, especially with a first baby. Labour tends to be prolonged, ABNORMAL PRESENTATION is more common, and postpartum haemorrhage (from weak uterine contractions after delivery) also occurs more often. Other hazards to the baby, apart from those named above, concern the greater likelihood of BIRTH DEFECTS. One genetic defect associated with older parents is DOWN'S SYNDROME (mongolism), the risk for which is ten times higher after the age of forty than it is for a woman in her twenties. Other chromosomal abnormalities also related to maternal age, along with nonchromosomal defects such as cleft lip and palate, congenital heart defects, spina bifida, hydrocephalus, and cerebral palsy. Since certain defects can be detected by AMNIOCENTESIS, some obstetricians recommend that all pregnant women of thirty-five and older undergo this procedure. Age also affects the capacity of the uterus to sustain a foetus, so that with increasing age there is a higher risk of miscarriage and stillbirth. Young teenagers, on the other hand, are at high risk as well. They have a higher incidence of pregnancy-induced hypertension, pre-eclampsia and eclampsia, and their babies tend to have a low birth weight. Anaemia is also more common, perhaps as a result of poor nutrition. However, since there are important considerations besides physical ones for parenthood, ideally all factors should be examined and weighed before undertaking a pregnancy. See also PREGNANCY COUNSELLING.

Agoraphobia An irrational fear (phobia) of open spaces, which for most sufferers usually means any place other than their own home. A person with agoraphobia who leaves home (for a shop, a street, an airport – almost anywhere) will often experience an *anxiety attack*, that is, a sense of overwhelming panic, with such physical manifestations as nausea, sweating, rapid heartbeat, and dizziness. (See also ANXIETY.) Agoraphobia is much more common in women than men, and tends to strike early, often beginning in the late teens or early twenties. It has been variously explained. According to traditional psychoanalytic theory, patients develop phobias in order to avoid certain objects or situations. They often have the feeling that something terrible, but usually nameless will happen to them. In extreme cases of agoraphobia fear may keep a person a virtual prisoner in the home, afraid of venturing outdoors at all. Psychoanalytic treatment of agoraphobia, directed at having the patient discover the roots of the fear in her past, has not been very successful. More patients seem to benefit from a behaviourist approach, which is less concerned with the source of the fear than with conditioning a person not to be afraid.

Albumin, urinary Also *albuminuria*. The principal protein found in the urine of persons suffering from a variety of kidney diseases. It is not present in normal urine. In pregnant women it is a warning sign of PREECLAMPSIA, and for this reason testing the urine for albumin is a standard part of each antenatal check-up.

Alcohol use The drinking of alcoholic beverages, which in moderation – a drink or two a day – is generally thought to be harmless for most individuals, but which in larger quantities can be harmful and become addictive, so that a person becomes severely dependent on alcohol. While the moderate use of alcohol is actually thought to be of some physical benefit to the heart, heavy drinking can damage the heart and blood vessels. Heavy drinking is also associated with cancer (particularly when combined with heavy cigarette smoking), especially of the mouth, throat, larynx, and oesophagus, as well as with liver disease. Alcohol increases the body's need for two B vitamins, niacin and thiamine, which are used in its metabolism, and for folic acid, with whose absoprtion and storage it interferes. Other disorders associated with alcoholism (alcohol addiction) are peptic ulcer, severe anaemia, and a variety of mental and emotional disorders.

Heavy drinking during pregnancy can cause serious and irreversible birth defects. Babies born of alcoholic mothers are at risk of developing the *foetal alcohol syndrome*, a pattern of physical and mental defects that includes severe growth deficiency, heart defects, malformed facial features, a small head, abnormalities of fine motor co-ordination, and mental retardation. Since it is not known exactly how much alcohol intake will endanger a foetus, it generally is recommended that a pregnant woman limit herself to two mixed drinks (each containing 1½ ounces of 86-proof alcohol) per day, *or* two five-ounce servings of table wine, *or* two twelve-ounce servings of beer. These amounts represent a maximum of daily consumption; one cannot safely have four drinks a day and none the next, since it is the concentration of alcohol (which passes through the PLACENTA) that damages the baby. Furthermore, some authorities warn that even two drinks can be detrimental in some individuals, and to be absolutely safe no alcohol should be consumed during pregnancy.

Alopecia See HAIR LOSS.

Amenorrhoea 1 Failure to menstruate at an age when regular menstruation is the norm and in the absence of pregnancy or lactation. *Physiological amenorrhoea* refers to lack of menstruation at times when it normally does not occur, that is, before puberty, during pregnancy and lactation, and after menopause.

2 **Primary amenorrhoea** Failure to begin menstruating by the age of eighteen. Although many adolescent girls worry if they do not yet menstruate when most of their peers have begun, the course of puberty and the age of MENARCHE vary so widely that there need be no real concern until the age of sixteen, *provided* there are other signs of early pubertal changes (growth spurt, underarm or pubic hair, breast development). Many doctors carry out some preliminary tests on a girl who has never menstruated by the age of sixteen, as much to reassure the patient as to rule out serious disease. One phenomenon that may be ruled out is *cryptomenorrhoea*, in which menstrual

bleeding does occur but is retained inside the vagina by some anatomical obstruction, such as an imperforate HYMEN. Another is the presence of a pituitary tumour, which can be investigated by means of a skull X-ray. Treatment for primary amenorrhoea is not usually undertaken until the age of eighteen.

Primary anenorrhoea is most often caused by some disturbance in the relationship between the pituitary gland and the ovaries (see MENSTRUAL CYCLE for further explanation), and only rarely by some anatomical problem (such as lack of a vagina, uterus, or ovaries). Amenorrhoea is not a disease but a symptom. However, it may be *idiopathic*, that is, the most thorough examination and extensive tests may uncover no discernible physical or emotional cause. Diagnosis is nevertheless directed at finding an organic cause, usually by process of elimination. It begins with taking a very detailed history, including acute or chronic illness of any kind, the possibility of unsuspected pregnancy, recent weight gain or loss, symptoms of other metabolic disease (thyroid, diabetes, etc.), and both the patient's early developmental history and the family history relating to menstruation, fertility, metabolic disease, and tuberculosis. It is followed by a careful physical examination, preferably including a pelvic examination. However, the position, size, and shape of the uterus and ovaries can be often determined by rectal examination if a vaginal examination seems difficult or disturbing. A skull X-ray may be taken to rule out pituitary tumours, and tests made of both vaginal and buccal (inside the mouth) smears and of the urine for the presence of hormones and for chromosomal abnormalities. An X-ray of the hands may show

whether or not the long bones of the fingers show pubertal changes indicating that menarche is likely to occur in a few months.

If the physical examination reveals no abnormalities, the laboratory findings are close to normal, and there are no symptoms and signs of other disease, the diagnosis is probably *delayed puberty*, a matter of slow maturation that will eventually correct itself. Sometimes it is simply a matter of a girl's attaining the CRITICAL WEIGHT apparently needed for menarche. Many doctors, therefore, recommend a wait-and-see approach, with follow-up scheduled every six to twelve months.

3 **Secondary amenorrhoea** Ceasing to menstruate for more than three months after normal menstrual periods have been established but well before the usual age for menopause. It must first be distinguished from *oligomenorrhoea*, infrequent periods with intervals of more than thirty-eight days but less than ninety days between periods, and *hypomenorrhoea*, fewer days of menstrual flow, or scanty flow, or both. There is so much variation in cycles among perfectly healthy women, as well as considerable variation in the same woman, that unless symptoms are extreme or there is another problem, such as inability to conceive, there is no pressing need to investigate. Especially during the first months or even years following menarche, many young women have very irregular cycles. Naturally, pregnancy and early menopause must both be ruled out before proceeding with diagnostic tests.

Diagnosis again involves a detailed history, physical examination (including pelvic examination), skull X-ray, and laboratory tests of urine and vaginal smears. An endometrial biopsy may be indicated if hormone patterns show a high risk of endometrial cancer. If no serious disease is suspected, secondary amenorrhoea may need no treatment unless a woman wishes to become pregnant. In that even hormone therapy, particularly stimulating the pituitary gland with progesterone alone or in combination with oestrogen to establish bleeding, and then stimulating ovulation by means of the FERTILITY PILL, is often effective.

Causes of secondary amenorrhoea include, *in addition* to those listed for primary amenorrhoea (see definition 2 above), damage to the pituitary resulting from postpartum haemorrhage and/or shock (SHEEHAN'S DISEASE); destruction of the endometrium by overvigorous curettage (ASHERMAN'S SYNDROME), radiation therapy, or an abnormally adherent placenta in a prior pregnancy; ovarian cysts and/or tumours; and drugs, including oral contraceptives (see definition 4 below). Extreme weight loss and/or very vigorous physical activity, such as that of ballet dancers or professional athletes, also may lead to amenorrhoea, (see also CRITICAL WEIGHT).

In addition, following childbirth there may be postpartum amenorrhoea and lactation amenorrhoea (it is considered amenorrhoea if it persists for more than three months after delivery in a non-breast-feeding mother, or longer than six weeks after nursing is discontinued), in which the continued production of PROLACTIN by the pituitary is not inhibited in the normal way by the hypothalamus; this condition may be self-correcting in time or be corrected by hormone therapy.

For herbal remedies used to bring on a delayed period, see EMMENAGOGUE.

3 See POST-PILL AMENORRHOEA.

Amniocentesis A technique of removing fluid from the AMNIOTIC SAC surrounding a foetus in order to detect certain genetic disorders and birth defects (including Down's syndrome, or mongolism, and Tay-Sachs disease), Rh disease of pregnancy, and to assess the baby's maturity. First developed in 1966, the procedure takes only a few minutes to perform under local anaesthetic and is usually done on an outpatient basis. However, it cannot be performed until a pregnancy has advanced to sixteen weeks. Usually the position of placenta and foetus is first determined by ULTRASOUND. A needle is introduced through the abdomen and uterine wall into the amniotic sac, and 10 to 20 cc. (millilitres) of amniotic fluid are removed for analysis. Because of the foetal cells contained in the fluid must first grow in a special nutrient medium, chromosome analysis usually takes from two to four weeks, and metabolic studies, which require a larger number of cells may take even longer. It is advisable to undergo amniocentesis with an obstetrician who is experienced with the procedure and has access to a laboratory accustomed to dealing with foetal cell analysis. Even then, in about 10 per cent of cases the cells do not grow the first time, especially if taken earlier than sixteen weeks, so that the procedure must be repeated.

The risk of amniocentesis to the mother is minimal. The risk to the foetus is somewhat greater, principally because the test may bring on premature labour, which, however, occurs in few than 1 per cent of cases. The procedure does not detect all birth defects. By 1987 it was useful only for discovering chromosomal abnormalities, some inherited metabolic disorders, and certain structural defects of the spine, notably SPINA BIFIDA and anencephaly (absence of the cerebrum, which precludes survival). It could not detect birth defects caused by the mother's exposure to RUBELLA, X-rays, drugs, or other harmful substances. Despite its limitations, it is widely recommended as a routine procedure for women carrying a child after the age of thirty-five, when the risk of chromosomal defects is substantially higher; for all women who have a high risk for trans-mitting a specific inherited disorder, such as SICKLE CELL DISEASE; and for all women who previously have borne a child with an inherited or chromosomal disorder. In addition, since amniocentesis also identifies the sex of the foetus, it is useful for women carrying a trait for sex-linked genetic disorders, such as MUSCULAR DYSTROPHY and HAEMO-PHILIA. Finally, in women who face some special problem in carrying a baby to full term, such as risk of uterine rupture, amniocentesis can help determine the maturity of the foetus, particularly its lungs and indicate when a Caesarean section can be safely performed (See also AMNIOGRAPHY; FOETOSCOPY.) Currently researchers are experimenting with methods of examining foetal genes by taking tissue samples from the CHORION, which can be done as early as eight weeks but has not yet been perfected.

Amniography A special X-ray procedure whereby structural defects in a foetus can be detected. Usually not possible to perform until late in preg-nancy lest the X-ray itself harm the baby, the procedure involves injecting a special dye into the AMNIOTIC SAC and then taking an X-ray; the dye outlines the shape of the foetus much more clearly than an ordinary X-ray. However, because it must be done so late in pregnancy,

abortion of a severely malformed foetus is usually much more difficult, so that the technique has limited use. See also FOETOSCOPY.

Amnioinfusion Also *amniocentesis abortion, intra-amniotic infusion, second-trimester abortion, late abortion, premature induction of labour.* A method of ending a pregnancy of fifteen to twenty-four weeks that involves the injection of a foreign substance into the amniotic sac surrounding the foetus, which after several hours induces regular uterine contractions that expel the foetus. The substance injected may be a strong salt solution (*saline abortion*), urea (a nitrogen waste product; *urea abortion*), or prostaglandins (a hormone; *prostaglandin abortion*).

Amnioinfusion can rarely be per-formed before fifteen weeks of pregnancy (counting from the first day of the last menstrual period) and is always done in a hospital so that emergency problems arising during the drug injection or during expulsion can be managed with safety. The average time needed for the proce-dure is twenty-four hours, but there is considerable variation among women in the time it takes for contractions to begin and for the foetus to be expelled, so that one should allow for a hospital stay of at least forty-eight hours. The procedure begins with administering local anaes-thetic to a small area in the lower abdomen. The doctor then inserts a slender hollow needle through the abdominal wall into the AMNIOTIC SAC, and introduces saline, urea, or prosta-glandins over a period of ten to fifteen minutes (even more slowly with saline, and then some amniotic fluid always must be withdrawn first). The woman must be fully awake during this procedure, so that she can immediately report any sensation of warmth, pain, dizziness, or other unusual feeling that might indicate an adverse drug reaction. The needle is then withdrawn and the area covered with a plaster; the patient then waits until contractions begin. Sometimes the cervix is dilated by inserting LAMINARIA, usually twenty-four hours prior to infusion, to ease the passage of the foetus, and occasionally OXYTOCIN is given intravenously to promote and strengthen uterine contractions. Prostaglandins tend to work faster than saline but may give rise to nausea and/or diarrhoea; saline works more slowly (it takes at least eight to twelve hours for contractions to begin, sometimes up to twenty-four hours) and may make the patient very thirsty.

The contractions begin gradually and increase in intensity. The cervical canal gradually dilates and eventually the amniotic sac breaks, releasing fluid through the vagina. After two to fifteen hours, the foetus is expelled. During the last few hours of expulsion painkillers and sedatives may be administered as needed, but general anaesthesia is not used. With saline abortion the foetus usually dies while still in the uterus; with prostaglandins it very occasionally emerges alive, and the hospital is then legally obliged to treat it as a premature infant (although its chance of survival is very small). Usually the placenta emerges after the foetus, but in some cases it must be extracted, and in still others, portions remain inside the uterus, necessitating a curettage (scraping) for removal.

Another method of late abortion is extra amniotic infusion in which prostaglandins are injected, by means of a tube, through the canal of the cervix into the space outside the amniotic sac. This avoids some of the risks of intra amniotic infusion.

Medically and emotionally, amnio-infusion is a far more traumatic procedure than other abortion procedures performed earlier in pregnancy. There DILATATION AND EVACUATION is, if possible, preferable.

The risks to the patient undergoing amnioinfusion are somewhat greater than those of normal childbirth. If saline solution is accidentally injected into a blood vessel, there is danger of shock and even death. The risk of haemorrhage and retained placental material is higher than for earlier abortion. The greater duration of the pregnancy, so that women frequently have felt the movements of the foetus, and the occasional delivery of a live foetus make amnioinfusion emotionally painful. Finally, the similarity of the experience to labour and delivery makes it traumatic for both patient and hospital staff.

Increasingly a new method of late abortion is being used in which pessaries containing prostaglandins are placed high in the vagina. This induces expulsion of the foetus although sometimes an evacuation of retained material must be carried out as well. As alternative to these methods is HYSTEROTOMY but this requires major surgery.

Amniotic sac Also *bag of waters*, *membranes*. A sac made of a membrane, called the *amnion*, that develops around a fertilized egg about one week after fertilization and eventually surrounds the entire embryo (later called 'foetus'). As it grows it fills with a clear fluid called *amniotic fluid* (or *waters*). The amount of fluid increases rapidly, to an average amount of 55 cc. (millilitres) at twelve weeks, 400 cc. at twenty weeks, and approximately 1 litre (about 2 pints) at thirty-eight weeks (near term). The volume then decreases as term approaches and, if the pregnancy is prolonged, may become relatively scanty. An excess of amniotic fluid, or HYDRAMNIOS, is sometimes associated with foetal malformations, multiple pregnancy (especially identical twins), and maternal diseases such as diabetes.

The make-up of the amniotic fluid changes during the course of the pregnancy. During the first four-and-a-half months it is made up of much the same components as the mother's blood plasma. Thereafter, however, particles of foetal tissue are shed into the fluid, which enable detection of some abnormalities in the unborn child (see AMNIO-CENTESIS).

The amniotic fluid serves several important functions. It provides a medium in which the foetus can readily move, cushions it against possible injury, and helps it maintain an even temperature. The foetus also drinks large amounts of amniotic fluid and excretes into it. During labour, if the presenting part of the foetus is not applied closely to the cervix, as with a BREECH PRESENTATION, the hydrostatic action of the fluid may be important in helping to dilate the cervix.

During the course of labour, usually towards the end of the first stage or early during the second stage, the amniotic sac ruptures by itself and the amniotic fluid gushes out through the mother's vagina. Occasionally the membranes rupture before labour begins, or sometimes they remain intact until the infant has been delivered so that it is born surrounded by them; the portion of membrane covering its head is sometimes called the *caul*. Surgically or manually rupturing the membranes during early labour (or before) is one way of inducing labour (see AMNIOTOMY).

Amniotomy Also *membrane rupture, breaking the bag of waters*. Deliberate rupture of the membranes, or AMNIOTIC SAC, in order to induce or hasten labour. Usually the obstetrician inserts an index finger or two fingers encased in a sterile glove through the partially dilated cervix until the baby's head is felt. Then, with the aid of an amniohook or other surgical instrument, the protective amniotic membranes are punctured, torn, or stripped from the uterine wall in the area near the cervix. The baby's head is then held up slightly with a finger to allow the amniotic fluid to escape. If the cervix is favourable, labour usually begins within an hour or two of amniotomy, although it may take as long as six to eight hours. If labour does not begin within twenty-four hours, it may be stimulated further with oxytocin administration (see INDUCTION OF LABOUR). No anaesthesia is needed for amniotomy. The principal risk of the procedure to the mother is bacterial infection; the risk to the baby is loss of the cushioning effect of the amniotic fluid during the early part of labour, which is lost anyway if the membranes rupture spontaneously at an early stage.

Anabolic steroids A group of synthetic hormones that resemble male sex hormones, such as testosterone, in that they increase muscle mass and have other body-building properties. Sometimes used in the treatment of breast cancer and certain endocrine and blood disorders, anabolic steroids have also been used to build up both men and women athletes, especially in sports requiring considerable strength (such as weight-lifting and wrestling). Not only is this use considered unfair (and illegal in some competitions, such as the Olympics), but it can give rise to serious side effects. In men the side effects include enlargement of the penis, sterility, breast growth and milk secretion, gastrointestinal complaints (nausea, vomiting, appetite loss), jaundice, and abnormal retention of fluids and electrolytes. Women athletes who take steroids may develop facial hair growth, voice deepening, clitoral enlargement, and menstrual irregularities. Because of their increasing use, urine tests to detect the presence of such steroids have been developed, and they are mandatory for athletes entering certain competitions. See also CHROMOSOME TEST.

Anaemia A shortage of red blood cells, diagnosed by means of a blood count (see under BLOOD TEST). If red blood cells make up less than 37 per cent of total blood volume, or the blood's haemoglobin value is below 12 grams power 100 cc. (millilitres) of blood, a woman is said to be anaemic. (The normal values are somewhat higher for men.) General symptoms of anaemia include undue fatigue, lightheadedness, frequent headaches, dizziness, spots before the eyes, ringing of the ears, and paleness of the skin under the fingernails. By far the majority of cases of anaemia are caused by iron deficiency. Other causes are unusual blood loss (through haemorrhage or major surgery, for example), vitamin deficiency (usually of vitamin B_{12} and/or folic acid), bone marrow disease, and a group of hereditary blood disorders that includes SICKLE CELL DISEASE.

Under certain conditions women in particular are apt to become anaemic.

Among these are pregnancy, which makes heavy nutritional demands on the body, particularly for iron and folic acid; the use of an intrauterine device (IUD), which often causes heavy menstrual flow and may therefore call for supplementary iron (either in the diet or in pill form); and use of oral contraceptives, which in some women creates a folic acid deficiency. There is disagreement as to whether or not all menstruating women require supplementary iron. Although some iron is lost with every menstrual period, it is normally restored between periods. Women with poor diets and/or exceptionally heavy periods run a higher risk of iron-deficiency anaemia, but most women with average flow who eat well-balanced diets need no supplements. In pregnancy, however, most authorities agree that iron and folic acid supplements are advisable.

The best dietary sources of iron are eggs, red meats, liver, and dried fruits. Folic acid (and also iron) is found mainly in green leafy vegetables (lettuce, spinach, cabbage, broccoli, watercress, parsley, escarole) and kelp (seaweed). Vitamin B_{12} is present in liver and organ meats, as well as in beef, pork, eggs, milk, and milk products. (See also DIET). Numerous herbs contain iron, among them red raspberry leaf (*Rubus ideaeus*), strawberry leaf (*Fragaria vesca*), comfrey leaf (*Symphytum officinalis*), burdock root (*Arctium lappa*), dandelion root (*Taraxacum officinalis*), and yellow dock root (*Rumex crispus*).

Anaesthesia 1 Loss of feeling induced by chemical agents called *anaesthetics*, affecting a limited surface area (*topical anaesthesia*), or a specific circumscribed area (*local* or *regional anaesthesia*), or, with loss of consciousness, the entire body (*general anaesthesia*). It is used to block sensations of pain from minor wounds and trauma, as well as pain from surgery, dentistry, and other traumatic medical procedures, and in childbirth. Topical anaesthetics are available in the form of throat lozenges, eardrops, mouthwash, ointments, rectal suppositories, and so on; many of these are very mild and are available without prescription.

Local and general anaesthesia, in contrast, must be administered by a doctor or dentist. When it is used for procedures major enough to require a hospital or clinic setting, it is preferable to have it administered either by an anaesthetist or doctor with advanced training in its use. Local anaesthesia is always given by injection; general anaesthesia is either inhaled or injected (see also under definition 2).

The choice of anaesthetic agent and of the kind of anaesthesia is usually dictated by the condition or operation involved – its nature, how long it takes to perform, the area affected – as well as by the patient's state of health. The major exception is childbirth, where a woman's preferences also may be taken into account.

2 In childbirth The earliest anaesthesia used in childbirth was chloroform, discovered in 1847. The first woman in labour who inhaled chloroform fumes was made unconscious and delivered within half an hour; she herself did not awaken for three days and had no memory of delivering the baby. At first the new method was denounced, but after it was used by Queen Victoria herself for delivery, opposition died down. In time, other kinds of *inhalation anaesthesia* came into use, principally ether, cyclopropane, and halothane. These general anaesthetics, as well as thiopentone,

which is injected intravenously, all have one serious disadvantage in childbirth; they pass through the placenta and anaesthetize the baby as well as the mother. They tend to produce sleepy babies with delayed sucking response and weight gain, and sometimes with serious respiratory problems as well. Nor is general anaesthesia without risk to the mother. The most serious is vomiting, which may cause material to be aspirated (breathed into the lungs). Also, general anaesthesia slows down uterine contractions, so today it is used quite rarely, and then only near the end of labour, just before expulsion of the baby. (Nitrous oxide, which is inhaled, induces an altered consciousness and pain relief but not loss of consciousness or true anaesthesia; it is usually administered together with oxygen in concentrations below 80 per cent.)

Most of the problems of general anaesthesia in childbirth have been eliminated with REGIONAL ANAESTHESIA, also called *conduction anaesthesia*, which does not blot out consciousness but only blocks the conduction of pain sensations to the brain from a specific region of the body. Relatively little of a regional anaesthetic is absorbed into the mother's bloodstream or crosses the placenta, so it does not affect the baby and can be used to relieve pain during labour as well as delivery. The anaesthetic agents injected for this purpose include procaine, lignocaine (Xylocaine), and various related compounds. However, those agents, too, can create some problems, such as lowered blood pressure in the mother, impairment of contractions, and, with spinal anaesthesia, headache. after delivery. Because no anaesthetic is totally risk-free, since the 1950s there has been increasing emphasis on various psychological methods of pain control, ranging from hypnosis to breathing exercises (see under PREPARED CHILDBIRTH), to replace or supplement anaesthetics.

Anal fissure A deep crack or split in the mucous membrane of the anal canal, which often is extremely painful because it can cause spasm of the anal sphincter (muscle). It is caused by the passage of large, hard stools, or may result from anal surgery, anal intercourse, or other trauma. The pain is particularly acute when the anus is stretched by a bowel movement or for examination. A superficial fissure will usually heal by itself, but some become chronic. Treatment includes a low-fibre diet, stool softeners, and the use of anaesthetic ointment before and after a bowel movement. A warm SITZ BATH immediately after a bowel movement may help ease the spasm. Chronic fissures that do not respond to treatment may require surgical repair.

Analgesic Any pain-relieving drug or remedy. Analgesic drugs are either narcotic or non-narcotic. The principal narcotics are opium and its alkaloids (morphine, codeine) and synthetic narcotics, including pethidine and methadone. All narcotics are potentially habit-forming; that is, a person becomes physically and emotionally dependent on using them, and experiences severe withdrawal symptoms when they are discontinued. The principal non-narcotic analgesics, most of which not only relieve pain but also reduce fever and inflammation, are the salicylates, such as aspirin; the pyrazolone derivatives, such as phenylbutazone and indomethacin and the aniline derivatives, such as paracetamol, which are not anti-inflammatory. Numerous herbs have also

been used as analgesics; indeed, opium itself is obtained from the poppy plant. Among HERBAL REMEDIES, a mild analgesic is catnip (*Nepeta cataria*), drunk as a tea prepared from its leaf sprays and flowers.

Anal intercourse, anal sex See under ANUS

Androgen A general name for any hormone that has a masculinizing effect on either sex. The principal androgen is TESTOSTERONE, produced by the testes in men and, in much smaller quantities, by the ovaries and adrenal glands in women. Other androgens secreted by the ovaries and female adrenal glands are androstenedione and dehydroisoandrosterone, but except in certain diseases the amounts are not large enough to have a masculinizing effect. During pregnancy the placenta converts these two androgens into oestrogens (female hormones). Synthetic androgens are used mainly to treat men with disorders caused by failure of the testes to produce androgen. They are not effective in treating sterility or impotence unless these conditions are the result of underdeveloped testes. Androgens are believed to be responsible in part for the sex drive (see LIBIDO), but the exact relationship is not totally clear. See also ANABOLIC STEROIDS.

Androgen insensitivity syndrome Also *testicular feminization*. A congenital condition in which girls or women appear to have normal external female genitals except for a swelling or lump in each groin, little or no pubic or underarm hair, and a vagina usually not deep enough for sexual intercourse. They also lack a fully developed uterus and Fallopian tubes, do not menstruate and cannot become pregnant. The condition occurs when a foetus develops so that the internal masculine organs begin to form but are never completely developed, and their rudimentary presence prevents the development of female organs. At puberty the breasts do develop, because the female hormone oestrogen is produced by the rudimentary testes (seen as lumps in the groin), and the shape of the body becomes decidedly female. The disorder is named after the fact that it is due to the lack of sufficient androgen-binding protein in the cells; the sex chromosomes are all XY, as in normal men. Many women with this condition lead normal lives – an operation to lengthen the vagina can be performed to permit vaginal intercourse – except that they cannot bear children.

Anorexia nervosa A form of self-starvation with both physical and psychological symptoms. It affects mostly girls in their teens and early twenties from a middle-class or affluent background, and it may be fatal in as many as 10 to 15 per cent of cases. Its principal characteristic is the patient's refusal to eat. The eating behaviour for any food that is consumed is often bizarre; eating may be followed by repeated self-induced vomiting and diarrhoea (see BULIMA-REXIA). Consequently, there is extreme weight loss (more than 20 per cent of body weight), accompanied by any or all of the following: secondary amenorrhoea (cessation of menstruation), hyperactivity, hypothermia (intolerance to cold), low blood pressure, slowed heartbeat, lanugo (extensive growth of downy body hair), fear of weight gain, an obsessive pursuit of thinness, denial of hunger, sense of ineffectiveness, and struggle for control over one's life. Anorexic patients, 90 to 95 per cent of whom are female, have a grossly distorted body image, regarding themselves as obese when in reality they are emaciated. They also may suffer from severe depression and attempt suicide.

The cause of anorexia is unknown but has long been thought to be psychological rather than organic. Numerous causes have been suggested: a desire to avoid sexuality (fear of pregnancy, denial of femininity); a caricature of conventional femininity (desire to conform to social norms by becoming slender); a sense of helplessness when faced with impending adulthood, and thus a means of avoiding independence. The parents of anorexic girls have also been blamed: the mothers for being dominant and intrusive, the fathers for being passive and emotionally withdrawn. Recently researchers have begun to investigate the possibility of organic disease, perhaps in the HYPO-THALAMUS, which controls appetite.

With the cause unknown, treatment is directed largely at preventing death from starvation; usually it is carried on in the hospital and in conjunction with psychotherapy. In less severe cases therapy – often family therapy – alone may be tried. In general, the disease is either self-limiting – the girl resumes eating, which after months of starvation may itself cause gastrointestinal and other physical problems – or the patient starves to death.

Anovulatory bleeding Also *anovulation*. Vaginal bleeding, often on a regular basis, without release of an egg (see OVULATION). In a physically mature woman, there is a regular monthly cycle during which oestrogen stimulates the buildup of the uterine lining (endo-metrium), an egg is released from the ovary, the remnant of the egg follicle produces progesterone, and either the egg is fertilized and becomes implanted in the endometrium, or it and the extra endometrial tissue are sloughed off in menstrual flow (see MENSTRUAL CYCLE for a more detailed description). Without ovulation, no progesterone is produced and the hormonal feedback system is thrown out of kilter. The extra endometrial tissue built up under oestrogen stimulation is eventually shed, but not at the regular rate and time that would have occurred with ovulation. Progesterone regulates the timing of the menstrual cycle, and without it menstruation becomes irregular or may cease altogether, or may may involve heavy, long-lasting menstrual periods.

Anovulatory bleeding is quite common in the first two or three years following MENARCHE, and again in the five or so years preceding MENOPAUSE. Also, women taking oral contraceptives that suppress ovulation have anovulatory cycles, which in their case are regulated by externally administered hormones. During a woman's reproductive years, lack of ovulation usually causes no problem unless she is trying to become pregnant or is distressed by menstrual irregularity. The administration of oral progesterone will often stop heavy bleeding but cannot reinstate ovulation. Some authorities maintain that lack of ovulation is responsible for practically all DYSFUNCTIONAL BLEEDING (vaginal bleeding not caused by an organic disease or lesion). Also see ENDOMETRIAL HYPERPLASIA.

Antenatal care Medical care for a woman from the time she suspects that she may be pregnant until the birth of the baby. In large measure, antenatal care is preventive, its chief purpose being to assure the delivery of a healthy baby without danger or harm to the mother. It is designed to detect at the onset conditions that may, if unchecked, adversely affect mother and/or child. Many such conditions can, if recognized early, be corrected or controlled. Among them are signs or symptoms of urinary infection, genital HERPES INFECTION and other kinds of infection, ECTOPIC PREGNANCY, PREECLAMPSIA, and abnormal uterine growth, all conditions requiring prompt treatment to prevent serious damage.

Antenatal care is available from general practitioners and obstetricians. Since a pregnant woman will be seeing her health-care provider for nearly a year, it is advisable to select one with some care. Among the factors to be considered in this choice are location (can the person/place be readily reached? Are the surgery hours convenient?); qualifications (see also MIDWIFE; OBSTETRICIAN); general orientation (approve of PREPARED CHILDBIRTH? willing to consider and/or attend HOME BIRTH?) and personality (willing to answer questions? give adequate individual attention?).

The initial visit usually takes place at the time when pregnancy is confirmed, or soon after, and ordinarily takes longer than subsequent ones. It should include a complete medical history with special attention to previous obstetric history (for example, complications in previous pregnancies, birth defects in the family, etc.); a complete physical examination, including pelvic examination, breast examination, height and weight, blood pressure; and a number of laboratory tests. Chief among the tests are a full blood count (including haemoglobin and haematocrit) and blood tests for syphilis, blood type (should transfusion be needed), RH-FACTOR, and possible antibody levels (including RUBELLA); a PAP SMEAR; a test for gonorrhoea; and a urine test (for protein and sugar) and urine culture. Further, black women should routinely be tested for SICKLE CELL DISEASE and Jewish women for TAY-SACHS DISEASE. Following the examination the doctor should advise the woman concerning, diet, exercise, general hygine, and sexual activity, and answer any questions she may have. Either then or later in the pregnancy, suggestions may be made concerning childbirth education of one kind or another.

After the initial visit, most women require monthly visits through twenty-eight weeks, every two weeks until twenty-six weeks, and weekly thereafter. These visits generally involve only a check for blood pressure (a rise may warn of possible PRE-ECLAMPSIA), weight, and urine, along with external examination of the abdomen, listening for the foetal heartbeat, and measuring the uterus to check on the growth of the foetus. See also DIET; PELVIMETRY; HIGH-RISK PREGNANCY; PREGNANT PATIENTS' RIGHTS; WEIGHT GAIN (definition 2).

Antibody A specific substance in the blood that detects and reacts to a material foreign to the body, called an ANTIGEN, and neutralizes it. Antibodies are one of the body's two chief defences against invading organisms; the other consists of cells, such as white blood cells, that surround and break up foreign matter. Antibodies are produced only when the appropriate antigens are present; each kind of antibody is effective only against a specific antigen. When an infection (invasion) ends, the blood levels of the appropriate antibodies fall, but if the same invader attacks again, antibody build-up is more rapid and effective than the first

time. It is this enhanced response that constitutes *immunity*. See also AUTOIMMUNE DISEASE.

Anti-cancer drugs See CHEMO-THERAPY.

Antidepressants Also *mood elevators*. A class of drugs used to relieve serious DEPRESSION. Because the majority of British psychiatric patients are women, and depressive illness is far more common in women than in men, they are more likely to be treated with antidepressants than men. There are two main kinds of antidepressant, the tricyclic antidepressants and the monoamine oxidase (MAO) inhibitors. The tricyclics have a mood-elevating effect but generally must be used for two to five weeks before their benefits are felt. They are often effective, but do not work in every case. Also, they must be used with great caution in patients with a history of glaucoma, phlebitis, heart disease, thyroid disease, epilepsy, or prostate disorders. Moreover, they can cause such unpleasant side effects as dry mouth, drowsiness, blurred vision, constipation, and urinary hesitation, although these effects often disappear after a few weeks' use or when dosage is lowered. Finally, they should never be discontinued abruptly; once the symptoms subside, the dose should be reduced very gradually.

The MAO inhibitors, which generally are tried only in severe cases of depression not helped by the tricyclics, are more potent drugs. They both elevate the mood and lower the blood pressure. However, they can have serious side effects, may not be used in the presence of asthma, or heart, liver, or kidney disease, or in conjunction with some drugs, and require the avoidance of certain foods and beverages.

Finally, a third kind of drug – lithium – is used specifically for MANIC-DEPRESSIVE ILLNESS, which differs from depression in that periods of manic behaviour alternate with periods of depression. Lithium, which controls the manic phase of the illness, may also cause serious side effects; furthermore, the dosage of the drug required to be effective can be very close to the level that can cause adverse reactions, so that regular and careful monitoring of blood levels is mandatory. No antidepressant should be taken without a careful evaluation of its benefits compared to its risks. See also TRANQUILLIZERS.

Antigen Any substance that stimulates the body to produce antibodies and reacts specifically with them. Such substances include toxins (poisons), foreign proteins, bacteria, and foreign tissue. See also ANTIBODY.

Anus The opening of the rectum to the outside of the body, through which solid body wastes (faeces) are expelled. The *anal canal*, a short passage about one and one-half inches long, leads from the external opening to the rectum. The skin around the anus is highly sensitive, both to irritation (as from diarrhoea or vaginal discharge) and to erotic stimulation, as in oral-anal sex (*analingus*, or 'rimming').

Anal intercourse, with the partner's penis inserted into the anus, requires more gentleness than vaginal intercourse, because the anus is not as elastic as the vagina and the delicate mucous membranes inside it may tear. Use of a lubricant (saliva, vaginal mucus, or water-soluble jelly) therefore is recommended. Also, because anal bacteria can cause serious vaginal infection, a penis or finger inserted in the anus during lovemaking should always be washed before being inserted in the vagina (or a condom may be used for anal intercourse and then removed for vaginal penetration). For the same reason, girls and women are urged to wipe from front to back after a bowel movement, so as to avoid wiping anal bacteria toward the entrance of the vagina or urethra. Both LYMPHOEDEMA VENEREUM and GONORRHOEA can affect the anus, and syphilis and herpes infection are other VENEREAL DISEASES that can give rise to perianal lesions (near the anus). See also ANAL FISSURE; HAEMORRHOIDS.

Anxiety Also *anxiety neurosis, panic disorder.* An emotional disorder characterized by prolonged feelings of profound fear and apprehension that have no appropriate cause. Everyone feels anxious at one time or another, but the feeling is usually of short duration and is directly related to an external cause; when the cause is removed, the anxiety disappears. Furthermore, if the source of anxiety is repeated again and again (as with stage fright, the fear of appearing before an audience), usually less and less fear is felt as a person gains experience with the situation. With neurotic anxiety, however, a person may feel increasing panic with each repetition, leading him or her to avoid the situation entirely. Anxiety relating to a specific situation or object is sometimes called a *phobia*; for an example, see AGORAPHOBIA. Sometimes it takes the form of obsessive-compulsive behaviour, that is, recurrent persistent ideas or repetitive compulsive actions, such as incessant hand-washing.

The symptoms of anxiety are both physical and emotional. There are feelings of tension and apprehension; making a decision becomes difficult, and one cannot concentrate. There is little tolerance of frustration, and there are usually sleep disturbances, such as difficulty in falling asleep, restless sleep, and nightmares. Physical symptoms, which can be acute during an anxiety attack (or attack of panic), include dizziness, palpitations, shortness of breath (panting), and sweating. Nausea and vomiting, or diarrhoea, may occur. No organic cause of such anxiety has been identified. Prolonged and debilitating anxiety is usually treated with psychotherapy and psychoactive drugs, principally the minor tranquillizers and antidepressants. A highly successful kind of psychotherapy for anxiety has been behaviour therapy, which in effect teaches the sufferer how not to become anxious.

Apocrine glands Scent glands in the pubic and axillary (underarm) areas that emit a milky, organic material with an erotically stimulating odour during sexual excitement. The scent is trapped by the pubic and axillary hair. Women have 75 per cent more apocrine glands than men. They develop during puberty, and are also present around the labia minora, nipples, and navel.

Appendectomy Surgical removal of the vermiform appendix, a small appendage of the caecum, the upper end of the large intestine. It can become inflamed and infected, usually with the bacterium *Escherichia coli*, which is normally resident in the healthy intestine. This condition is called *appendicitis* and calls for removal of the appendix because, should the infection become severe, peritonitis readily develops. *Peritonitis* is inflammation of the membrane that lines the abdominal cavity and constitutes a life-threatening emergency. The appendix serves no real function, and a healthy appendix is sometimes removed during other abomdinal surgery, especially hysterectomy and Caesarean section, as a preventative measure.

Appendicitis can also develop during pregnancy – in fact, it is the most common acute surgical condition occurring in pregnant women – and then calls for especially prompt treatment. Treated early, it rarely interferes with the pregnancy. Should treatment be delayed and the appendix perforate (burst), labour is often brought on, regardless of the length of the pregnancy.

Pregnancy makes appendicitis more difficult to diagnose. The usual symptoms and signs – pain in the lower right quadrant of the abdomen, an elevated white blood cell count, nausea, and vomiting – are similar to some of the sensations of normal pregnancy, and the locus of pain is harder to determine because of the enlarged uterus. Surgery is usually the best course of treatment. If peritonitis has already developed, powerful antibiotics must also be used to control the infection.

Areola The ring of pink or brownish skin surrounding the nipple of the breast. Like the nipple itself, the areola has nerve endings and blood vessels that extend from larger connections within the breast itself. Within the areola are some rudimentary sebaceous (oil) glands, called *areolar glands, tubercles of Montgomery,* or *Montgomery's follicles,* arranged in a circular fashion around the edge; during pregnancy these small roundish elevations are somewhat more prominent. Also, during pregnancy the areola's colour becomes deeper, and some women develop a *secondary areola,* a circle of faint colour that is seen just outside the true areola from about the fifth month on. Following delivery, the secondary areola becomes fainter or disappears. See also NIPPLE.

Arteriosclerosis Also *hardening of the arteries*. A group of diseases characterized by thickening and loss of elasticity of the arterial walls, impairing the flow of blood through the arteries. The principal diseases are arteriosclerosis itself, in which there are changes in the small arteries and which is usually secondary to HYPERTENSION (high blood pressure) and, most common of all, *atherosclerosis*, in which the arteries are thickened by *atheroma*, localized accumulations of fatty substances. Atherosclerosis often obstructs the arteries that nourish the heart and brain, and its complications are a major cause of death in Britain.

Atherosclerosis may begin early in life and usually gives rise to no symptoms for years. Gradually the walls of the arteries become thicker and the flow of blood is restricted. Eventually atheroma may completely block a major artery, which can, depending on its location, lead to dramatic and sometimes fatal results – a heart attack or cerebral vascular accident. Atheroma also promotes the clotting of blood in arteries, and when clots create a blockage in a vital artery (supplying heart or brain), a similar crisis may result.

Although the causes of atherosclerosis are not known, there are definite predisposing factors. Chief among them are hypertension, high blood levels of cholesterol and triglycerides, stressful living, cigarette smoking, and diabetes, and possibly also obesity. The risk increases with a family history of early atherosclerosis, and also with age. Preventive measures include periodic checks of blood pressure and, after middle age, of blood levels of cholesterol and triglycerides, followed by appropriate treatment if any of these levels rise beyond safe limits. Stopping smoking, weight control, and control of diabetes also may help. Precautionary dietary measures are also recommended – some doctors advise them for everyone, regardless of history – particularly reducing salt intake, to avoid high blood pressure, and reducing intake of foods that raise serum cholesterol and replacing those foods high in saturated fats, such as butter and pork products, with polyunsaturated fats, found in corn and other vegetable oils.

Some researchers believe that arteriosclerosis does in fact have a single cause, a protein in the blood called homocysteine, which causes profound disruptions in the growth of the arterial wall cells in test animals. This protein is created in the body when a certain amino acid commonly found in animal protein is inadequately metabolized. To metabolize it properly, adequate amounts of vitamin B_6 are needed, and therefore these researchers hypothesize that daily supplements of this vitamin (or its inclusion in the vitamin supplements already added to flour) might prevent the disease altogether. However, their theory has not yet been sufficiently verified to win wide acceptance.

Artery One of a system of thick-walled, elastic muscular tubes that carry blood away from the heart. The major arteries lead to all structures of the body, branching and re-branching into smaller and smaller arteries, and finally *arterioles* and *capillaries*, as they reach the organs they serve. Every contraction of the heart's ventricles forces a quantity of blood into the arteries, whose muscular walls stretch to accommodate these sudden surges. Each surge is followed by a contraction of the artery wall, which serves to push the blood along and so supplements the pumping work of the ventricles. Blood thus flows through the arteries in regular spurts rather than a steady stream.

The distention of the arteries as blood surges through them can be detected in those vessels close to the surface of the body, such as the radial artery in the wrist, and is called the *pulse*. The rate of the heart's pumping can thus be determined by the pulse rate. The adult resting pulse is, on average, somewhere between 50 and 90 beats per minute, but the normal range is wider still. A rapid heart rate – anywhere from 100 beats a minute or more (except in an unborn baby, where 140 beats per minute is not at all abnormal) – is called *tachycardia* and may be symptomatic of numerous disorders, but the heart rate normally increases with vigorous exercise, sexual excitement, fear, and under numerous other circumstances. The principal disease of the arteries is ARTERIOSCLEROSIS, whose cause and cure are not known and whose most serious complications are fatal. See also VEIN.

Arthritis Also *rheumatism* (pop.) General name for a number of inflammatory diseases characterized by swelling, redness, and/or tenderness of one or more joints. Not all joint aches, pains, or stiffness constitute arthritis, a term usually reserved for conditions that are more or less chronic. A notable exception, however, is arthritis caused by infection, which generally can be totally cured by appropriate antibiotic treatment, although if it is not treated in time the affected joints can be permanently damaged. Among the infectious agents that can cause such arthritis are streptococci, staphylococci, pneumococci (which causes pneumonia), gonococci (which cause GONORHOEA), and the organisms that cause influenza, hepatitis, bacterial endocarditis, and rubella. Another arthritic disease is *rheumatic fever*, which begins as an infection, usually by streptococci, and develops into an AUTOIMMUNE DISEASE. Both RHEUMATOID ARTHRITIS and SYSTEMIC LUPUS ERYTHEMATOSUS afflict women far more often than men; OSTEOARTHRITIS, the most common kind of arthritis is more common in women than men when it strikes after the age of forty-five, as is usually the case.

Artificial insemination Inserting sperm into a woman's vagina by means other than sexual intercourse, in order for her to become pregnant. It is generally considered a last resort for a couple who want a baby when the man is infertile and the woman is fertile. Occasionally it is used when the man is fertile but the woman has a disorder preventing the passage of sperm through her cervix; her partner's sperm then is directly introduced into the uterus (*intrauterine insemination*). In recent years it has been occasionally used when a woman wishes to remain single or avoid heterosexual intercourse but wants to bear a child.

In *homologous* artificial insemination the sperm is the husband's or regular partner's, and in *heterologous* it is that of an unrelated donor. Some doctors consider the latter a form of adoption – it has been called 'semiadoption' – and most reputable doctors insist that a couple considering donor insemination undergo lengthy interviews over a period of time and/or psychological evaluation, so that their emotional stability both individually and as a couple can be assessed. In addition, most insist that the woman be demonstrably fertile (based on basal temperature chart to show she is ovulating, a Rubin test or some other test to show that her tubes are not blocked, and sometimes also an endometrial biopsy), and that the man have undergone extensive medical investigation for the cause of his infertility and any available treatment for it. Other criteria are that the man will have been aware of his infertility for at least one year and that he really wants the procedure performed – especially if it is donor insemination – and is not just being pressed to agree by the woman.

Homologous artificial insemination is sometimes successful when a man has healthy sperm but in insufficient numbers (see OLIGOSPERMIA). Heterologous insemination is indicated when there are either no sperm (azoospermia) or no live sperm (necrospermia) or when the male partner has a hereditary disease carrying too great a risk for natural offspring. The choice of donor is, of course, very important. The main criteria are that he is fertile, as shown by semen analysis (see under SPERM for further details); that he is free of any illness, transmittable disease, and history of hereditary diseases; that his intelligence is equal to that of the couple and that he is emotionally stable; that his physical proportions are similar to those of the husband or male partner; and that his blood group and type are compatible with those of the woman. For extra safety, some doctors prefer to use only married donors with two or more healthy children of their own.

Doctors often use *multiple donors*, that is, semen is inserted two or more times during a single ovulatory period with a different donor's used each time. Insertion is by syringe into the vagina; generally a speculum is inserted first in order to expose the cervix. The woman is asked to remain prone for twenty minutes after insertion, with her pelvis somewhat higher than her head and shoulders, and before rising may insert a tampon or a cervical cap over the cervix to help retain the semen longer and enhance the chances of conception. Artificial insemination is usually performed twice a month (on the twelfth and fourteenth days of a twenty-eight-day menstrual cycle, or at comparable times for longer or shorter cycles) for about four months. If the woman does not conceive, there may be further testing of her fertility and, if no abnormality is discovered, the process is continued for another six months. Statistics indicate that about half of all women conceive during the first three months, and about 90 per cent do so within six months, but in practice the rate of success may be lower.

Human artificial insemination dates from the mid-19th century. It was first successfully performed by Dr. James Marion Sims in 1866; the first insemination using a donor's sperm was performed in the 1890s by Dr. Robert L. Dickinson. See also SPERM BANK; TEST-TUBE BABY.

Acheim-Zondeck test See under PREGNANCY TEST.

Asherman's syndrome The presence of scar tissue (see ADHESION) in the uterine wall in amounts sufficient to prevent regular menstruation and cause infertility. Such scar tissue can result from repeated infection, as in chronic PELVIC INFLAMMATORY DISEASE, or from repeated or overstrenuous curettage (see D AND C), or from an abnormally adherent placenta in a previous pregnancy. Although rare, Asherman's syndrome can cause AMENORRHOEA (see definition 3) and lead to permanent infertility. Therefore, if a D and C must performed in the presence of infection (as, for example, when infected placental tissue must be removed after a miscarriage or abortion), the curettage (scraping) of the endometrium must be done exceptionally gently and cautiously to avoid this condition. For women who wish to become pregnant, the usual treatment for Asherman's syndrome is to break up the scar tissue surgically (generally requiring an abdominal incision) and insert an INTRAUTERINE DEVICE (IUD) for a few months, so as to keep the uterine walls open and prevent adhesions from re-forming while the endometrial tissue grows back. After normal menstrual periods have been reestablished, the IUD is removed.

Aspermatogenesis See under STERILITY.

Aspiration See VACUUM ASPIRATION. For needle aspiration, see BIOPSY, definition 3.

Asymptomatic Without symptoms, that is, without signs of a particular disorder or disease. For example, a man may have a *Trichomonas* infection without knowing it because he experiences no itching, discharge, or other symptoms, and then may unwittingly transmit it to his partner.

Athletic ability, women's The strength, co-ordination, speed of reflexes, and other qualities and skills required in various sports as found in women, compared to those of men. Until the age of about ten, boys and girls are much the same in physical strength. The amount of oxygen a boy or girl can deliver to the muscles, known as *maximal oxygen uptake*, is identical, as are strength and endurance. By the age of fifteen, however, when sex hormones affect the body's development, there is considerable difference between the two sexes. Although female and male hormones are present in both, the comparative amounts are vastly different. The longer-term growth spurt and increased testosterone (male hormone) levels in boys make for a great increase in upper-body (arm and shoulder) strength, and the entire body becomes taller and heavier. After PUBERTY the female, in contrast, has a much larger percentage of fat to total body weight (25 per cent compared to 14 per cent in males) and less potential for developing muscle mass. In adulthood in the 1980s the average British man was four inches taller than the average woman, and thirty to forty pounds heavier. Women have smaller bones, smaller lungs, and less muscle mass than men. In sports where strength, height, and speed are called for, therefore, as in basketball, the best women athletes are necessarily inferior to the best men. The same is true for sports requiring largely upper body strength, such as the racket sports (tennis, squash, etc.). Where other qualities are required, however, such as flexibility for gymnastics, women excel. In some activities, moreover, women have been closing the gap between their performance and that of men, notably in swimming (both speed and long-distance) and in long-distance running.

One problem for women athletes who train very hard is that they may stop menstruating (see AMENORRHOEA, definition 3). Preliminary results of studies currently underway suggest that when the ratio of a woman's body fat to lean weight drops below a certain threshold, as it does with vigorous training, a signal is sent to the pituitary gland to stop ovulation, causing menstrual periods to stop; when these women regain weight their periods usually resume. What is still not known is the effect of training and exercise on hormones, raising questions such as whether, with heavy exercise, a woman's adrenal glands will, like her muscles, become larger, like those of men, and might then produce more androgens (male hormones), which in turn are linked with more aggressive behaviour, higher bone density, and muscle-protein synthesis.

Automanipulation See MASTURBATION.

Axillary Of or in the armpit. Breast cancer that has begun to metastasize (spread) often involves the axillary lymph nodes, which are usually examined very carefully whenever the disease is suspected. The growth of axillary hair is one of the early signs of puberty.

Azoospermia A total absence of sperm in the seminal fluid, rendering a man sterile. See STERILITY.

B

Back labour During childbirth, discomfort from uterine contractions that is felt principally in the lower back. It often occurs with a POSTERIOR PRESENTATION, presumably because the back of the baby's head is pressing against the mother's back. It may be eased by leaning forward or crouching on the hands and knees, and by having the birth attendant apply firm hand pressure against the lower back.

Ballottement See under QUICKENING.

Band-aid surgery See LAPAROSCOPY.

Barrier methods Contraceptive methods or devices that depend largely or entirely on blocking the passage of live sperm through the cervix. Among them are the CERVICAL CAP, CONDOM, CONTRACEPTIVE SPONGE, DIAPHRAGM, and various kinds of spermicide.

Bartholin cyst See CYST, definition 3.

Bartholin's glands Also *vestibular glands*, *vulvovaginal glands*. A pair of pea-sized glands on each side of the introitus (vaginal entrance) that open into the vagina. They are believed to secrete minute quantities of mucus to lubricate the vagina during sexual intercourse. Normally small and inconspicuous, these glands can become greatly enlarged when they are infected, a not infrequent occurrence. The infecting organism is often the gonococcus, which causes gonorrhoea, but other bacteria may also be responsible. The first sign of infection usually is a hot, extremely tender lump near the introitus. It can become as large as a lemon. With severe infection an abscess forms, which usually must be opened surgically and drained. Antibiotic therapy alone is not likely to work quickly enough because the abscess is circumscribed and its blood supply reduced, so antibiotics cannot reach it in sufficient amounts. Following surgery a small drain is left in place for several days.

Repeated infections of the glands can cause the formation of scar tissue that blocks the ducts, leading to accumulation of the secretions in a large cyst (see also CYST, definition 3). This, too, requires drainage to avoid repeated infection. Sometimes *marsupialization* – surgery that in effect converts the gland into a pouch – may prevent repeating infection, but if the condition continues to recur the gland may have to be removed. Both marsupialization and gland removal usually require general anaesthesia. Recovery from these procedures tends to be rapid, although local tenderness and swelling may persist for several weeks afterward.

Basal body temperature Also *BBT*, *temperature method*. The lowest

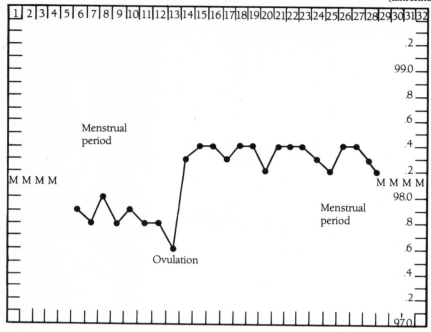

Basal Body Temperature Chart

temperature of a normal healthy person during waking hours, which can be used as a means of determining whether or not a woman ovulates, and when. During the MENSTRUAL CYCLE the hormone progesterone, released after ovulation, causes a measurable increase in basal body temperature. A slight drop in temperature usually (but not always) occurs twelve to twenty-four hours before ovulation, and a sustained rise follows for at least three days, and sometimes until the beginning of the next cycle. In order to use this phenomenon for either birth control or conception, a specially marked thermometer (marked in tenths of degrees and available in most chemist shops) is used to take a woman's temperature every morning immediately upon waking (before rising, eating, etc.). It remains

inserted for a full four minutes, orally, vaginally, or rectally, but always in the same way. The temperature is noted on a graph. When it rises more than 0.1 degree (Celsius) or 0.4 to 0.8 degrees (Fahrenheit) and remains elevated for three days, ovulation presumably has occurred and the fertile period is over. Records made over a period of six to eight months usually give a good indication of the pattern of ovulation, which can be used either to prevent or time a pregnancy. For birth control the temperature method is more accurate than the calendar method but still is far from totally reliable (see NATURAL FAMILY PLANNING). When combined with the CERVICAL MUCUS METHOD (and then called *sympto-thermic method*) it is somewhat more dependable. However, results may be made inaccurate by a cold or other infection, fatigue, emotional stress, and other factors. Further, some women have no clear identifiable pattern of basal body temperature, even when they ovulate regularly.

Benign Describing a growth or tumour that is not cancerous. Although its presence means that a group of cells have multiplied more rapidly than normal, so that a mass of extra tissue has formed, a benign tumour differs in three ways from a malignant (cancerous) tumour: it cannot metastasize (spread) to a different part of the body; it cannot invade and destroy surrounding normal tissue; and it cannot recur (although a new benign tumour can develop). Benign tumours can usually be removed completely if they are not too close to vital organs, and the outlook for total cure is very favourable. See also CANCER.

Bilateral Affecting both sides. A *bilateral oophorectomy*, for example, means surgical removal of both ovaries.

Billings method See CERVICAL MUCUS METHOD.

Bimanual examination See under GYNAECOLOGICAL EXAMINATION.

Biopsy 1 Also *surgical biopsy, incisional biopsy.* The surgical removal of tissue from a living person for evaluation and diagnosis by a pathologist. It is the primary diagnostic technique for breast cancer and most other solid growths. Surgical biopsy can be performed under local anaesthetic in a doctor's surgery, or under general anaesthetic in a hospital on either an inpatient or an outpatient basis. The excised tissue specimen can be examined in two ways either quickly by a *frozen section*, while the patient is still anaesthetized, or by a *permanent section*, a forty-eight-hour process in which the tissue is fixed in formalin, embedded in paraffin blocks, and then sliced, stained, and studied microscopically. A frozen section permits biopsy and surgical treatment to be combined in one operation; a permanent section allows for a more definitive analysis and time for both patient and doctor to consider alternative treatments. See also Definition 5, 6, 7, and 8 below.

2 **Excisional biopsy** The removal of an entire growth, rather than a portion of it, for evaluation (see definition 1 above).

3 **Needle biopsy** Also *needle aspiration.* The removal of tissue or fluid from a growth (tumour or cyst) by means of a hollow needle to determine whether or not it is cancerous. Technically, if only fluid is removed the procedure is called 'aspiration'; if tissue is removed it is a 'biopsy'. In practice the terms are used interchangeably. Needle biopsy is sometimes performed in a doctor's surgery (rather than a hospital) and requires either local or no anaesthesia. The doctor first inserts a fine needle with a hypodermic syringe into the growth. If fluid can be withdrawn, it is analyzed for benign and malignant (cancerous) cells. If it is a benign cyst, it may be drained of fluid, surgically removed, or simply observed. If no fluid can be withdrawn, a needle of wider bore is used to remove a small amount of tissue for similar analysis. A positive biopsy (indicating cancer cells in the sample) is always conclusive, but a negative one may not be, because the needle may have missed the malignant portion of a growth. Thus, while needle biopsy is easier and less expensive than surgical biopsy, it is open

to a wider margin of error. Nevertheless, it may be preferable to surgical biopsy when a patient cannot undergo even minor surgery owing to poor health or because the recuperation period would interfere with other necessary treatment. Other tests involving the removal of fluid for diagnostic purposes but not related to cancer tests are AMINOCENTESIS, CULDOCENTESIS, and various kinds of BLOOD TEST.

4 Punch biopsy The removal of a small wedge of suspicious tissue with a special instrument that, in effect, punches rather than cuts it out. *Multiple punch biopsy* (involving several punches) is almost always used to diagnose possible cancer of the cervix based on an abnormal PAP SMEAR.

5 Breast biopsy A surgical biopsy (see definition 1 above) of breast tissue. An incision three to four centimetres (one to one-and-a-half inches) long is made over the nodule if the tumour or lump is near the surface. If the lump is deeply embedded, the incision may be made under the breast and the breast lifted up to expose the growth. The growth is then excised, together with surrounding tissue, and the small blood vessels in the area are closed off so that little or no blood is lost. In the case of a large or deep mass, a drain may be inserted and removable sutures (stitches) used to close the incision. See also CANCER, BREAST.

6 Vulvar biopsy The removal and analysis of a small patch of skin from the vulva in order to test for skin cancer. It usually requires only local anaesthesia, and if the incision is small, not even sutures will be required.

7 Cervical biopsy The removal and examination of a small amount of tissue from the cervix, usually performed if a PAP SMEAR has indicated abnormality.

Examination by COLPOSCOPY may pinpoint the area from which tissue should be taken. Cervical biopsy is often an outpatient procedure and requires no anaesthesia; usually only a mild cramp or two are felt when the specimen is taken. If the suspicious area extends up into the cervical canal (see CERVIX) the doctor may recommend an *endocervical curettage*, in which tissue from the cervical lining is scraped off and evaluated. In CONIZATION, a cone-shaped piece of tissue is cut from the cervix.

8 Endometrial biopsy Also *uterine biopsy.* The removal and analysis of tissue from the uterine lining, or endometrium. There are two ways of obtaining the tissue. The first is by means of *curettage*; that is, a small scraper, called a curette or curet, is inserted through the cervical canal into the uterus and is scraped downward along the endometrium to remove shallow strands of tissue. A local anaesthetic in the cervix may be used to minimize the pain, which ranges from moderate to strong cramping. An outpatient procedure, endometrial curettage is often used to evaluate abnormal bleeding, especially in women over thirty-five or in those who have a family history of endometrial cancer, and to evaluate fertility problems (the lining gives evidence of ovulation and of normal endocrine activity). The second principal method is by *vacuum aspiration* (suction) and resembles the procedure used for an early vacuum abortion. A narrow tube is inserted into the uterus through the cervix and the application of suction removes a portion of the endometrial tissue. Vacuum scraping, like curettage is used to make sure there is no abnormal thickening of the lining (endometrial hyperplasia) or cancerous tissue. Local anaesthesic may be used to minimize cramping. Vacuum aspiration has largely replaced other techniques that use a salt solution to wash cells from the uterine cavity.

Birth attendant A person who assists a woman during labour and delivery. The term is usually used for a person trained to do this work, such as a midwife or obstetrician. See also MIDWIFE; PREPARED CHILDBIRTH.

Birth canal The corridor, or passage, through which a baby passes during childbirth, from the uterus down and out through the vagina. Some confine the use of the term to the vagina itself; others apply it more broadly to the entire bony pelvis, the cervix, and the vagina, since constriction at any point in this area can prevent the passage of the baby.

Birth control A term invented by Margaret Sanger (1879-1966), a pioneer in the early 20th-century movement to help women prevent unwanted pregnancies, for the means and methods so used. In the early 20th century condoms and diaphragms were available in Britain although in 1909 a bill was put before parliament to ban the sale of all contraceptives. However campaigners such as Marie Stopes who wrote *Married Love* (1918) helped to change views of the legislators. Until 1967 voluntary organizations such as the Family Planning Association played a leading role in providing clinics for women seeking contraceptive advice and supplies. The 1967 NHS (Family Planning) Act allowed local authorites to give advice and supplies but a fee was charged. In 1974 free family planning services were made available.

Though the term 'birth control' is relatively new, various modes of birth control have been practiced since ancient times, despite the fact that understanding of the human reproductive system was very limited until the late 19th century. Over the years, animal dung, serpent fat, honey, lemon juice, silk paper, and many other substances have been placed inside the vagina to prevent conception. Today a variety of tested contraceptives and methods are available. Most of them involve only the woman's body, although there are a few MALE CONTRACEPTIVES. All have advantages and disadvantages, and none is entirely risk-free, although methods of NATURAL FAMILY PLANNING carry only the risk of pregnancy. Moreover, even today, birth control, which implicitly acknowledge that sexual activity without intent of reproduction is healthy and normal, is frowned on by certain groups, notably the Roman Catholic Church and other religious bodies, and some forms of it are expressly forbidden by them. The availability of birth control also implies a changing attitude toward female sexuality, acknowledging that – contrary to Victorian and earlier ideas – women as well as men were concerned with the pleasure of sex and may have a sanctioned role other than that of motherhood.

Ideally, choosing a method of birth control should precede any heterosexual activity, except when pregnancy is desired. A woman's first birth-control check-up, which can be performed at a family planning clinic or by a family doctor, should involve a breast and pelvic examination, blood pressure, urine and blood tests, and a PAP SMEAR. If ORAL CONTRACEPTIVES are being considered, further tests may be needed. An important part of the check-up is the interview, during which the doctor tries to identify any relevant diseases and habits (for example, liver problems, high blood pressure, smoking) and educates the woman concerning the kinds of birth control available (see the discussion under CONTRACEPTIVE) and which of them might best suit her way of life. The interview should include a history of her reproductive life, including menstrual cycle, pregnancies and their outcome, sexual experiences and frequency, and previous contraceptive experience, and for oral contraceptives, family history concerning certain diseases. A follow-up visit should be made three months later to make sure that the method chosen is satisfactory. See also PREGNANCY COUNSELLING.

Birth defects Also *congenital abnormalities (defects)*. Physical abnormalities in babies that are present from birth, which may or may not be hereditary. Some of them, such as phenylketonuria (PKU), can be detected and treated immediately, with a high chance of complete recovery. Others, such as Tay-Sachs disease and sickle cell disease, may not be detected for months or years and may be not only untreatable, but fatal. Still others, such as mental retardation, occur in widely varying degrees, from very slight to very severe.

There are two principal sources of birth defects. One is outside influences during pregnancy and delivery, which include the mother's exposure to radiation, drugs (including alcohol and nicotine), virus infections, malnutrition, various chronic diseases, and damage during labour and delivery. The other is abnormalities of the baby's genes or chromosomes, which are sometimes called *genetic disorders*. Some genetic disorders, such as Gaucher's disease, are hereditary; others, such as Down's syndrome (mongolism) are not.

The number of known *teratogens* – agents with injurious effects on the development of a foetus – is large and growing quickly (as more is learned about various chemicals and their effects). Among them are methyl mercury (found in contaminated fish), which can cause CEREBRAL PALSY; the hormones oestrogen and progesterone, which when administered during pregnancy can produce cardiovascular defects; the antibiotic tetracycline, which can produce hypoplasia (underdevelopment) of the teeth and stained dental enamel; the RUBELLA (German measles) virus, which can lead to early foetal death as well as serious abnormalities; the tranquillizer THALIDOMIDE, which prevents normal development of arms and legs; and various kinds of radiation, including high-dosage X-rays, which can produce an assortment of disorders. Rubella is by no means the only common infectious disease that causes damage. Other viruses also are dangerous, among them those causing chicken pox, herpes simplex, hepatitis, influenza, syphilis, smallpox, and some kinds of encephalitis. (See also CONGENITAL INFECTION.) For this reason, it is highly recommended that women who are pregnant (or who *could* be pregnant) avoid all live vaccines (made with attenuated live organisms), anaesthesia, chemicals, exposure to X-ray and other kinds of radiation, and drugs – not only prescription drugs but over-the-counter remedies such as aspirin. They should also greatly restrict (if possible, stop) smoking and limit their intake of alcohol. (See also DRUG USE AND PREGNANCY; ALCOHOL USE; SMOKING.)

It is estimated that more than 4 per cent of the population carry some kind of genetic disorder, of which there are three basic kinds: chromosome defects, single-

If You Are Pregnant,
Protect Your Unborn Child by Avoiding

- All nonessential medication (including antacids, laxatives, over-the-counter painkillers) unless prescribed by a doctor who knows you are (or might be) pregnant

- Alcoholic beverages (keep to bare minimum or abstain entirely)

- Excessive caffeine (reduce or stop consumption of coffee, tea, cola drinks, etc.)

- Immunization with any live virus vaccine, including flu vaccines

- Infection, especially with rubella, measles, mumps, herpes simplex, syphilis, gonorrhoea, viral hepatitis, cytomegalovirus, influenza, and toxoplasmosis

- Tobacco (reduce or, preferably, stop smoking)

- X-rays unless essential (in that case, be sure to shield pelvic area with lead apron)

gene disorders, and multifactorial or polygenic disorders. *Chromosome defects* involve either an excess or lack of chromosomal DNA. Unlike the other genetic defects, they are seldom *familial*, that is, they usually constitute an isolated instance in a family. The most common chromosomal disorder is DOWN'S SYNDROME, usually caused by the presence of an extra chromosome. Like other chromosomal defects, it is often associated with maternal age, that is, the older the mother, the greater the risk of this birth defect. A special category of chromosomal defects are those affecting only the sex chromosomes, which produce ambiguities of sex differentiation in the child. Among these are TURNER'S SYNDROME and KLINEFELTER'S SYNDROME. The latter is associated with paternal age, that is, the older the father, the greater the risk. Chromosomal defects in prospective parents are readily detected by examining the nuclei of white blood cells scraped from the lining of the mouth (a *buccal smear*), since they are present in every body cell. (See also CHROMOSOME.)

Single-gene defects occur when there is one or a pair of *mutant* genes. If the gene is *dominant*, its presence in either father or mother gives each of their children a 50 per cent chance of contracting the disorder. (The terms gene, mutant, dominant, and recessive are explained under CHROMOSOME.) More than 1,200 dominant-gene disorders have been identified, among them Huntington's chorea, a progressive and fatal neurologic disorder, and primary hyperlipidaemia, a predisposition to premature arteriosclerosis. If the gene is *recessive*, its presence in both parents gives each of their offspring a 25 per cent chance of having it. Among the 950 or so such disorders known are TAY-SACHS DISEASE, SICKLE CELL DISEASE, and PHENYLKETO-

NURIA. If the gene is recessive and *X-linked* (present on the X chromosome only), it is transmitted only by mothers principally to their sons (their sons carry a 50 per cent risk). Among the 150 disorders of this kind that have been identified are HAEMOPHILIA A, which is characterized by lack of the clotting factor in blood; DUCHENNE MUSCULAR DYSTROPHY, progressive weaking and degeneration of the muscle fibres; and a form of mental retardation associated with a 'fragile X' chromosome, in which the X chromosomes are marred by constrictions that make them fragile or easily broken.

Multifactorial or *polygenic disorders* come from the interaction of pairs of genes with each other and with environmental factors. This kind of birth defect includes many congenital malformations, among them cleft lip and cleft palate, club foot, and SPINA BIFIDA. Some of these, too, seem to be associated with older parents. In addition, it is believed that genetic factors are partly responsible for the development of arthritis, gout, stomach ulcers, high blood pressure, schizophrenia, diabetes, manic-depressive illness, and some kinds of cancer.

Since 1968 AMNIOCENTESIS has been used to diagnose chromosomal abnormalities in the foetus, as well as a few biochemical disorders and some brain and spinal-cord defects. Also, GENETIC COUNSELLING can be valuable for suggesting tests to determine the presence of a disease and assessing the risk of its transmission to children. In 1981 a baby who might have died because of its inability to use the vitamin biotin (a genetic defect) was diagnosed early, before birth, and was treated successfully by giving the mother large daily doses of the substance for the final three months of pregnancy, an unusual instance of antenatal therapy.

Birth stool A backless seat used during childbirth to keep the mother in a sitting position. This position serves to shorten and widen the pelvis, assists gravity in expelling the baby, and helps avoid the discomfort of BACK LABOUR. It is said to be particularly useful during the second (expulsion) stage of LABOUR. At least one American manufacturer now produces a motorized *birthing chair* that enables the woman to sit upright or recline and also gives the birth attendant full access to the pelvic area.

Birth weight The weight of a newborn baby, which is often directly related to its relative maturity and chances of survival. The average weight for a full-term white baby in Britain is 7 pounds (3,200 grams). Most PREMATURE babies, that is, babies born before thirty-seven weeks of gestation, weigh less than 2,500 grams (5½ pounds) and are often not well enough developed to survive without special care (sometimes not even then). Therefore the birth weight of 2,500 grams was considered a mark of adequate maturity, and any baby weighing less was considered a high risk. However, weight alone is not the only indicator of maturity, and some full-term or even postmature (past term) infants weight less than 2,500 grams and are in no special danger. Today, therefore, babies tend to be evaluated in terms of both weight and gestational age, and their care is based on these criteria as well as other factors.

The cause of low birth weight may be genetic (parents who are of short stature themselves or transmitting a genetic disorder associated with short stature) or, more often, malnutrition. Malnutrition of the baby in turn may be caused by a disease of the mother, such as hypertension, kidney disease, or severe diabetes, that prevents the passage of sufficient nutrients through the placenta. Cigarette smoking and drug addiction in the mother also appear to be associated with low birth weight, as is inadequate diet. Some researchers maintain that efforts to keep a pregnant woman from gaining too much weight – a popular strategy of obstetricians for many years – result in inadequate protein intake, which contributes to low birth weight (and other problems). See WEIGHT GAIN, definition 2; also under DIET.

Bisexual   The desire and/or practice of having sexual relationships with a person of either sex, that is, engaging in both HOMOSEXUAL and HETEROSEXUAL activities.

Bladder   Also *urinary bladder.* A sac in the front of the pelvis that serves as a reservoir for urine, which it receives through the ureters from the kidneys and discharges through the uretha. Roughly triangular in shape when empty, the bladder is capable of considerable distention as it is filled, taking on an ovoid form. The inside of the bladder is lined with mucous membrane covering layers of involuntary muscle fibres, which are kept in a state of relaxation at the same time that the urinary SPHINCTER is contracted. The kidneys deposit urine in the bladder at the rate of about thirty drops a minute. When the bladder is full, there is a sensation of pressure, perceived as the need to void. The female bladder is very prone to inflammation and infection, usually caused by bacteria transported upward from the urethra (see CYSTITIS). Relaxation of the muscles

following pregnancy and childbirth occasionally causes loss of support, so that the bladder projects down, sometimes all the way into the vagina; see CYSTOCELE. See also FREQUENCY, URINARY; STRESS INCONTINENCE.

Bladder infection   See CYSTITIS.

Bleeding, vaginal   After menarche and before menopause, bleeding that usually represents either normal MENSTRUAL FLOW or some disturbance of the menstrual cycle, called BREAKTHROUGH BLEEDING. Strictly speaking, the blood nearly always just passes through the vagina and exits from it, having originated in the uterus. Before menarche (the first menstrual period) and after menopause (defined as one year after the last period), any vaginal bleeding should be considered abnormal and, because it can be a symptom of cancer or some other serious disease, should be promptly investigated. Vaginal bleeding during pregnancy is also not normal and should be checked without delay. Some vaginal infections give rise to a blood-tinged discharge (see VAGINITIS). For other causes and kinds of vaginal bleeding, see ANOVULATORY BLEEDING; DYSFUNCTIONAL BLEEDING; ENDOMETRIAL HYPERPLASIA; FUNCTIONAL BLEEDING; HAEMORRHAGE, VAGINAL; POSTMENOPAUSAL BLEEDING; POSTPARTUM HAEMORRHAGE.

Bloating   See OEDEMA.

Blood clot   See THROMBUS.

Blood count   See under BLOOD TEST.

Blood pressure   See under HYPERTENSION.

Blood test Test of a sample of blood to detect disease or some abnormality. There are blood tests for syphilis, rubella and its antibodies, thyroid function, liver damage, and hundreds of other conditions. The most common kind of blood test is a *blood count* to detect ANAEMIA, which can be performed by taking a small amount of blood from the finger or earlobe. (For most other blood tests a larger specimen must be drawn from a vein, in the arm or elsewhere.) Two techniques for a blood count are in common use. The *haemoglobin method* measures the concentration of haemoglobin (red pigment) in the blood; any haemoglobin value below 12 grams per 100 cc. (millilitres) of blood indicates anaemia. The *haematocrit method* measures the percentage of red blood cells in total blood volume; anything below 35 per cent is considered anaemia. Many authorities believe a blood count should be part of every standard medical check-up.

A more extensive test used for routine screening of all hospitalized patients is the *full blood count*, or *FBC*, which measures the number, size, and oxygen-carrying capacity of the components that make up blood. In adults the number of mature red and white cells remains fairly constant, with old cells being replaced by new ones created in the bone marrow. The FBC determines whether this process is functioning smoothly. Haemoglobin, which transports oxygen from the lungs to other body cells, is checked for its efficient functioning. The number of white blood cells per sample is counted; an elevated number may indicate the presence of infection. The blood's smallest particles, the platelets, which aid in clotting, are also counted, and a description is presented of all the blood cells found (especially the structure of the red blood cells).

Blood Chemistry Profile

Glucose (sugar) acts as the major fuel for bodily processes. Determining the amount of glucose in one's blood may be useful in diagnosing diabetes (high blood sugar) or hypoglycaemia (low blood sugar).

BUN (Blood Urea Nitrogen) is the end point of protein breakdown in the body. One's BUN level varies with the amount of protein intake. Determining the amount of BUN in the blood may be useful in discovering diseases related to the kidneys or the urinary tract.

Creatinine is the waste material from the breakdown of creatine phosphate, which interacts with other substances to produce energy used by the body. The level of creatinine in the blood remains fairly constant and is a good indicator of kidney function. An elevated level of creatinine may suggest that the kidney's ability to filter and remove waste from the bloodstream is damaged, or that there is reduced blood flow to the kidneys due to blockage.

Enzymes are different proteins which function as biochemical catalysts aiding the processes of the body. Enzyme levels are checked to determine if the heart muscle and the liver are functioning properly.

Bilirubin is the waste product from the breakdown of haemoglobin. The substance exists in a nonsoluble (indirect) and a soluble (direct) form. Determining the levels of bilirubin may be used to discover disorders of the liver, bile ducts (ducts through which a digestive juice secreted by the liver is poured into the small intestine), or red blood cells. An elevated level of direct bilirubin may indicate that red blood cells are breaking down at an excessive rate. An elevated level of indirect bilirubin may indicate that the substance is building up because the liver can't do its job effectively.

Calcium/Phosphorus By weight, calcium is the most plentiful mineral in the body; it is stored in the blood and bones. Phosphorus unites with calcium to form an insoluble combination that gives the skeleton its shape and structure. Proportions of calcium and phosphorus are delicately balanced, and testing the levels of these minerals may determine problems in muscle contraction, carbohydrate metabolism, kidney malfunction, or the presence of kidney stones.

Uric acid is the endpoint of the breakdown of nucleic acids, which store genetic information needed to encode individual characteristics of each cell. Elevated levels of uric acid can be seen in a variety of conditions, one of which is gout – a condition in which a large amount of uric acid is being deposited in the vicinity of cartilage tissues such as joints.

Cholesterol is the basis for the synthesis of compounds that regulate many important bodily processes. The body manufactures cholesterol, mainly through the liver. Cholesterol is also available in foods such as fatty cuts of meat, dairy products, and egg yolks. Two types of cholesterol exist: high-density lipoprotein (HDL) and low-density lipoprotein (LDL). A high reading of HDL is considered 'good'; a low reading of HDL may indicate that plaque is being deposited in arteries which may clog them.

Proteins are the major solid portions dissolved in the liquid portion of blood (serum). Varying amounts of proteins may indicate how well the body's metabolic processes are functioning, how well the blood is transporting nutrients to various parts of the body, and how well the body can defend itself against infection. Generally, tests for protein include specific tests for albumin and globulin, two types of protein vital for effective transportation of chemicals through the bloodstream.

Bloody show Also *show.* See MUCUS PLUG.

Bone loss Also *bone resorption.* See under OSTEOPOROSIS.

Braxton-Hicks contractions Irregular contractions of the muscles of the uterus that occur during pregnancy. During the last weeks a woman becomes aware of the fact that her abdomen periodically becomes tense and firm (not painful). Actually, these contractions begin to occur early in pregnancy but are not noticeable until a few weeks before term, when they contribute to the dilation of the cervix. They are named after the doctor who first observed them. Occasionally they are strong enough to be mistaken for true labour (see FALSE LABOUR).

Breakthrough bleeding   Also *spotting, staining, metrorrhagia.* Bleeding from the vagina between regular menstrual periods. One common form of breakthrough bleeding is *midcycle spotting*, light staining that occurs in about 10 per cent of women for about two days halfway through the menstrual cycle, at the time of ovulation. It is harmless and requires no treatment.

In women of reproductive age who are not ovulating, the principal means of dealing with irregular bleeding are the administration of hormones (usually progesterone alone or combined with oestrogen), or a curettage—either a surgical D AND C or VACUUM ASPIRATION. In women who are ovulating, removing part of the endometrium (uterine lining) by curettage often stops heavy bleeding, at least for a time, and in the case of endometrial polyps serves to remove the cause as well. In either instance the tissue removed should be examined by a pathologist to rule out other, more serious conditions. Bleeding in girls before puberty and in women after menopause is definitely indicative of a possible serious disorder and should be investigated without delay. See also POSTMENO-PAUSAL BLEEDING.

Breast   One of a pair of modified sweat glands located in the superficial tissue of the chest wall, which in men have no function but in women are able to secrete milk. In women the breast usually extends from the second or third rib to the fifth or sixth rib; underlying it are the pectoral muscles. Each breast contains about twenty separate lobes, arranged like the spokes of a wheel. Each lobe consists of many smaller lobules and ends in tiny milk-producing glands called ACINI. The lobes, lobules, and acini are connected to the NIPPLE by a complex network of ducts. The remainder of the breast is composed of fat and fibrous tissue.

Two kinds of fibrous structure support the breast and maintain its form. One is a layer of connective tissue that runs immediately under the skin of the breast. The second is made up of multiple fibrous bands, called *Cooper's ligaments*, which begin at the layer of connective tissue and run through the breast to attach loosely to the fascia over the muscles of the chest wall. Many women also have crescent-shaped areas of thickened tissue at the lower border of each breast; these are called *inframammary ridges* or *folds* and have no known significance. The bulk of each breast's gland tissue is in the upper outer quadrant (closest to the armpit), and this is also the most common site for breast tumours. In fact, often a little breast tissue projects from this quadrant into the armpit, or axilla; it is called the *axillary tail*, or *tail of Spence.*

The growth and development of the breast are regulated by hormones. Chief among them are oestrogen and progesterone, from the ovaries, and prolactin, from the pituitary. Oestrogen promotes growth of the milk duct system, stimulates the growth of glandular buds at the ends of the ducts, causes the deposit of fat and proliferation of fibrous tissues within the breast, and increases the pigmentation (colouring) of the nipple and AREOLA. Progesterone stimulates the growth and maturation of the gland tissues of the breast and causes the gland buds to develop into acini, but it can exert this effect only when the breast tissue has first been prepared by oestrogen. Prolactin acts directly on the breast to stimulate gland growth and is responsible for the production of milk. Two other hormones, growth hormone (somatotrophin or somatomammatrophin) and adrenocorticotrophin, are necessary for breast tissue to respond to oestrogen, progesterone, and prolactin, but the mechanism whereby this operates is not understood.

Breast development in girls usually begins around the age of ten or eleven. If it occurs much before the age of nine or if none has occurred by the age of sixteen, it is advisable to check for possible abnormalities. At first only the nipple begins to protrude from the chest, and then gland tissue begins to grow under it; this is sometimes called a breast bud, and may occur on one side much sooner than on the other. A woman's breasts rarely are identical in size, but if the difference is very great one should check for abnormality caused by a tumour or other problem.

The size of the breasts depends on heredity, the influence of oestrogen and progesterone, and nutrition, weight gain or loss often affecting breast size. Almost any size is considered normal. Some women who are very unhappy about the appearance of their breasts undergo surgery to enlarge or reduce them (see MAMMAPLASTY). Massive breast growth may occur during puberty or pregnancy as the result of abnormal sensitivity of one or both breasts to increased oestrogen levels; some women find that oral contraceptives have a similar effect although usually to a lesser extent. The shape of the breasts depends on heredity, fat deposits, and the strength of the Cooper's ligaments; changes in shape occur primarily as a result of stretched ligaments, which occurs sooner or later with age. The use of a bra for heavy breasts may delay such stretching, but the main purpose of wearing bras is for comfort and appearance.

The breast is subject to a number of disorders, ranging in seriousness from an occasional cyst or minor infection to cancer. The three most common lesions are CYSTIC DISEASE, FIBROADENOMA, and cancer (see CANCER, BREAST). See also BREAST-FEEDING; BREAST SELF-EXAMINATION; CYSTOSARCOMA PHYLLODES; DUCTAL PAPILLOMA; LACTATION; LIPOMA; MAMMALGIA; MAMMARY DUCT ECTASIA; MAMMARY DUCT FISTULA; MASTITIS; PAGET'S DISEASE, definition 1.

Breast augmentation, reduction, reconstruction See MAMMAPLASTY.

Breast cancer See CANCER, BREAST.

Breast-feeding Also *nursing.* Suckling an infant, the oldest form of feeding human babies and a method shared by all mammals. (See LACTATION for an explanation of milk production.) In Western civilization breast-feeding has from time to time fallen into disrepute. Wealthy women who did not wish to be tied down to regular feedings of an infant would employ a *wet-nurse*, a woman lactating after having given birth herself, who was willing and able to breast-feed another woman's child. Wet-nurses were indispensable when a mother died during or soon after childbirth, a frequent occurrence until sterile methods of childbirth were introduced in the 19th century. In the 20th century, with the development of a special baby-food industry that also manufactured milk formulas to be fed to newborn babies, an alternative to the wet-nurse became available in grocery shops and chemists. Various means were employed to stop lactation in mothers not planning to breast-feed, such as breast-binding and ice-packs. These do not actually stop lactation (only lack of suckling does), and one method, the administration of hormones (particularly DIETHYLSTILBOESTROL, or DES), is dangerous to the mother.

Most authorities agree that breast-feeding is the ideal form of nourishing an infant. Breast milk is highly digestible and transmits an arsenal of immunological weapons (both antibodies and anti-allergens) to an infant's still immature body, immoblizing otherwise harmful infectious organisms and allergens. Breast-feeding is regulated by the infant; the amount of milk produced is directly proportionate to the amount the baby suckles, and hence overfeeding and early obesity are prevented. Breast milk is always warm, fresh, sterile, and conveniently available.

Breast-feeding has advantages for the mother as well. Suckling after childbirth stimulates the pituitary to release oxytocin, the hormone that makes the uterus contract during labour and afterward helps it return to its normal state. Extra weight gained during pregnancy is more easily lost; the nursing mother needs only about 500 extra calories a day and need not follow any special diet other than making sure she drinks enough liquids – almost any liquid. Breast-feeding usually delays the resumption of ovulation and menstruation, but birth control must still be used to avoid pregnancy since one is never sure when ovulation resumes until after the fact. The principal disadvantage of breast-feeding is that it ties down the mother. Usually, however, substitute bottles can be given as often as once a day – more often if they are made with her breast milk, expressed manually and refrigerated – and of course she can discontinue breast-feeding whenever she wishes.

There are a few contraindications to breast-feeding. Among them are active tuberculosis and chicken pox in the mother, both of which can be transmitted to an infant through her milk. Also, women taking anti-cancer drugs, radio-active medications of any kind, or hormones are advised not to breast-feed. Barbiturates, large amounts of alcohol (more than six ounces a day), and some antibiotics and tranquillizers should be avoided. On the other hand, women who had had breast reconstruction surgery with silicone implants may be able to breast-feed, as can women who have had breast reduction surgery (unless very large amounts of secretory tissue have been removed or several mammary ducts have been cut). Women who have had a mastectomy can usually nurse with the remaining breast. Breast engorgement and local infection – even a breast abscess – need not interfere with nursing; indeed, the pain of these conditions may be relieved by nursing, which reduces the pressure of fluids on the affected parts. A woman can continue to nurse while pregnant with another child; although nursing does trigger the release of oxytocin, it does not induce miscarriage. However, some authorities warn that, since dietary calcium tends to go to the breast milk first, the foetus may thus be deprived of it, leading to a low birth weight and impaired development.

Following the birth of another child a woman can continue to nurse both the new baby and a toddler. Many women have successfully nursed twins and triplets. A premature infant who must be placed in an incubator can be fed milk expressed from the mother's breasts by hand or with an electric breast pump, which will maintain her milk supply and give the child the benefits of breast milk until it can nurse.

There is no evidence that breast-feeding has any permanent effect on the size and shape of the breast (see BREAST). Although for a time it was believed that women who breast-fed had a lower risk of developing breast cancer, there is no clear-cut evidence that breast-feeding affords such protection.

Breast-feeding may be begun immediately after delivery (even before the umbilical cord is cut), although many hospitals delay the initial feeding for eight hours or longer. Some also offer one or two feedings of water first, to help the infant regurgitate any mucus or other secretions swallowed during delivery. Those who strongly favour breast-feeding oppose this practice, believing a baby should be put to the breast as soon as possible after delivery. *Colostrum*, a protein-rich yellow fluid that precedes milk secretion (see under LACTATION), is the chief source of nourishment for the first three or four days, but suckling stimulates earlier milk production. To breast-feed effectively the infant must place the NIPPLE well back in the mouth, close the lips tightly around the AREOLA, and squeeze the nipple against the palate with the tongue. This procedure compresses the lactiferous sinuses behind the areola and draws milk into the mouth. (Complicated as this may sound, most infants accomplish it almost immedi-

ately.) For the first few weeks, until the milk supply is well established and the baby is growing at a normal rate, most authorities recommend letting the baby nurse whenever it wants to, approximately every three or four hours or even more often, a method called *demand feeding*. After this initial period of adjustment, the mother can to some extent regulate the feeding schedule according to her convenience.

A number of HERBAL REMEDIES have been used to help women with the problem of sore nipples. Among these are rubbing the nipples with resin of balsam fir or with sweet almond oil; simmering three tablespoons of common spurge or milk purslane (*Euphorbia maculata*) in a cup of olive oil or glycerine for fifteen minutes and then rubbing on the nipples. The herb milkwort (*Polygala vulgaris*), eaten raw or made into a tea, has been used to increase the milk supply but may be toxic.

Breast self-examination A systematic examination by a woman of her own breasts in order to detect any abnormalities. Ideally it is carried out every month, but if one forgets it is better to do it occasionally than not at all. Breast cancer is the most common malignancy in women (current statistics estimate that one in every sixteen women in Britain will develop it) and carries the highest fatality rate of all cancers in women. Since early detection makes it much easier to treat breast cancer successfully, breast self-examination is the first and best line of defence. Approximately four out of every five breast lumps so detected turn out to be a cyst or other benign (noncancerous) lesion. If a lump is found, however, it is essential to determine as quickly as possible if it is cancerous or not.

The best time to perform breast self-examination is within a week after each menstrual period ends. Women who menstruate very irregularly, or who are pregnant, or who no longer menstruate, should select a particular day (the first, the fifteenth, payday) of each month to perform the examination. There are two parts to self-examination, inspection (looking) and palpation (feeling). Inspection is performed in front of a mirror, first with the arms at the sides and then with both arms raised over the head. Look for changes in size or shape, sores or scaling on the nipple or areola, discharge from the nipple, change in position of one or both nipples, redness or other skin discolouration, inward puckering or dimpling of the skin or nipple, enlargement of skin pores, or any other change from previous appearance. Placing the hands on the hips and pressing to contract the muscles of the chest wall makes dimpling more obvious.

Palpation is done in two positions, first standing and then lying down. Standing – preferably in the bath or shower because it is easier to feel when the skin is wet and slippery – raise the right arm high and with the left hand, with fingers flat, gently explore the right breast in a clockwise motion. Feel for any unusual lump, mass, knot, thickening, area of tenderness, or other change from previous examination. Then repeat the process for the opposite side. Lying down, place the right hand behind the head and a small pillow or folded towel under the right shoulder. Then examine the right breast with the left hand, with fingers flat and close together, pressing gently in small circular motions around the breast as though it were the face of a clock. Begin at the outermost top edge of the breast and keep circling to examine every part of the breast, including the nipple. Then repeat the process for the other side.

For pendulous breasts, palpation should be done with both hands together. Place one hand under the breast, palm up, and the other above the breast, palm down. Then palpate between the fingers of both hands, slowly rotating the hands. The pendulous portion can thus be examined between the two hands rather than between one hand and the chest wall.

Breech presentation Also *breech birth*. In childbirth, the position of the baby when its buttocks (breech) are the presenting or leading part (that is, leading its descent into the birth canal). Breech presentation occurs in 3 to 4 per cent of all deliveries. Occasionally the breech is *incomplete*, with one foot or knee presenting (sometimes called a *footling breech*). In the far more common CEPHALIC PRESENTATION (head first), after the baby's largest part – the head – passes through the birth canal, the rest of the body follows with little difficulty. In a breech birth, successively larger portions of the baby are born: first buttocks, then shoulders, and last the head. Moreover, in cephalic presentation the head, which is still very malleable, is moulded by the forces of the contractions pushing it through the birth canal, as a result of which it may decrease as much as half an inch in diameter. In breech presentation there is no such opportunity, so that a larger pelvic diameter is needed to accommodate the passage of the head.

Opinion differs as to whether breech labours are more prolonged than cephalic ones – many obstetricians believe they are – but all agree that their risk to the baby is almost four times greater. Part of the reason for this is that breech babies are often premature; indeed, this may be the main cause of breech presentation, the smaller (premature) foetus having room to turn upside down inside the uterus. Another risk is the danger to the baby's head; intracranial haemorrhage, pressures on the head, the obstetrician's attempts to pull the head through the cervix, which has closed somewhat before the head can emerge – all contribute to this danger. Also, there is danger of compressing the umbilical cord, thus cutting off the baby's oxygen supply. In view of these risks, most obstetricians try to prevent breech presentation. If it is recognized in the last few weeks of pregnancy (from palpating the mother's abdomen), attempts may be made at *external version*, that is, gently but firmly manoeuvering the baby's position from the outside of the abdomen. Unfortunately, even when such version (turning) can be readily accomplished, the baby will often turn back to breech presentation.

In spontaneous delivery there is usually no problem until the baby's umbilicus is reached. From that point on, the doctor must be extremely watchful. If the head is larger than the pelvic girdle, a CAESAREAN SECTION must be performed. While dangerous in itself, Caesarean section is safer than a difficult extraction and should be used if there is a small pelvis, a very large baby, or uterine dysfunction (weak contractions). X-ray PELVIMETRY before or during labour may shown whether a baby's head is too large for the pelvis and help in weighing the risks and benefits of vaginal versus surgical delivery.

Brow presentation In childbirth, the position of the baby when its brow (forehead) is the presenting or leading part (the part that leads the baby's descent into the birth canal). Often a brow presenta-

tion will convert itself into either a vertex or a face presentation as the baby moves down the birth canal, forcing the baby to flex its chin into its chest (see CEPHALIC PRESENTATION). If brow presentation persists, vaginal delivery may be possible with a very small baby, but with a full-term baby of average size it usually is not, and a CAESAREAN SECTION will have to be performed. Brow presentation is, however, the least common of abnormal presentation.

Bubo a painful inflammation or swelling of a lymph gland, usually in the groin, developing especially in the course of a venereal infection. See under CHANCROID and LYMPHOGRANULOMA VENEREUM.

Bulimarexia A cycle of alternate gorging (*bulimia*) and self-starvation (*anorexia*) that continues over a period of time. The name was coined by an American psychologist, Marlene Boskind-White, in the 1970s. Bulimarexia occurs chiefly in young women who have abnormally low self-esteem and become obsessed with attaining an ideal figure, which they perceive as an extremely thin body. They tend to view themselves as fat when in fact they often are already very thin. The cycle frequently begins with an eating binge, in which the woman eats anything and everything available until she literally feels ill. It is followed by feelings of self-disgust and shame, which she deals with by extreme dieting or complete fasting, and sometimes also by purging (self-induced vomiting, laxative abuse, use of amphetamines). This aberrant behaviour then becomes a regular routine. Unlike ANOREXIA NERVOSA, bulimarexia rarely prohibits functioning in day-to-day life or requires hospitalization, although the bizarre eating pattern takes up considerable time and energy. It 'is not known how widespread the condition is, partly because it was recognized only recently and partly because one of its characteristic features is that the binging and purging take place secretly. Attempts to cure the condition usually involve some form of psychotherapy. Group therapy in particular appears to show promise, since it forces patients to acknowledge that neither their behaviour nor the feelings prompting it are unique. Therapy is directed largely at building up self-esteem.

Bulimia   See under BULIMAREXIA.

C

Caesarean section Also *abdominal delivery, surgical delivery.* Delivery of a baby through a surgical incision in the uterus. Although this kind of surgery dates from ancient times, until recently it was performed only to save the life of the child because it almost invariably caused the death of the mother (unless she was already dead; Caesareans were and still are performed to extract live infants from dead mothers). Today the use of blood transfusions and antibiotics has enormously reduced the death toll from haemorrhage and infection, making Caesarean section one of the safest of major operations. By 1980 it also had become, at least in North America, one of the procedures performed so frequently that many began to consider it unnecessary surgery. In Britain, the Caesarian section rate is not so great (about 10 per cent) but has shown an increase over the last ten years.

The principal indication for a Caesarean section is SYSTOCIA, that is, abnormal labour, caused by a contracted (too small) pelvis, too large a baby, abnormal presentation, uterine dysfunction (too weak contractions), or a combination of these factors. In addition, many American doctors long maintained that vaginal delivery risks rupturing the scar of a previous Caesarean delivery. This belief, not held in most other countries including Britain, was increasingly questioned, and in 1982 the American College of Obstetricians and Gynecologists reversed a 75-year-old policy and announced that vaginal deliveries following a Caesarean were safe under certain circumstances. Other indications for surgical delivery are haemorrhage caused by either ABRUPTIO PLACENTAE or PLACENTA PRAEVIA, the presence of PRE-ECLAMPSIA or ECLAMPSIA, RH FACTOR incompatibility, serious infection, other serious maternal disease such as heart disease or diabetes, and foetal distress, principally asphyxia.

A Caesarean section is much safer than it used to be, but it still constitutes major surgery. The risk of death to the mother is two to four times greater than with vaginal delivery, and recovery from it is much slower than from a vaginal delivery. Two main kinds of operation are in current use, differentiated by the location of the uterine incision. A *cervical incision,* which may be either transverse (crosswise) or vertical (longitudinal), is made in the lower segment of the uterus, above the cervix and behind the bladder. The low transverse incision (*Kerr incision*) is used whenever possible because it involves less blood loss during surgery, less risk of rupture in subsequent pregnancies and subsequent vaginal deliveries, less postoperative infection, and easier repair. Sometimes, because of foetal size (very large or very small) or position, or lack of space, or other problems, the low vertical incision (*Kronig-Selheim incision*) is performed. It is generally thought to be associated with more morbidity than the low transverse technique but is still considered preferable to the classical Caesarean.

In the older *classical section*, a vertical incision is made in the body of the uterus (rather than its lower portion). It allows a greater length for the surgical opening and more room for delivery of the foetus. It is used when there are problems with the mother (as when the placenta covers the lower uterine segment) or, more often, problems relating to the foetus's size and position (such as a crosswise, or transverse, lie). This incision is associated with more bleeding at the time of surgery and more intra-abodominal infection postoperatively. However, it continues to be used, especially in emergency cases when time is of the essence, because it is quicker and easier to perform.

The incisions just described are into the uterus, not the abdomen, and therefore do not affect the visible scar. There also are two kinds of abdominal incision, a vertical one that extends from the umbilicus almost to the pubis, or a transverse (PFANNENSTIEL) incision, just above the pubic mound. With a vertical abdominal incision the uterine incision usually also is vertical, but with a transverse incision it may be either vertical or transverse. Either general or regional anaesthesia may be used.

For women who looked forward to a vaginal delivery and planned to use one or another method of PREPARED CHILDBIRTH, a Caesarean can be a very upsetting experience. Some classes for prepared childbirth include educational material to prepare a woman for surgical delivery if it should become necessary.

Calendar method See under NATURAL FAMILY PLANNING.

Cancer Also *carcinoma, malignancy, malignant tumour, neoplasm*. A general name for what is thought to be at least one hundred different diseases that have certain traits in common. All of them are characterized by *abnormal cell division*; instead of normal cells reproducing in an orderly fashion to carry on the process of tissue growth and repair, cancer cells begin an uncontrolled process of dividing, creating a mass of extra cells or tissue that, when it takes a solid form is called a TUMOUR. There are several different kinds of cancer cells, each with a different rate of growth and spreading ability, but virtually all of them behave in this way. Secondly, cancer is usually *invasive*, that is, it infiltrates and actively destroys surrounding healthy tissue (but see also CANCER IN SITU). Thirdly, cancer can metastasize, that is, it can spread to other parts of the body, forming new growths called *metastases*. It was long thought that metastasis takes place by means of cancer cells spreading through the blood or lymph (the clear fluid that bathes body cells), but some authorities believe that at least some cancers are a systemic disease – one that affects the entire body in the same way as a generalized infection. Finally, cancer tends to *recur*. After a period of improvement or seeming cure, it may strike again, in the same part of the body or elsewhere. Untreated, cancer usually is fatal, displacing healthy tissue and causing organs to cease functioning until the patient dies. Occasionally, however, the disease will go into spontaneous remission, with the symptoms decreasing or disappearing altogether.

Cancer can attack just about any of the body's organs—the respiratory system,

The American Cancer Society's Screening Guidelines, 1981 also in appropriate in Britain

Test or procedure	New recommendation			Previous recommendation
	Sex	Age	Frequency	
Chest X-ray (for lung cancer)		Not recommended		High-risk persons, annually[1]
Sputum cytology (for lung cancer)		Not recommended		Not recommended
Signoidoscopy (for bowel cancer)	M & F	Over 50	Every 3-5 years[2]	Persons over 40 annually
Stool guaiac slide test	M & F	Over 50	Every year	Persons over 40 annually
Digital rectal examination	M & F	Over 40	Every year	Same
Pap test (for cervical cancer)	F	20-65[3]	At least every 3 years[4]	Annual
Pelvic examination (for cervical cancer)	F	20-40 / Over 40	Every 3 years / Every year	Annual / Same
Endometrial tissue sample	F	At menopause for high-risk women only[5]	At menopause	Same
Breast self-examination	F	Over 20	Every month	Same
Breast physical examination	F	20-40 / Over 40	Every 3 years / Every year	Annual / Same
Mammography	F	Between 35-40 / Under 50 / Over 50	One baseline exam / Consult family doctor / Every year	No general policy
Health counselling and cancer check-up[6]	M & F / M & F	Over 20 / Over 40	Every 3 years / Every year	'Periodic'

1 Persons over 40 who smoke or are exposed to other lung carcinogens.
2 After two initial negative examinations a year apart.
3 Pap test should also be done on women under 20 who are sexually active.
4 After two initial Pap tests done a year apart are negative. High-risk women should have more frequent Pap tests.
5 History of infertility, obesity, failure of ovulation, abnormal uterine bleeding, or oestrogen therapy.
6 To include examination for cancers of the thyroid, testicles, prostate, ovaries, lymph nodes, oral region, and skin.

SOURCE: American Cancer Society

digestive system, reproductive system, bones, brain, skin, blood, lymph. Indeed, cancers are often named after the organ where they originated (lung cancer, breast cancer, etc.). Cancer may also be classified according to the kind of tissue in which they arise. Adenocarcinomas involve glandular tissue; sarcomas involve connective tissue; adenosarcomas involve both connective and gland tissue (see also ADENOCARCINOMA; SARCOMA); leukaemias involves the blood cells; lymphomas involve the lymph nodes.

In women, nearly half of all cases of cancer affect the reproductive system, breast cancer accounting for about one quarter and the rest attacking the pelvic area (vulva, vagina, cervix, endometrium, Fallopian tubes, ovaries). Of the latter, cervical cancer is the second most common malignancy in women after breast cancer, followed by endometrial cancer (of the lining of the uterus). Cervical cancer tends to strike women in their mid-forties, while endometrial and ovarian cancers are more common after menopause. Tubal cancers are very rare.

The cause of cancer is still not known, but it is known that certain substances, called *carcinogens*, seem to trigger the disease. It is recognized, for example, that exposure to high doses of radiation often leads to the development of cancer, both in laboratory animals and in human beings. Similarly, heavy cigarette smokers are more apt to develop cancer of the respiratory system. On the other hand, direct cause-effect relationships cannot be established, because some heavy smokers never develop cancer even over a long lifespan. Viruses definitely cause some cancers in animals, and perhaps also in human beings. Also, certain cancers have been linked to a single dominant gene, indicating that a susceptibility to these particular malignancies is hereditary.

Because many cancers are not associated with warning symptoms such as pain until they are far advanced – often too far for any treatment to be effective – early cancer detection is of prime importance. Thus all women are advised to examine their own breasts monthly for lumps or other irregularities, as we as to have regular tests of their cervical cells (see BREAST SELF-EXAMINATION; PAP SMEAR). With early detection, before a cancer has had time to destroy much surrounding tissue or to spread to other parts of the body, the chances for a complete cure (using surgery, radiation, drugs, or some combination of these treatments) are thought to be much greater. Newer diagnostic techniques, such as radionuclide imaging, also assist early detection. (See also CHEMO-THERAPY; IMMUNOTHERAPY; RADIATION THERAPY.)

Some patients reject surgical, radiation, and chemical treatment in favour of nutritional, manipulative, or psychological therapies, used alone or in combination (or together with medical treatment). The nutritional approaches, which regard cancer as a systemic disease, include fasting, said to eliminate poisons from the body and deprive developing cancer cells of nourishment; raw foods (after fasting), to encourage the body's elimination of toxins and continue to starve the cancer cells; eliminating or limiting salt, refined sugar, and caffeine from the diet; vitamin therapy, with large doses of vitamin A (to build immunity, fight infection, keep cells from ageing), the B vitamins (to cope with stress and facilitate oestrogen metabolism), laetrile (B_{17}), found in apricot pits, which allegedly kills cancer cells without harming normal cells, vitamin C, in massive doses, vitamin E, and such minerals as magnesium, selenium, and zinc. Manipulative techniques include acupressure, acupuncture, and shiatsu. None of these has been recognized as an effective treatment by any reputable medical organization or shown to be effective by careful controlled studies.

One kind of psychological therapy used in conjunction with traditional (surgical, chemical) therapies and/or nutritional treatment is *mind visualization*. It involves mentally confronting issues in one's life that may have 'provoked' the cancer and then focusing one's emotional and mental energies on combatting the malignancy. Patients are taught to visualize at regular daily intervals the destruction of cancer cells by their own immune cells (and by any other means of treatment they may be undergoing). While such therapy may seem farfetched, cancers sometimes regress or go into remission for no objective reason, and so little is known about biofeedback (the body's responses to inner mental processes) that it cannot be dismissed entirely.

Researchers have formulated seven warning signs of cancer and advise anyone who observes any of these symptoms to seek medical advice as quickly as possible:

1. A change in bowel or bladder habits.
2. A sore that does not heal.
3. Unusual bleeding or discharge.
4. A thickening or lump in the breast or elsewhere.
5. Persistent indigestion or difficulty in swallowing.
6. An obvious change in a wart or a mole.
7. A nagging cough or hoarseness.

Usually these symptoms will indicate some other condition than cancer, but it is safer to make sure. See also the entries below on specific cancers affecting women; also, PRECANCEROUS LESIONS.

Cancer, breast The most common kind of CANCER in women between the ages of twenty-five and seventy-five. In Britain it was expected to attack approximately one in every sixteen women at some time during their lives. The highest risk is for white women between thirty-five and sixty-five, who have not borne children or who postponed their first pregnancy until after the age of thirty, who began to menstruate fairly early (before the age of eleven), who stopped menstruating late (after fifty-five), and who have had CYSTIC DISEASE of the breasts. Women with a mother or sister who has had breast cancer may have a risk two or three times greater than other women, depending partly on when the cancer developed (before or after menopause) and if it affected one or both breasts. An injury or blow to the breast is not related to the development of breast cancer, nor is breast-feeding, but exposure to ionizing radiation increases the risk.

Breast cancer is not a single disease. There are probably at least fifteen different kinds, each with a different rate of growth and different tendency to metastasize (spread to other parts of the body). It is local only briefly, and can develop in many parts of the breast: in the milk ducts, between ducts, in fat, in lymph or blood vessels, in the nipple, in the lobes where milk is manufactured (see PAGET'S DISEASE, definition 1). Men can also get breast cancer, but they account for only 1 per cent of all cases.

Practically 95 per cent of breast cancers are first detected by women themselves, making regular self-examination one of the principal means of early detection (see BREAST SELF-EXAMINATION). Besides lumps (80 per cent of which turn out to be benign growths or cysts), other early symptoms are thickened areas, irregularities of shape, nipple discharge, redness, flaking, puckering, enlarged pores, or other skin changes. Pain is rarely a symptom until the cancer is quite far advanced. The principal means of diagnosis – and many believe the only definitive one – is BIOPSY (see definition 5), although such means as MAMMO-GRAPHY, TRANSILLUMINATION, ULTRA-SOUND (see definition 1), and THERMO-GRAPHY also are employed, mainly as screening devices. Breast cancers may or may not be hormone-dependent, so a positive biopsy should be combined with an OESTROGEN-RECEPTOR ASSAY.

Treatment, which is still controversial, generally involves surgery of varying degrees, ranging from removal of a tumour alone to removal of the entire breast, underlying muscle, and axillary lymph nodes (see MASTECTOMY). The rationale of surgery (and the choice of what kind of surgery) is based on different ideas concerning the nature and spread of cancer. The radical rationale, which calls for the most extensive surgery, holds that the bloodstream is not the important route of metastasis (spread). Rather, a cancerous tumour remains local at the site of origin, spreads to nearby LYMPH NODES, and then continues spreading through the body in a systematic fashion. If adjacent lymph nodes are removed with the tumour, it is reasoned, the route of spread is cut off. A different view is that cancer is a systemic disease involving a complex spectrum of host-tumour relationships, and therefore variations in local or regional therapy are unlikely to affect a patient's survival. Rather, the cancer must be attacked systemically, through the use of RADIATION THERAPY, CHEMOTHERAPY (anti-cancer drugs), endocrine manipulation (changing the body's hormone levels and balance), and IMMUNOTHERAPY. Whatever therapy is used, there is no doubt that it is most effective when the cancer has not advanced much beyond Stage I or II. Approximately three quarters of the women found to have axillary (underarm) lymph node involvement when they were first treated eventually die of cancer, as do about one quarter of those without evidence of cancer in the nodes.

Until the 1970s surgeons usually combined biopsy and mastectomy into one operation (the *one-stage approach*). When research began to indicate that less radical surgery or nonsurgical treatment sometimes was just as effective, women began to campaign for a *two-step procedure*. After biopsy (step 1) they would determine which of the available treatments was best for them.

See also CANCER, INFLAMMATORY BREAST.

Cancer, cervical A CANCER of the cervix, that is, the neck of the uterus. The most common kind of pelvic cancer in women, it is almost 100 per cent curable if it is caught in its early stages and treated surgically. However, because it typically gives no warning whatever, it may be present for as long as four to ten years before it invades the deeper cervical tissues and gives rise to symptoms. Even then it is curable in 80 per cent of cases. Thereafter, however, it spreads to the vagina, uterus, bladder, and even the rectum, usually quite rapidly, and the outlook for cure is much less hopeful. Because its presence is as a rule unannounced, it is extremely important that all women, from the age of twenty on or when they become sexually active (whichever is first), undergo regular screening for cervical cancer, which is done by a very simple procedure called a PAP SMEAR.

Cervical cancer attacks about 2 to 3 per cent of all British women, most between the ages of thirty-five and fifty-five. If it is diagnosed very early, as a severe DYSPLASIA, it may respond to treatment, the method chosen depending on the location. Inside the cervical canal it is treated surgically with CONIZATION, which removes only part of the cervix and preserves the patient's ability to bear children; on the outside (ectocervix) it may be treated with CRYOSURGERY or laser therapy. In the next stage, when it is confined to the surface of the cervix (sometimes called CANCER IN SITU), treatment usually consists of surgical removal of both cervix and uterus (a hysterectomy); the ovaries can be left intact, since cervical cancer does not spread to the ovaries and is not affected by the production of oestrogen. If the cancer has advanced to the deeper tissues of the cervix, it is usually treated with radiation, although sometimes extensive surgery may be undertaken. At this stage there is still a 75 to 85 per cent chance of cure. With more advanced cancers, radiation is always the treatment of choice.

Although the cause of cervical cancer, like that of other cancers, is not yet known, there is increasing evidence that a sexually transmitted virus, Herpes simplex II, might be involved in at least some cancers, since women with genital HERPES INFECTION develop cervical cancer far more frequently than women never so infected. Earlier observations of the high incidence of cervical cancer in women who had sexual intercourse from an early age and with many different partners, as well as the lower incidence in women whose mates were invariably circumcised (Jews and Muslims), appeared to bear out this view. See also ADENOCARCINOMA, definition 2).

Cancer, endometrial A CANCER of lining of the uterus. It appears most often after the age of fifty and is often associated with previous menstrual irregularity (irregular periods), sporadic ovulation, and difficulty in becoming pregnant. It is also found more in obese women, in women with high blood pressure, and in women with diabetes. The most common symptom of endometrial cancer is irregular bleeding, with or without abdominal discomfort. For this reason women past menopause – defined as no menstrual periods for one year – who experience any bleeding or spotting, even just a pink stain, should be checked immediately. They may require a suction curettage and biopsy, or, if strongly suspicious, surgical D and C followed by examination of the tissue scrapings by a pathologist. (See BIOPSY, definition 8.) A Pap smear is not reliable for detecting endometrial cancer because the abnormal cells shed by the endometrium usually degenerate before reaching the vagina. In women still menstruating, grossly irregular periods and/or bleeding or staining between periods are cause for suspicion and, since about one quarter of all endometrial cancers occur before menopause, should be promptly investigated.

Cancer, inflammatory breast A rare kind of CANCER of the breast in which a tumour grows very rapidly and the skin over it is swollen, red, hot, and painful, as though there were a bacterial infection (there is not). It occurs mostly during pregnancy, and a biopsy is needed to establish the diagnosis. Inflammatory breast cancer is treated with radiation (with or without a simple mastectomy, involving removal of just the breast), following by hormone therapy or chemotherapy. See also CANCER, BREAST.

Cancer, ovarian A CANCER of the ovaries, which is among the least common of pelvic cancers but is, the fourth most common cause of death from cancer in Britain (after breast, colon, and lung cancer). The most silent of the pelvic cancers, and the most difficult to diagnose, ovarian cancer is usually too far advanced for successful treatment by the time there are symptoms. There are usually no early signs, it tends to spread rapidly, and it generally involves both ovaries simulataneously. It can occur at any age; under five and over eighty are not uncommon. The first warning signs are persistent indigestion and abdominal discomfort, particularly a sense of pelvic fullness because the cancer produces fluid in the abdominal cavity. Pain during sexual intercourse may be another sign. The only early detection is by a pelvic examination, in which the doctor can feel the enlargement of either ovary. Such enlargement must then be distinguished from an ovarian cyst (see CYST, definition 6). If a cyst is suspected in a woman who still wants to bear children, she is usually given oral contraceptives at first, whereas in a woman approaching or past menopause an immediate exploratory operation might be performed. If the ovary is found to be cancerous, the uterus, both tubes, and both ovaries generally are removed immediately. However, if the cancer is quite small and localized, the other ovary sometimes may be spared (see OOPHORECTOMY). Surgery is usually followed by radiation and/or chemotherapy. Even then, the outlook is not very favourable, since only 30 per cent of patients survive for five years or longer. Unlike endometrial cancer, ovarian cancer is rarely oestrogen-dependent; therefore removal of the ovaries may be followed by oestrogen replacement therapy to relieve severe menopausal symptoms. See also STAGING.

Cancer, pelvic General name for any cancer of the reproductive organs in the pelvis, in women particularly the uterus (cervix and endometrium) and ovaries, but also the Fallopian tubes, vagina, and vulva. Of these, cancer of the cervix is the most common, followed by cancer of the uterine lining, or endometrium. Cancer of the Fallopian tubes and of the vagina is extremely rare. See CANCER, CERVICAL; CANCER, ENDOMETRIAL; CANCER, OVARIAN; CANCER, VAGINAL; CANCER, VULVAR; CHORIOCARCINOMA.

Cancer, skin See CANCER, VULVAR; MELANOMA.

Cancer, uterine A CANCER of the uterus. The most common kinds are cervical cancer and endometrial cancer (see CANCER, CERVICAL; CANCER, ENDOMETRIAL). Much rarer is CHORIOCARCINOMA.

Cancer, vaginal A CANCER of the vagina. Primary vaginal cancer (originating in the vagina) is quite rare except in daughters of women who were treated with DIETHYLSTILBOESTROL during their pregnancy. (See also ADENOCARCINOMA, definition 2.) Cancer may spread to the vagina from the cervix but then is still regarded as cervical cancer.

Cancer, vulvar A CANCER of the VULVA, usually affecting the labia (lips) surrounding the vagina. This type of cancer is essentially a skin cancer and appears as a lump or sore on the vulva that can be readily seen and felt. However, women often tend to ignore such a lesion, which, if it is malignant, can then grow considerably. Another kind of vulvar cancer is MELANOMA, also a skin cancer; although it is rare, it is the second most common kind of vulvar malignancy.

The warning signs of vulvar cancer are a persistent sore or wartlike growth on the skin of the vulva, and persistent itching, redness, or thickening of the vulvar skin, or change in a mole. The lesions sometimes look very much like those of CONDYLOMA ACUMINATA (genital warts), and the only way to distinguish the two conditions is by biopsy (see BIOPSY, definition 6). Treatment is surgical, consisting of vulvectomy (removal of the labia, clitoris, underlying glands in the groin, about one-half of the vagina, and several inches of skin on each side of the vulva). Despite such extensive excision, sexual intercourse is still possible afterwards and can be satisfactory. See also PAGET'S DISEASE, definition 2.

Cancer in situ Also *carcinoma in situ.* Literally, cancer 'in place'. A growth disturbance in which normal cells are replaced by abnormal-appearing cells that do not yet have two fundamental characteristics of advanced cancers: invasiveness and metastasis (see CANCER). Instead the lesion is confined to the site of origin and has not yet invaded neighbouring tissues or spread elsewhere. Some authorities regard it as a very early and localized (hence 'in place') cancer, also called Stage 0 (see STAGING), and

believe that it can become invasive and then spread. Further, since there is no way to predict which lesions will remain localized and which will spread, they recommend immediate surgical removal. See also DYSPLASIA; PRECANCEROUS LESIONS.

Candida albicans See YEAST INFECTION.

Carcinoma Strictly speaking, a malignant (cancerous) tumour of epithelial tissue, as opposed to one involving connective tissue (sarcoma) or lymph tissue (lymphoma). However, in general medical usage the term is often used interchageably with CANCER.

Carcinoma in situ See CANCER IN SITU.

Castration Surgical removal or destruction by radiation of both gonads (sex glands), that is, both ovaries in women or both testes in men. When those glands can no longer fill their function of hormone production, permanent sterility results. See also STERILIZATION.

Catheter, urinary A flexible tube inserted through the urethra into the bladder, either for obtaining a urine specimen uncontaminated by bacteria on the skin or in the urethra, or to ensure the flow or urine when the usual sphincter muscles are not working owing to trauma or disease. Since the insertion of a catheter itself can transport bacteria into the bladder, it is extremely important that sterile procedures be followed. Catheterization is often used after operations in the genito-urinary area, including

Caesarean section, to ensure emptying of the bladder; sometimes an indwelling catheter (commonly a *Foley catheter*) is allowed to remain inserted for several days, until normal function returns. Patients who catheterize themselves on a long-term basis – a procedure called *intermittent self-catheterization* that is used by some paraplegics and others – generally use only clean rather than sterile technique and develop surprisingly few urinary infections.

Caul   See under AMNIOTIC SAC.

Cauterization   Also *cautery, electro-cautery, electrodesiccation*. Destroying cells by applying chemicals or heat to them. Cauterization is commonly used to treat warts on the vulva (see CONDYLOMA ACUMINATA), inflammation of the cervix (see CERVICITIS), and precancerous lesions of the cervix (see DYSPLASIA). The heat that kills the cells is produced by a controlled high-frequency electric current at the tip of a cautery probe, which is touched to the desired area. The heat kills only the surface cells. The procedure is mildly to moderately painful, depending on the kind of tissue being treated, and creates an unpleasant odour of burning, but it takes only a few seconds. Before electrocautery was available doctors applied agents such as silver nitrate to the cervix, but these were far less effective. Cauterization may cause some swelling in the cervix, which might temporarily narrow the cervical canal. It usually causes a profuse watery vaginal discharge that lasts several weeks, and occasionally some staining or bleeding. Complications rarely occur. A newer treatment for similar disorders is freezing, or CRYOSURGERY. Cauterization is also used to close the Fallopian tubes in

TUBAL LIGATION and the vas deferens in VASECTOMY.

Cephalhaematoma   In a newborn baby, a blood clot under the scalp, between the bone and the membrane covering it (periosteum). Usually resulting from a difficult delivery, it may not appear for twelve to twenty-four hours after birth. It tends to enlarge more during the next few days, remains stable for a few weeks, and then begins to disappear. No treatment of any kind is needed, nor does any permanent damage result from it.

Cephalic presentation   In childbirth, any position of the baby in which its head presents (that is, will emerge first). The ideal and most common presentation is the *vertex*, that is, where the crown or top of the skull (called 'occiput') is the presenting part. This is by far the easiest position for delivery. All others are called 'abnormal', including other cephalic presentations, each of which raises special problems; see BROW PRESENTATION; FACE PRESENTATION; POSTERIOR PRESENTATION.

Cerebral palsy   General name for a group of motor disorders that result from damage to the central nervous system occurring before, during, or after birth (up to the age of six), often due to lack of oxygen to the brain. The symptoms, all stemming from lack of muscular control by the brain, range from mild to severe and include awkward or involuntary movements, lack of balance, irregular gait, guttural speech, facial grimacing, and drooling. The causes include a very difficult labour, birth trauma, neonatal asphyxiation, prematurity, severe childhood illness (such as meningitis), and lead or arsenic poisoning. Intelligence may or may not be affected, depending on which part of the brain was injured. A cerebral palsy patient's difficulties in communicating and inability to control the voluntary muscle do not necessarily mean he or she is deficient in understanding, or has impaired mental ability.

Cerebral palsy is not progressive; on the contrary, the handicaps can be considerably lessened by physiotherapy, speech therapy, and bracing and/or orthopaedic surgery. For women with cerebral palsy, menstruation and fertility are unaffected. Pregnancy is possible in the less severe forms of the disorder, although delivery may be complicated by muscle spasms and the woman's inability to bear down at will. Sexual stimulation and arousal may trigger spastic and other involuntary movements, which may also make sexual intercourse difficult in certain positions. Sensation and orgasm, however, are not affected.

Cerebral vascular accident Also *cerebrovascular accident, CVA, stroke.* A sudden disturbance of the brain's blood supply, usually caused by haemorrhage (uncontrolled bleeding), an EMBOLISM, or a blood clot (see THROMBUS) in a blood vessel supplying the brain. It is potentially fatal and may be permanently disabling. Deprived of oxygen-filled blood, some brain cells are either paralyzed or destroyed and cease to control the body functions that are normally under their direction. An accident in one side of the brain may cause *hemiplegia* (paralysis and numbness) of the opposite side of the head and body (face, arm, leg). Other manifestations of CVA include loss of bladder control, emotional instability, speech and language problems, memory impairment, and visual disturbances.

As the word 'accident' implies, the onset of this condition is usually abrupt and constitutes a medical emergency. Early symptoms include weakness on one side of the body, numbness, visual disturbance such as double vision, and/or seizures, weakness or numbness in an arm, leg, or on the face, usually just on one side of the body; double vision, or blurred vision in one or both eyes; deafness or ringing in the ears; dizziness or fainting; difficulty swallowing; difficulty speaking or understanding spoken language; sudden headache; and abrupt personality changes, impaired judgment, or forgetfulness.

Cerebral vascular accident accounts for approximately one-third of all causes of paralysis in women between the ages of seventeen and forty-four, as well as being the most common cause of neurological disability among men and women of all ages. The risk of stroke rises with age, since contributing factors such as atherosclerosis and hypertension also occur more often after the age of fifty. The outcome of a stroke is highly variable. About one-third of all hospitalized patients die. Of those who survive, about 30 per cent recover fully, slightly more than half are left partly handicapped, and the remainder are severely handicapped for life.

In general, the extent of neurologic recovery from stroke depends on a person's age and general health, the location and dimensions of brain damage, and rehabilitation therapy that is begun early and pursued aggressively. The sooner improvement begins, the better the outlook. About half of those with moderate or severe hemiplegia, and most of those with minor hemiplegia, recover partially by the time they leave the hospital and eventually are able to care for themselves. Rehabilitation therapy should begin almost immediately and be pursued even when it seemingly exhausts the patient. Physiotherapy and speech therapy can both be of great benefit. The extent of recovery is usually established by the end of six to nine months, but some patients continue to show steady improvement over a longer time.

For women who have had a cerebral vascular accident, there may be a period of lack of interest in sex for several months. Extreme fatigue is experience by nearly all stroke victims, sometimes persisting for as long as a year, and it frequently affects sexual responses. Spasms of the affected leg (in those with hemiplegia) and urinary incontinence (loss of bladder control) may hamper sexual intercourse, and orgasm may be more difficult to achieve. Menstruation and fertility are not affected at all. Pregnancy may lessen bladder control even more. Oral contraceptives are contraindicated, and if an intrauterine device (IUD) is used, one should be alert to any associated increases in menstrual bleeding.

Cervical cap A flexible rubber or plastic cap that fits tightly over the cervix and prevents sperm from entering the cervical opening. It is about 1½ inches long, is widest at the opening, and has a thick, semi-rigid rim. Plastic caps are somewhat larger than rubber ones and somewhat differently shaped; they are used much less often than rubber ones. The cervical cap is held in place by suction. Used together with a SPERMICIDE (preferably cream, but jelly also works), it works much as a DIAPHRAGM (see definition 2) does and must similarly be fitted to an individual woman. However, it may be left in place considerably longer (authorities differ on this point; see below) and therefore is more convenient to use. The cap should not be relied on

as a contraceptive during menstrual periods, because the menstrual flow breaks the suction holding it in place (although it can be used to collect the menstrual flow). Experiments are currently underway with a custom-fitted cap with a one-way valve that will open automatically to release menstrual flow and other secretions.

The cervical cap was invented in the early 1800s in Europe and by the end of the 19th century was fairly widely used there. It was originally used without spermicide, and indeed some claim it is theoretcially as effective without spermicide as a diaphragm is with spermicide (apparently the airtight fit constitutes a genuine barrier to sperm, whereas the looser spring mechanism of the diaphragm does not). However, conclusive evidence is not yet availabe, and to lessen the risk of failure the use of spermicidal cream is definitely recommended; cream adheres better and longer than jelly; and a smaller amount is needed than with a diaphragm because the cap is much smaller. The cap is filled two-thirds full with cream and carefully inserted so as to cover the cervix. It should not be removed for at least twelve hours after the last intercourse and may be left in place a maximum of seven days provided it retains enough cream. To make sure it does, a woman is advised to remove the cap three days after the first use; if it is

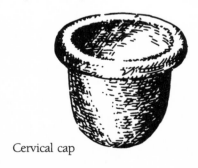

Cervical cap

still at least one-third full of cream it may be refilled and inserted for five days, checked again, and the next time inserted for seven days. After removal, which is accomplished by lifting the rim away from the cervix to break the suction, the cap should be washed with soap and water. Should it retain some odour, it can be soaked in rubbing alcohol for twenty-four hours, or in one cup of water with one tablespoon cider vinegar or lemon juice for twenty minutes; odour can also be avoided by inserting one drop of liquid chlorophyll on top of the spermicide before next inserting the cap.

The cap appears to have no side effects except possible irritation from the spermicide; when that occurs, a different brand may solve the problem. Occasionally the cap is dislodged during intercourse; if it happens more than once or twice the fit should be rechecked. because of this possibility, use of a CONDOM during the first eight times of intercourse with a cap is recommended. Also, some women do have marked cervical changes during their menstrual cycle, and have therefore found it necessary to use two sizes of cap to accommodate these changes. Finally the cap is somewhat harder to insert than a diaphragm, and therefore a higher proportion of women cannot learn to use it.

Cervical cyst See CYST, definition 4.

Cervical erosion See CERVICITIS.

Cervical mucus method Also *ovulation method*. A method of determining the time of OVULATION based on the fact that the cervical mucus secreted by most women changes in volume and consistency during the course of each menstrual cycle. After menstruation the mucus is scarcely noticeable in amount. It gradually increases in quantity and is thick, sticky, and opaque. Just before ovulation occurs the amount of mucus increases and it becomes clear and slippery, similar in consistency to raw egg white. It has a quality called *Spinnbarkeit* (a German word meaning 'ability to be spun'), meaning it is stringy and stretchable. Soon after it reaches a peak of stretchability, in a day or two, ovulation takes place. After ovulation the mucus again becomes thicker and stickier, though not as much as before, until menstruation, when the cycle begins again. The regular checking of cervical mucus consistency for purposes of preventing conception (birth control) is also called the *Billings method*, after two Australian doctors (husband and wife) who recommend it.

The cervical mucus method in its simplest form consists of having a woman check her mucus manually every day. If she becomes familiar with her own pattern and that pattern proves to be fairly regular, it is a fairly reliable method of birth control. Combined with taking BASAL BODY TEMPERATURE, it becomes even more reliable (see also NATURAL FAMILY PLANNING). However, the presence of seminal fluid (after intercourse), spermicides (creams, jellies, foam), douching, or any vaginal or cervical infection can obscure or remove natural mucus, making the method useless.

A woman can also perform simple tests on her own cervical mucus to determine what stage of the cycle she is in. At ovulation the mucus contains an abundant amount of glucose (sugar); by using chemically treated paper (special fertility kits for this purpose are sold over the counter in many chemists) and applying a small sample (fingertip) of mucus to the paper, she can determine by the colour the paper takes on how much glucose the mucus contains. Another test, the *fem test*, requires the use of a microscope. At ovulation the cervical mucus, placed on a slide under the microscope, shows a distinctive branching pattern resembling that of a fern. Before ovulation the mucus looks unfernlike, or has at most only a few branches. After ovulation, the fernlike appearance disappears within two or three days. The fern test, however, does not work in women who bleed slightly at ovulation or who have an inflammation of the cervix (cervicitis).

A number of mechanical devices to measure the consistency of cervical mucus more accurately are now being developed and tested. See also MITTEL-SCHMERZ; ill. Under MENSTRUAL CYCLE.

Cervical os See under CERVIX.

Cervical polyp See POLYP, definition 2.

Cervicitis Inflammation of the CERVIX, often caused by infection but sometimes by chemicals or a foreign body (tampon, IUD string, penis). Mild cervicitis has no symptoms at all. A more severe case will cause a heavy vaginal discharge, sometimes with a foul odour. It may be thin or thick in consistency, ranges from gray-white to yellow in colour, and occasionally is tinged with blood. Pain may be felt during vaginal intercourse or when the cervix is touched with a fingertip or tampon, and sometimes there is spotting or bleeding after intercourse. It is advisable to identify the cause of the infection, which may be yeast, trichomonas, gonococcus (which causes gonorrhoea), or some other organism,

and do a PAP SMEAR as well to make sure no precancerous condition exists. Once the cause is identified, specific treatment may be begun. If the cervicitis is caused by bacteria normally residing in the vagina, sulpha cream or suppositories may be tried and, if ineffective, followed by antibiotic treatment, usually in the form of vaginal creams or suppositories. In the case of trichomonal or gonorrhoeal infection, the woman's partner must also be treated. In instances where the condition persists and is bothersome, CAUTERIZATION or CRYOSURGERY, which destroys the abnormal tissue on the surface and helps induce healing and growth of new tissue, may be considered. Apart from the unpleasantness of chronic discharge, women who wish to become pregnant may not be able to conceive because a thick secretion is blocking the passage of sperm. In women using an intrauterine device (IUD) to prevent conception, treatment of cervicitis can usually proceed without removing the device, but in severe and recurrent cervicitis many doctors believe it should be removed and another mode of birth control used.

Among women who prefer more conservative therapy, a number of kinds have been tried. They include use of birth control jellies and creams (see SPERMICIDE); vitamin E capsules inserted as a vaginal suppository at bedtime; an acidic douche, made from crushed vitamin C tablets or vinegar or lemon juice diluted with water; and HERBAL REMEDIES, specifically an infusion made from rosemary (*Rosmarinus officinalis*), sanicle (*Sanicle europaea* or *mariandica*), comfrey (*Symphytum officinalis*), and heal-all or self-heal (*Prunella vulgaris*), used either as a douche or to soak a tampon that is then inserted into the vagina.

Cervix A cylindrical structure that is part of the UTERUS, specifically the narrow lower end, most of which protrudes into the vagina. It is often called the *neck* of the uterus, the rest being called the *corpus* or *body*. The bulk of its 2.5-centimetre (1-inch) length is the *cervical canal*, or *endocervix*. At the lower end, inside the vagina, is a small opening called the *external os*. Before childbearing the external os is a small regular opening about 5 millimetres in diameter. During labour it dilates to a diameter of 10 centimetres (2½ inches), and thereafter it never returns to its former shape, instead resembling a transverse slit about ¼ inch long. At the upper end of the cervical canal is another small opening into the body of the uterus, which is called the *internal os*. In non-pregnant women the cervix is pink; in pregnancy it assumes a bluish colour, a result of increased blood supply. This colour change is one of the earliest presumptive signs of pregnancy.

The cervix is lined with numerous small glands which furnish constant thick secretions. Occasionally some become blocked, forming a Nabothian cyst (see CYST, definition 4). The secretions change in response to stimulation by different hormones during the menstrual cycle, making it possible sometimes to determine when ovulation is taking place (see CERVICAL MUCUS METHOD). The cervix is subject to a number of disorders, the most serious of which is cancer, largely symptomless but detectable by a PAP SMEAR (see CANCER, CERVICAL). Less serious but often very annoying are POLYPS (see definition 2), CERVICITIS, and DYSPLASIA. See also INCOMPETENT CERVIX.

Chadwick's sign A change of colour in the tissues around the entrance to the vagina and the cervix that helps in the presumptive early diagnosis of pregnancy. Normally these tissues are pink, but in pregnancy they take on a purplish, dusky colour. The colour deepens in the course of the pregnancy, and it is most apparent in second and subsequent pregnancies.

Chancre A sore that is the first visible sign of SYPHILIS.

Chancroid Also *soft chancre, ulcus molle.* A VENEREAL DISEASE caused by a rod-shaped bacterium, *Haemophilus ducreyi*, that is most common in the tropics. It is transmitted by vaginal, anal, or oral-genital intercourse, and is most apt to invade the genitals through an existing lesion, such as a small cut or scratch. In most women chancroid gives rise to no symptoms, so they may be unknowing carriers of the disease. In men one or, more often, several small sores appear on the penis or in the urethra one to five days after the infecting contact. The sore is a raised bump surrounded by a narrow red border. It some becomes pimple-like, filled with pus, and then ruptures to form a painful open sore with ragged edges. Chancroid sores bleed easily when touched, and sometimes spread along a line to form a single long, narrow sore. In women the sores appear on the vulva, thighs, vagina, cervix, or inside the urethra, and may be centred at the base of pubic hairs. Sometimes the chancroid sores disappear by themselves within a few days. In half of untreated cases, however, the bacteria infect the lymph glands in the groin. Within five to eight days after the first sore appears, the glands on one or both sides of the groin become enlarged, hard, and painful. They fuse together to form a single rounded swelling called a *bubo*. The overlying skin is red. If untreated the bubo may push to the surface and rupture, oozing pus. A large open sore results, which is highly susceptible to infection by other organisms as well.

Diagnosis of chancroid is often confused with other venereal diseases, especially SYPHILIS and LYMPHOEDEMA VENEREUM (the latter also characterized by bubos). A culture of pus forming an open sore will reveal the causative organism. Treatment is with tetracycline for seven to ten days; for patients who are pregnant, breast-feeding, or allergic to tetracycline, sulpha drugs may be substituted. Bubos about to burst should be incised and drained. Occasionally plastic surgery may be needed if they have disfigured the genital area. After treatment, there should be follow-up tests every three months for a year to make sure the disease has been eradicated.

Change of life   See MENOPAUSE.

Chastity   Sexual purity, referring either to abstinence from unlawful sexual intercourse (that is, outside of marriage) or to total abstinence (celibacy). See also VIRGINITY.

Chemotherapy   Also *anticancer drugs*. Strictly speaking, any treatment with chemical substances, or drugs, but generally the term is reserved for drugs used to treat CANCER. Anticancer drugs are very powerful agents that kill cancer cells shed into the bloodstream and lymph system by the original tumour, as well as the tumour itself, especially when injected directly into it. They also affect healthy cells. The drugs presently in use are most effective against tumours whose cells are actively growing (making DNA and dividing). For this reason they also destroy certain normal tissues that have a high proportion of actively growing cells, such as white blood cells, hair roots, and various gastrointestinal tissues, especially mucous membranes. Because they are so toxic, it is especially important (but difficult) to establish dosages for these drugs sufficient to kill a tumour but not to damage too much normal tissue. Other considerations in planning chemotherapy include timing, so as to attack cells while they are dividing, and monitoring toxicity.

Chemotherapy is mainly used in three ways: (1) as an attempt to cure a cancer when metastasis (spread) is openly present; (2) as an attempt to cure a cancer when there is no obvious metastasis but the prognosis following removal of a tumour is guarded, as a form of prevention; (3) to reduce symptoms and prolong survival when cure is not possible.

Different cancer drugs work in different ways. Some inhibit cell growth, much as radiation does, and others prevent cell division altogether. Others block cell division by interfering with enzymes needed for the synthesis of RNA and DNA building blocks, and still others adhere to DNA and therefore interfere with cell reproduction. Certain kinds of cancer respond better to one drug than another. For example, CHORIOCARCINOMA is one of the few cancers that respond very well to drugs that block cell division. In some cancers combinations of several drugs work more effectively than any one drug; each attacks a different stage of the cancer's growth. Among these are certain cancers of the blood and lymph, notably acute lymphocytic leukaemia and Hodgkin's disease. In breast cancers with lymph node involvement, surgical removal of the affected breast and all the lymph nodes, plus radiation treatment, does not yield as high a rate of recurrence-free survival as the same treatment combined with a drug that prevents cell division.

Chemotherapy is administered orally or by injection into a muscle or vein, weekly or monthly, occasionally daily, or in special cycles. In most cases a combination of drugs is used. The most common side effects are nausea and vomiting, ulcers in the mouth, skin rashes, and the loss of hair; the last usually a temporary problem. Menstrual periods may become irregular or cease. In men the sperm count may be reduced, either temporarily or permanently; therefore some oncologists (cancer specialists) advise men to deposit some sperm in a SPERM BANK before undergoing chemotherapy; it can be stored there for ten years or longer. Sometimes intravenous administration will cause a burning sensation at the site of the injection for several days. More serious possible toxic effects, not apparent for some time, include bone marrow depression (a reduction in the bone marrow's production of white blood cells), which reduces resistance against other diseases; a decrease in blood platelets (thrombocytopaenia); cystitis; hepatic fibrosis (death of liver tissue); and, after long-term use, the development of acute leukaemia. Indeed, one of the major problems of chemotherapy – and all other cancer treatment – is that agents potent enough to treat a cancer sometimes cause another cancer elsewhere in the body. However, since most cancers have a very long latency period (take long to develop), the risk of carcinogenic drugs is considered worthwhile for many patients.

Childbearing, age for See AGE, CHILDBEARING.

Childbed fever See PUERPERAL FEVER.

Childbirth education See PREPARED CHILDBIRTH.

Chlamydia infection See under PELVIC INFLAMMATORY DISEASE; URETHRITIS; VAGINITIS.

Chloasma Also *mask of pregnancy, melasma.* Irregular brownish patches of varying size that appear on the face during pregnancy, often in a wing-like pattern over the cheeks, forehead, and upper lip, giving rise to the name 'mask of pregnancy'. They usually disappear, or at least fade considerably, after delivery. Similarly, ordinary freckles tend to become darker during pregnancy. Women who experience such pigment changes in pregnancy may also experience them when they take oral contraceptives, supporting the theory that they result from increased melanin production triggered by higher levels either of oestrogen and/or progesterone or of melanocyte-stimulating hormones. Because oral contraceptives are associated with a higher risk of developing MELANOMA (a fast-growing skin cancer), women who have chloasma in pregnancy or while taking oral contraceptives are advised to discontinue such drugs permanently. Women with chloasma in pregnancy should also avoid or minimize their exposure to the sun and always use a sunscreen outdoors, since sunlight tends to aggravate the pigmentation and may make it less likely to fade.

Chocolate cyst See under ENDOMETRIOSIS.

Choriocarcinoma A kind of cancer resulting from a HYDATIDIFORM MOLE (after it has been expelled) or, more rarely, following normal delivery, when it develops from tissues of the baby. The chief symptom is bleeding, often very heavy and sometimes so profuse that the haemorrhage is fatal. This kind of cancer spreads very fast, to the lung, brain, bone, and even skin, so that prompt treatment is essential. Fortunately choriocarcinoma has been found to respond very well to anticancer drugs, which have largely replaced the surgical treatment (hysterectomy) formerly necessary.

Chorion The outermost membrane covering the fertilized egg, part of which—the chorionic villi—will develop into the PLACENTA. The chorionic villi become embedded in the uterine lining and are bathed in a pool of maternal blood where the exchange of nutrients and waste products takes place.

Chromosome A microscopic body in the nucleus of almost every living cell containing coded instructions that tell the cell what it can produce and do during its life and that are transmitted to its offspring. A chromosome can be regarded as a strand of *genes* each of which governs a different trait, such as eye colour, in the organism. The genes are arranged on the chromosome in linear order, and a given gene normally occupies the same place on its chromosome in each cell within the living organisms of its species. The chromosomes in a cell occur in pairs, each of which has genes for the same trait. However, although the pairs of genes govern the same trait, they are not necessarily identical; thus a person can have one gene for brown eyes and one for blue eyes. When there are a number of possible genes for a given trait, some

are usually *dominant* over others, which are said to be *recessive*. For example, brown eyes are dominant and blue eyes recessive; therefore a person who has one gene for each will have brown eyes, but a person with two genes for blue eyes will have blue eyes. Since some genes are associated with specific diseases, such as sickle cell disease, or with a tendency to develop certain disorders, such as diabetes, whether they are dominant or recessive is important in determining the chances of their being transmitted to offspring.

The traits an organism inherits from its parents are governed by the way their genes are passed down. In normal cell division, called *mitosis*, each chromosome – and therefore each gene – is duplicated before the cell divides, so that each of the two new or 'daughter' cells receives an identical set of genes. Sexual reproduction, however, involves the fusion of two special cells called *gametes*, the egg cell of the mother and the sperm cell of the father. In order for offspring to have the correct number of chromosomes (and genes) for their species, each gamete must provide *half* that number. Therefore, in a chromosome-reducing process called *meiosis*, the pairs of chromosomes are separated, with one member of each pair going to a particular egg or sperm. Thus the parent with one trait for brown eyes and one for blue can give either the brown-eye gene or the blue-eye one to his sperm (or her egg). The second gene for eye colour will come from the other parent. In human cells, which normally have forty-six chromosomes, twenty-three come from each parent.

Normally, children resemble one or another of their parents or grandparents in most of their basic physical features.

Occasionally, however, a totally new characteristic appears, one that cannot be traced back even several generations. In effect there has been a sudden accident, resulting in a changed gene or genes. Such a change is called a *mutation*, and the organism showing the change is a *mutant.* Usually just a gene is affected, but sometimes the change affects a chromosome. In either case the changed genetic material is passed on to that organism's offspring. Mutations can be caused by environmental factors, some of which have been identified although many are still unknown. With the development and use of many new chemicals and the increased use of high-energy radiations, mutations have become far more common. They have been experimentally produced in test animals by means of exposure to high doses of X-rays, gamma rays, extremely high temperatures, and a growing variety of chemical agents. Most mutant genes are recessive – the offspring with dominant ones do not survive – so in effect they are masked by the normal gene of their pair. They do not appear until two parents with the same mutant genes have offspring. (For more about recessive-gene disorders, see under BIRTH DEFECTS.)

Significant abnormalities in chromosomes occur in approximately one of every 250 live human births, and an estimated three-quarters of these genetic 'errors' are considered undesirable. In addition, about one-third of all miscarriages are believed to be caused by chromosomal abnormalities. Most facts about genetic defects have been discovered quite recently; indeed, only in 1955 was it determined that human beings normally have forty-six chromosomes. Today, research is focusing on such pursuits as *mapping* genes, to determine the location of genetic particles on each chromosome strand; *splicing* genes, changing their arrangement to learn what changes will result; deciphering *genetic markers*, that is, indications of genetic tendencies to develop certain diseases when specific environmental factors are encountered, such as the tendency for some heavy smokers to develop serious lung disease (such as emphysema) while others do not; *synthesizing* genes in the laboratory; and transplanting foreign genes (from plants, animals, human beings) into bacteria, a pursuit called *recombinant DNA research*. Researchers are also developing methods for examining the genes of the foetus in the early weeks of pregnancy to test for the presence of inherited disorders such as sickle cell disease or Huntington's chorea.

Chromosome test   A test sometimes administered to women athletes to determine whether or not they are in fact biologically female. The test consists of taking a buccal smear (a tiny scraping from inside the mouth) and examining the cells for their chromosomes. The chromosomes of particular interest are the so-called *sex chromosomes*, two X chromosomes in every female and one X and one Y chromosome in every male (see under CHROMOSOME for an explanation). The use of the test was allegedly made necessary by the increasing use of ANABOLIC STEROIDS to increase athletic strength, as well as by the performance of TRANSSEXUAL surgery.

Chronic   Developing over a period of time and having a long duration. The opposite of chronic is ACUTE.

Circumcision   Surgical removal of the

foreskin, or PREPUCE, of the penis in men and the clitoris in women. This operation was sometimes performed on women in order to curb MASTURBATION (to some extent it replaced clitoridectomy; see under CLITORIS), and is still performed in some non-Western cultures. There is no valid medical reason for ever performing it on women. For a good part of the 20th century circumcision was almost routinely performed in British hospitals on boy babies, usually a few days after birth, for purposes of hygiene and, as some experts believed, to prevent penile cancer. Both purposes are now in question. Circumcision is also a ceremonial ritual in certain religions, mandatory for all males in Judaism and Islam, and used for women and/or men among other groups.

Climacteric See MENOPAUSE.

Climax See ORGASM.

Clitoris A small cylindrical structure at the upper front of the VULVA, between the *labia minora* (see under LABIA), which form its prepuce (hood), or foreskin. Lying just above and in front of the urethral opening, it resembles the male penis in that it contains many nerve endings and erectile tissue (capable of stiffening). Like the penis, it is extremely sensitive, especially at the glans (tip), and becomes engorged with blood during sexual stimulation. However, it is much smaller, usually less than 1 inch (2½ centimetres) long, even when it is erect. Highly responsive to touch, so much so that many women find its direct stimulation painful, the clitoris is the primary focus of ORGASM in a woman; indeed; its only known function is for sexual pleasure.

The importance of the clitoris in sexual response was long overlooked. Even as late as the 1950s some doctors and alleged experts on sex differentiated between what they called a 'clitoral' and 'vaginal' orgasm, maintaining that the former was an 'immature' response and the latter the only one appropriate for adult women. This differentiation was based on where the source of stimulation was located – vaginal penetration, not manual stimulation – rather than on a genuine difference in response, and has been largely discounted as a misconception.

In 19th century Europe (and in other parts of the world even today) the clitoris was sometimes surgically removed—an operation called *clitoridectomy*—for a variety of purposes. In 1858 this operation was first performed in England to check female 'mental disorders'. Later it was performed to check MASTURBATION. Today the operation is considered, in most advanced countries, to be a cruel and unnecessary mutilation, except in those rare cases where cancer has spread to the external genitals (see CANCER, VULVAR).

Clonidine Also *antihypertensive pill*, *blood pressure pill*. A drug used primarily to relieve HYPERTENSION (high blood pressure) but that has also been found helpful by some women in relieving the HOT FLUSHES of menopause because it functions by producing transient vaso-constriction. Available only by prescription it is a potent drug and must be used with caution.

Coitus Also *copulation, sexual intercourse.* Vaginal sexual intercourse, with the man's penis placed inside the woman's vagina. See also *anal sex* under ANUS; ORAL SEX; SEXUAL RESPONSE.

Coitus interruptus Also *French method, pulling out, withdrawal method.* A Latin term meaning 'interrupted intercourse', and referring to a method of BIRTH CONTROL in which the male pulls his penis out of his partner's vagina before he ejaculates ('comes'). It is one of the oldest and simplest methods of preventing conception, requiring no equipment of any kind, but it also has the highest failure rate. Some seminal fluid may leak from the penis before ejaculation, and even a drop or two can contain thousands of sperm. Furthermore, many men are unable to withdraw completely in time, and the spilling of even a little seminal fluid on the outer female genitals may deposit sperm that migrate up inside the vagina. In any event, this method requires great self-control and is considered, at best, 75 per cent effective, and often far less so. Many couples also find it unsatisfactory, the man because he must constantly be watchful of his level of excitement in order to withdraw in time, the woman because she may not trust his ability to withdraw and also may not be ready for orgasm at the same time and consequently have to rely on other means of stimulation for gratification.

Colostomy A surgical opening of the colon (large intestine) through the abdomen for discharge of solid waste (faeces), which is made when a diseased or injured colon and/or rectum cannot be treated medically. The principal cause of such disease is cancer of the colon and/or rectum; other causes are diverticulitis, familial polyposis, birth defects, and severe injury. Occasionally a *temporary colostomy* is performed in order to allow the lower part of the colon and/or rectum to heal; in such cases there are usually two stomas (openings), one to discharge waste and the other only mucus, and when the injured parts have healed the openings are closed. In a *permanent colostomy*, usually part of the colon and all of the rectum are removed, and the end portion of the remaining colon is brought through the abdominal wall to form a single stoma.

Colostomies are performed in different parts of the colon, depending on where it is diseased, and are generally named after the relevant portion. A *sigmoid colostomy* is an opening in the upper end of the sigmoid colon. In a *descending colostomy*, the opening is somewhat higher, in the descending colon. Most colostomies are in the sigmoid or descending colon, and stomas for either type are on the left side of the abdomen. Sigmoid colostomies are usually permanent. Evacuation of faecal matter is often controlled by irrigation, that is, periodic enemas, so that no collection appliance is needed. A *transverse colostomy* is an opening in the transverse colon, and the stoma is located on the upper abdomen, in the middle or on the right side. Evacuation can sometimes be controlled by irrigation, but more often an appliance (bag) is used to collect faecal matter. A transverse colostomy is usually a temporary procedure, with two stomas. Occasionally, however, it is an end colostomy with a single opening, with most or all of the colon beyond it removed. For the operation's significance for a woman's reproductive and sexual functioning, see under OSTOMY.

Colostrum See under LACTATION.

Colposcopy A technique for examining the cervix and vagina with a *colposcope*, a low-power microscope that has a strong light source with a green filter.

It is generally undertaken when a PAP SMEAR indicates areas of abnormal cells in order to locate and identify the area of abnormal structure, but it can also be used to examine external sores or other abnormalities on the vulva. The colposcope mangifies the cervix ten to twenty times, enabling a view of the area where squamous epithelial cells join columnar epithelial cells on the face of the cervix (see CERVICAL EVERSION for further explanation), called the *transformation zone*, and also showing the pattern of blood vessels and white patches. These areas – the transformation zone, white patches, and blood vessels – can indicate precancerous changes and the actual presence of cancer. If any area viewed looks suspicious, a biopsy (tissue sample) can be taken and examined in the laboratory with the assurance that the specimen actually comes from the most abnormal area. If abnormalities extend upward into the cervical canal where they cannot be seen, even when using a tiny speculum to dilate the cervix, the doctor may recommend further investigation, either endocervical curettage (scraping tissue from inside the cervical canal) or possibly CONIZATION. Colposcopy is quite painless (the instrument does not actually touch the body) but usually requires the patient to lie still for fifteen or twenty minutes with a speculum in place.

Colpotomy See under CULDOSCOPY.

Compression fracture Also *crush fracture*. A bone that is broken by compression, that is, simple pressure with a severe injury of any kind. It most commonly occurs as a complication of OSTEOPOROSIS in the weight-bearing vertebrae of the spine. The pain is usually acute, as with any other fracture, and is aggravated by weight-bearing (any upright position). There may be local tenderness as well. Usually the pain goes away in a few days or weeks. Persons with numerous compression fractures of the vertebrae may develop exaggerated curvatures of the spine (see DOWAGER'S HUMP), may lose several inches of height, and may experience chronic, dull, aching back pain. For acute severe back pain caused by a compression fracture, treatment includes use of an orthopaedic support, analgesics, and, if there is muscle spasm, heat and massage.

Conception See FERTILIZATION.

Condom Also *prophylactic, rubber, safe*. A delicate sheath, usually made of rubber, that is used to cover the penis during sexual intercourse and prevent the sperm that are ejaculated from entering the vagina. The oldest and most common form of mechanical MALE CONTRACEPTIVE, it is still widely used for BIRTH CONTROL. It also reduces the spread of sexually transmitted diseases, such as gonorrhoea, syphilis, herpes, and condyloma acuminata (see VENEREAL DISEASE). A condom is placed on the penis while it is erect but before it is put into the vagina. In order to make sure the device does not break, about half an inch of empty air space should be left at the tip in order to allow enough room to hold the ejaculated seminal fluid (some condoms are made with nipple-shaped tips to hold the ejaculate). After ejaculation the man or his partner must hold on to the condom rim as he slowly withdraws his still erect penis, taking care not to spill any seminal fluid on the woman's external genitals. For lubrication, either water-soluble jelly or saliva can be used; petroleum jelly (Vaseline) should be avoided because it makes the rubber of the condom break down. Some prelubricated condoms are available. Condoms are readily obtainable in chemists without prescription; purchases of condoms from vending machines in petrol stations or men's toilets is not recommended, because these condoms may be old or outdated, and consequently leak or break readily. A condom can be stored in its package up to two years before use but should not be kept in a warm, moist place (such as a wallet or pocket), because heat makes it disintegrate.

A condom should be used for only a single act of intercourse. Should it tear or break while the man is withdrawing, the woman should immediately insert contraceptive foam or jelly in order to be protected (see SPERMICIDE). She should *avoid* douching, which might serve to spread the sperm. Used alone, a condom theoretically is 85 to 90 per cent effective in preventing pregnancy; if the woman also uses foam at the same time it is said to be 95 per cent or more effective. There are no side effects from using condoms for either man or woman. Their only disadvantage is that there is some interruption in lovemaking while the condom is put on, and some men believe they lessen penile sensation.

Most condoms are made of latex rubber. Early condoms were made from animal intestines (most often sheep caecum); some condoms of this material are still available, but there is no advantage in using them, they are more expensive, and some authorities maintain that the manufacturing standards for them are less well defined that those for rubber condoms, and hence they may be less reliable.

Condoms were used in ancient Egypt as an adornment. They were revived to prevent conception and venereal disease in the 18th century. Rubber condoms were developed early in the 19th century and were soon being mass-produced.

Today there is little difference among brands of condom. Most are 7½ inches long, and the open end has a wider ring of stronger latex to help keep it in place. Some brands come in different colours or with ribbing. Most condoms are prerolled. When they are not, they should be rolled up just before use, and then unrolled onto the erect penis up to its base. Air should be expelled from the tip before the condom is rolled on.

Conduction anaesthesia See REGIONAL ANAESTHESIA.

Condyloma acuminata Also *genital warts, venereal warts*. A virus infection that causes small benign tumours to grow around the moist folds of the vulva and inside the vagina in women and on the shaft of the penis in men (sometimes also around the anus in both sexes). They are caused by a papilloma or papova virus – they were the first tumour in human beings definitely known to be caused by a virus – that is usually transmitted by sexual contact. Poor hygiene is also a contributing factor. The virus has a long incubation period, so that the warts may not appear until one to six months after one has been exposed to them. They begin as tiny, discrete, pinkish or tan growths about the size of a rice grain, either singly or in clusters (looking somewhat like cauliflower), and they grow rapidly. They sometimes itch, and scratching helps spread them. Because they resemble cancerous growths a biopsy may be taken (see BIOPSY, definition 6) to establish the diagnosis.

Treatment for small warts consists of

applying podophyllin to them two or three times at weekly intervals, taking extreme care to avoid touching the surrounding healthy tissue, and washing off the medication after six to eight hours. If the warts are large or the patient is pregnant, cryosurgery (freezing), cauterization (burning), or surgical excision is preferable; the warts are limited to the superficial layers of the skin and can be readily removed in this way. (Podophyllin must be avoided by pregnant women because it can damage the foetus if applied inside the vagina.) Even if podophyllin treatment is effective, the warts tend to recur, and treatment must then be resumed. The sexual partner, too, should be examined to avoid a cycle of reinfection. Oral contraceptives and pregnancy both appear to stimulate the growth and spread of warts. See also VENEREAL DISEASE.

Cone biopsy See CONIZATION.

Congenital abnormalities (defects)
See BIRTH DEFECTS.

Congenital infection An infection present in a baby at birth, having been acquired from the mother before or during delivery. It is caused by an organism transmitted to the foetus across the placenta or to the baby as it passed through the birth canal. Various infectious diseases, notably rubella and chicken pox, can be transmitted to a baby in this way, and even when they are mild in the mother they can be very serious – sometimes fatal – in the infant. Venereal diseases such as HERPES INFECTION can also be transmitted to a baby as it passes through the birth canal. In addition to such additions, a baby can be born *addicted* to an opiate such as heroin, or to alcohol, and suffer withdrawal symptoms when the source of supply – the mother's body – is removed. See ALCOHOL USE; DRUG USE.

Congestive Referring to an abnormal accumulation of blood in the body's tissues. In *pelvic congestion syndrome*, a catchall term for a combination of symptoms including painful menstruation, lower abdominal and lower back pain, and other pelvic discomfort, the term 'congestion' refers to engorgement of the blood vessels of the pelvis. See also DYSMENORRHOEA, definition 5.

Conization Also *cone biopsy*. The surgical removal of a cone-shaped piece of tissue from the cylindrical cervix. Formerly used principally as a diagnostic tool to make sure abnormal tissue was not actually cancerous, conization today is used more cautiously, since COLPOSCOPY for a directed biopsy usually affords an adequate diagnosis. Conization requires general anaesthesia and therefore is nearly always performed in a hospital. The surgeon cuts a cone-shaped wedge out of the cervix, removing the upper portion of the cervical canal along with the entire outer surface of the cervix. After the centre cone is removed, the cut edges of the cervix are sutured (stitched).

Conization is a major surgical procedure, with the risk of several complications. Of these, the most common is heavy bleeding, during or immediately after surgery, or even a week or so later, when the stitches are absorbed. Haemorrhage may require further treatment (transfusion and/or other surgery). Less common complications are perforation of the uterus and infection. Long-term complications include cervical incompetence (see INCOMPETENT CERVIX), leading to miscarriage in future pregnancies; infertility, owing to inadequate cervical mucus production (the portion of cervix removed contains a susbstantial number of mucus-producing glands); and narrowing or stenosis of the cervical canal by scar tissue, which can interfere with later delivery or even, in the case of blockage, trap menstrual flow. For these reasons colposcopy is now performed instead of conization whenever possible. See also BIOPSY, definition 7.

Constipation Infrequent or difficult bowel movements (elimination of faeces and/or hard stools). Contrary to earlier thought, a daily bowel movment is not essential to good health. Although regular evacuation of faeces is important, what is regular for one person is not for another; some individuals normally have three bowel movements a day while others have one every three or four days. Occasional constipation usually presents no great problem, nor does the occasional use of a mild laxative. It is only when constipation becomes chronic, so that a person becomes largely or wholly dependent on laxatives, that serious disease needs to be ruled out. Organic causes of constipation include an intestinal obstruction, a tumour, diverticulitis, or some other gastrointestinal disorder, and can usually be readily diagnosed. Most constipation, however, is functional, due either to a mistaken belief that a daily movement is essential or to an inactive colon (especially in the elderly, the bedridden, or a younger laxative-dependent person) or to irritable bowel syndrome (spastic colon).

Some women regularly have trouble with constipation during pregnancy, especially during the latter months, when the enlarged uterus presses on the descending colon. Others experience it monthly during the few days preceding a menstrual period (see under DYSMENORRHOEA definition 5), and still others are troubled with it during menopausal years, suggesting that changing hormone levels may affect the muscle tone of the intestinal tract. For the most part, functional constipation is best treated with regular exercise, a diet high in bulk (bran cereal, fresh fruit, raw vegetables), and plenty of water. Some medications cause constipation, among them oral contraceptives, iron, some antacid preparations, and narcotics such as codeine. If proper diet and exercise do not relieve constipation, a bulk stool softener (usually a seed preparation with psyllium or cellulose that creates a softer, bulkier stool) may help. There are numerous over-the-counter laxatives, some of them based on herbs such as cascara. Various HERBAL REMEDIES for constipation range from mild (liquorice root, or *Glycyrrhiza lepidota*) to quite strong (senna pods, or *Cassis acutifolia*). Dependence on these, however, is no more desirable than dependence on an inorganic laxative.

Contact dermatitis An inflammation of the skin resulting from contact with irritating agents or substances. Any part of the skin may be involved. For contact dermatitis of the genital area, see under VULVITIS.

Contraceptive Any device, substance, or method used to prevent pregnancy. This includes abstaining from intercourse, either entirely (celibacy) or during a woman's fertile period (after ovulation; see NATURAL FAMILY PLANNING); withdrawing the penis from the vagina before ejaculation (see COITUS INTERRUPTUS);

Estimated Effectiveness of Common Contraceptives

Method	Theoretical Effectiveness*	Practical Effectiveness*
Coitus interruptus (withdrawal)	91%	75 to 80%
Condom	97%	85%
Diaphragm with spermicide (jelly)	97%	85 to 90%
Douche	?**	50%?**
Foam	97%	80%
Hysterectomy	100%	100%
Intrauterine device (IUD)	97 to 99%	93 to 96%
Lactation (breast-feeding for 2 months)	75%	60%
Oral contraceptive (combination-type Pill)	99.66%	96 to 98%
Tubal ligation (minilaparotomy)	99.5%	99.5%
Vasectomy	99.5%	99.5%

* Theoretical effectiveness is the effectiveness when the method is used without error and exactly according to instructions; practical effectiveness takes into consideration all the users of a method – those who use it correctly (and perfectly) and those who are careless.
** Comparable test results are not available to estimate theoretical effectiveness; practical effectiveness believed to be 50% *at best*.

breast-feeding a baby, which temporarily delays ovulation (but note that one never knows for how long until after menstruation has resumed, indicating ovulation did occur); destroying sperm or making them inactive (see SPERMICIDE; THERMATIC STERILIZATION; ULTRASOUND, definition 2); imposing a physical and/or chemical barrier to prevent the passage of sperm through the cervix (see CERVICAL CAP; CONDOM, CONTRACEPTIVE SPONGE; DIAPHRAGM; SPERMICIDE); flushing sperm out of the vagina after intercourse (see DOUCHING); making the uterine lining unreceptive to a fertilized egg (see INTRAUTERINE DEVICE); suppressing ovulation and/or sperm production by means of hormone medications (see ORAL CONTRACEPTIVE; PEPTIDES; PROGESTIN) or by STERILIZATION. Their

effectiveness varies widely, from virtually 0 per cent (douching) to nearly 100 per cent (sterilization). Safety and freedom from side effects also vary, the diaphragm, cervical cap, contraceptive sponge, and condom being considered freest of risk to the user (other than accidental pregnancy) and oral contraceptives and intrauterine devices (IUDs) carrying the highest risk of side effects. For safety from unwanted pregnancy the ratings are exactly the reverse, oral contraceptives having the lowest failure rate (2 per cent) followed by IUDs (4.2 per cent), and then all other forms. Improved modes of contraception are still being investigated among them reversible sterilization and vaccines against sperm. Most contraceptive devices are available only by prescription, the principal exception being some barrier methods (spermicidal cream, jelly, foam, and condoms). See also BIRTH CONTROL; MALE CONTRACEPTIVE.

Contraceptive sponge A sponge made of polyurethane foam and containing a spermicide that is inserted in the vagina to trap sperm and prevent their passage through the cervix. It is available without prescription from chemists and is marketed under the name 'Today'. It comes in one size only. For insertion the sponge is wetted and placed high in the vagina where it can be left for up to 24 hours. It has a loop attached to it to allow it to be pulled out easily. After intercourse it should not be removed for at least 6 hours. As a means of preventing pregnancy it is probably not as effective as the diaphragm.

Contraction, uterine Also *labour pain*. The temporary shortening of the muscle fibres of the UTERUS, which occurs involuntarily during labour and serves to push the baby down through the birth canal. The uterine muscles actually begin to contract periodically early in pregnancy, but these contractions are usually perceived only in the ninth month or so and are painless (see BRAXTON-HICKS CONTRACTIONS). When labour begins, the contractions become regular. During the first stage of LABOUR they are short, mild, and separated by intervals of ten to twenty minutes. Often they are first felt as discomfort in the small of the back, but soon they begin to be felt in the lower abdomen as well. The contractions gradually recur at shorter intervals and become stronger and longer in duration. As the cervix dilates to about 4 to 7 centimetres, they last approximately sixty seconds and occur every four to eight minutes. At the end of the first stage of labour, or with 7 to 10 centimetres dilation, they may last as long as one and one-half minutes, with intervals as short as thirty seconds between contractions. After the cervix is fully dilated, during the second stage of labour (the expulsion of the baby), contractions last fifty to one hundred seconds and occur at intervals of two to three minutes. At this point the muscles of the abdomen are brought into play, and most women (if anaesthesia does not prevent it) feel an urge to strain or bear down strenuously and thus assist the uterus in expelling the baby. Following delivery, there may be a few minutes' wait and then uterine contractions resume at regular intervals until the PLACENTA separates from the uterine wall and is expelled. After delivery of the placenta, the attending doctor or midwife usually massages the woman's abdomen at regular intervals to make sure the uterus continues to contract. If it does not there is danger of excessive bleeding (see POSTPARTUM HAEMORRHAGE). Thereafter the uterus continues to contract periodically, the contractions sometimes giving rise to somewhat painful sensations called *afterpains*. In some women these are severe enough to require mild analgesics and may last for a number of days. They are particularly noticeable when the baby is put to the breast, probably because of the release of oxytocin (see LACTATION for further explanation). Usually, however, they decrease in intensity and become quite mild within forty-eight hours after delivery. The afterpains further reduce the uterus to its former, pre-pregnant size and also help stop bleeding.

Uterine contractions are involuntary. They occur in labouring women who receive a regional anaesthetic, such as

CAUDAL or EPIDURAL ANAESTHESIA, as well as in women who have no control over other muscles in their pelvis, such as paraplegics. They occur not only in labour, but sometimes during menstruation (cramps; see DYSMENORRHOEA, definition 4) and, in much milder form, during ORGASM. Why strong contractions hurt is not known; some authorities believe the pain comes from the stretching of the cervix and perineum, others that it comes from hypoxia (oxygen lack) in the contracted muscles, and still others from compression of nerves in the pelvis. See also ANAESTHESIA, definition 2.

Contraindication Any condition that makes a particular treatment or procedure undesirable. An *absolute contraindication* means the treatment is hazardous to the patient and should not be used; a *relative contraindication* means that the risks must be carefully weighed against the benefits before undertaking the treatment. For example, a history of cardiovascular disease (blood clots, heart attack, stroke) is an absolute contraindication to taking oral contraceptives; a history of diabetes or gall bladder disease is a relative contraindication to oral contraceptives. Similarly, pregnancy is an absolute contraindication to the insertion of an intrauterine device (IUD); a history of severe anaemia is a relative contraindication, because the IUD makes many women bleed more heavily.

Cosmetics also *make-up*. General name for products that are designed to improve the appearance of the face, skin, eyes, hair, and other features, but are not absorbed in amounts significant enough to alter body functions. Lipstick, nail polish, mascara, eye shadow, perfume, hair dye, powders, and lotions are generally harm-less but occasionally can cause health problems. The most common is an allergic reaction (marked by itching, swelling, tearing of the eyes, and/or rash), usually but not always caused by the perfume in the product. So-called *hypoallergenic* cosmetics are virtually odourless. Some face make-up aggravates acne, and some hair dyes and tints contain aniline, a common allergen. Mascara that does not contain sufficient preservatives may contain bacteria that, if they come in contact with the eyes, can cause serious infection and even permanent eye damage. See also DEODORANT.

Occasionally manufacturers have added oestrogen to cosmetics on the theory that it prevents signs of ageing such as wrinkles. There is no evidence that it does; moreover, oestrogen can be absorbed through the skin, possibly leading to dangerous side effects.

Counselling See PSYCHOTHERAPY; FEMINIST THERAPY; PREGNANCY COUNSELLING; GENETIC COUNSELLING.

Crabs See PUBIC LICE.

Cramp A sudden, painful contraction of a muscle or group of muscles. *Menstrual cramps* are uterine contractions like those of labour (labour pains) but both milder and less regular (see DYSMENORRHOEA, definition 4.). *Leg cramps* are common during pregnancy and childbirth. Often a pregnant woman will wake in the night to find the muscles of one calf or foot in painful spasm; it is best relieved by local massage, kneading the muscles until they relax, or by lengthening the muscle by pointing the toes toward the head, or by standing on the affected foot. Leg cramps may also occur during the second stage of labour, when the baby's head presses on the pelvic nerves; they can be relieved by massage.

Critical weight The proportion of body fat tissue to lean tissue that appears to be necessary for both menarche (the first menstruation) and the maintenance of more or less regular menstrual cycles. Before the adolescent growth spurt that precedes menarche (the first period), most girls show a 5 to 1 ratio of lean to fat tissue; by menarche this ratio has changed to 3 to 1, or 24 per cent fat and 76 per cent lean, an increase in fat tissue of 125 per cent in two to three years. The average critical weight at menarche in Britain in the early 1980s was between 95 and 105 pounds; this may explain why plump girls tend to menstruate earlier than very slender ones.

The first year or two of menstrual cycles are usually ANOVULATORY (there is no ovulation). By the time OVULATION begins (at an average age of fifteen in 1980), fat tissue makes up 28 per cent of the body composition. Many adolescent girls contintue to gain weight during the two years following the growth spurt (their average weight in 1980 was 121 pounds), for reasons not wholly understood.

Before the early 1970s many reasons were advanced for what triggers the onset of menstruation: climate, genes, education, height, weight, diet. An American doctor, Rose Frisch, then suggested that critical weight was the necessary factor, but exactly how the higher proportion of fat tissue stimulates hormone production is not completely understood. One theory is that metabolic changes signal the hypothalamus to begin producing the factors that trigger menstruation (see MENSTRUAL CYCLE). Whatever the mechanism, it also operates in girls with ANOREXIA NERVOSA (self-starvation) as well as in professional athletes and dancers, who, when their body makeup is less than about 15 per cent fat (in some cases even below 22 per cent), have either very irregular periods or none at all, but whose menses resume regularity when they gain weight.

Cryosurgery Also *cryotherapy.* Destroying abnormal cells by freezing. Cryosurgery is commonly used to treat warts on the vulva (CONDYLOMA ACUMINATA), some precancerous lesions of the cervix (DYSPLASIA), and occasionally inflammation of the cervix (CERVICITIS). Many doctors prefer it to CAUTERIZATION (burning), because it is less painful, produces a more even level of tissue destruction, and causes less scarring and narrowing of the cervical canal.

Cryosurgery is performed with a handheld metal-tipped instrument, a *cryoprobe,* connected to a tank of compressed nitrous oxide, carbon dioxide, or freon. When the compressed gas is released into the cryoprobe, it expands rapidly and produces intense cold, about −60° Fahrenheit (−51° Centigrade). The metal tip of the instrument, cooled by conduction, is held to the affected area, such as the outer surface of the cervix, for two minutes or so, in order to freeze the tissue thoroughly. The procedure is virtually painless; the only sensations are a feeling of coldness and, sometimes, mild cramping. LIke CAUTERIZATION, cryosurgery can cause temporary swelling that narrows the cervical canal for a time, as well as a profuse watery vaginal discharge that lasts for a few weeks. The flow at first is heavy enough to require using a pad (tampons should not be used). If the discharge smells, powdering the labia with cornstarch may eliminate odour.

Cryosurgery should be performed soon after the end of a menstrual period so as to avoid contact with menstrual flow during the early stage of healing. Also, infection is more apt to occur near the time of ovulation or menstruation. Nothing should be placed inside the vagina for two weeks afterwards, and tampons should not be used for six to eight weeks. An IUD need not usually be removed for cryosurgery on the cervix.

Cryptomenorrhoea See under AMENORRHOEA, definition 2.

Cryptorchidism Also *undescended testes*. The incomplete or improper descent of one or both testes at birth. In *total cryptorchidism* the testis remains within the abdominal cavity as a result of mechanical or hormonal abnormalities. In *incomplete descent* it lies within the inguinal canal but is obstructed by mechanical factors. In *hypermobile testes*, the most common such condition, the testes lie within the scrotum sometimes (as during a hot bath) but then retract into the inguinal canal. In most cases of hypermobile testes descent will occur of its own accord before or during puberty. In the other kinds, however, surgical repair – preferably before the age of three or four – is indicated, with simultaneous repair of the inguinal hernia that often accompanies the condition. Delay beyond the age of five may impair sperm formation after puberty and be a cause of eventual infertility.

C section See CAESAREAN SECTION.

Cul-de-sac Also *Douglas cul-de-sac, rectouterine pouch*. A blind pouch that lies between the lower back portion of the vagina and the rectum. It is through the cul-de-sac that CULDOCENTESIS and CULDOSCOPY are performed.

Culdocentesis Placing a needle through the vagina into the CUL-DE-SAC portion of the abdomen, behind the uterus, in order to determine the presence of blood. If non-clotting blood is withdrawn, there is a strong possibility of a ruptured ECTOPIC PREGNANCY, and further diagnostic procedures such as CULDOSCOPY or LAPAROSCOPY, should follow. Culdocentesis can be performed in an outpatient clinic. Occasionally it is performed in cases of PELVIC INFLAMMATORY DISEASE in order to identify the infecting organism.

Culdoscopy Also *colpotomy*. The insertion of a special instrument, a *culdoscope*, through a small incision in the vagina, just behind the cervix, into the CUL-DE-SAC, which enables visual examination of the pelvic organs and performance of tubal ligation. The Fallopian tubes can be examined through the culdoscope for any blockage that prevents conception or for the presence of a tubal pregnancy (see ECTOPIC PREGNANCY; also CULDOCENTESIS). By inserting instruments, each of the Fallopian tubes can be pulled out through the incision, a portion of them removed, and the cut ends ligated (tied), rendering the woman sterile. This operation can be performed under either local or general anaesthesia and, because the incisions made through the vagina, leaves no visible scar. However, it is difficult to perform on women who have scarring or adhesions from previous surgery, pelvic infection, or severe endometriosis. It carries a relatively high risk of post-operative infection and haemorrhage. Furthermore, it is an awkward procedure because the patient must be placed on her knees, with her head down and her buttocks up toward the surgeon, a position difficult to maintain under either general or local anaesthesia. Consequently, for purposes of sterilization culdoscopy has been largely replaced by other forms of tubal ligation, principally LAPAROSCOPY and MINILAPAROTOMY.

Culture The growing of microorganisms, such as bacteria or living cells, in the laboratory, in a medium designed to encourage them to reproduce. Also, the product of such a procedure. Cultures are frequently made from samples of sputum, urine, blood, spinal fluid, stools, and cells from the throat, vagina, or other organs in order to determine what organism is causing an infection. Under favourable conditions the organism usually multiplies in a matter of hours or days and can then be readily identified, but cell cultures often take three to five weeks.

Cunnilingus A form of oral sexual intercourse in which a woman's partner uses his or her mouth (lips, tongue) to stimulate her genitals. Some authorities believe it should be avoided when a woman is in the advanced stages of pregnancy, at least in any form that might involve blowing air into her vagina, lest it cause an air embolism (potentially fatal). See also FELLATIO; ORAL SEX.

Curettage Literally, scraping, referring to the removal of thin strands of tissue from the uterus or some other organ. The instrument used for this purpose is called a *curette* or *curet*. See D AND C; also BIOPSY, definition 8; VACUUM ASPIRATION.

Curvature of the spine See SCOLIOSIS.

Cushing's syndrome A disorder of the adrenal glands that is characterized by overproduction of the hormone cortisol. Originally discovered in 1932 by Dr. Harvey Cushing, who believed it resulted from pituitary tumour or other growth, it has been found to occur also in the absence of such a tumour but in the presence of an adrenal tumour, or of malfunction of the hypothalamus. The disease occurs mostly in women of childbearing age and is characterized by rapidly developing obesity affecting the face, neck, and trunk, oligomenorrhoea or amenorrhoea (infrequent or no menstruation), a moon face, hirsutism (excess body hair), acne, purplish striae (stretch marks) of the skin, especially on the abdomen, a tendency to bruise easily, and hypertension (high blood pressure). Diagnosis is based on the presence of a large amount of corticoids in the urine. Treatment depends on whether the cause lies in the pituitary or the adrenals, and usually involves radiation therapy to the pituitary and/or removal of one or both adrenal glands (and subsequent cortisone replacement therapy for life).

Cycle See MENSTRUAL CYCLE; for the ovarian cycle, see OVULATION; for the cervical cycle, see CERVICAL MUCUS METHOD.

Cyst 1 A small, fluid-filled sac of tissue that can develop in various parts of the body, including the breasts, ovaries, and cervix, as well as the skin. Some cysts contain semisolid material.
2 **Sebaceous cyst** A slow-growing tumour of the skin, frequently found on the scalp, ears, face, back, scrotum, vulva, or breasts. It rarely causes discomfort unless it becomes infected, but then it may form an abscess. The treatment, if

any is needed, consists of applying moist heat every few hours until it comes to a head and drains. If this is not effective, the cyst is drained, either through a small stabbing incision or, in the case of larger cysts, through surgical incision. An infected cyst generally requires the insertion of a drain for a week or so; thereafter the wall of the cyst must be removed if the cyst is not to recur.

3 **Bartholin cyst** A cyst that develops when a duct of one of the BARTHOLIN'S GLANDS, located near the opening of the vagina, becomes blocked. If the cyst is small, no treatment is needed. However, if it is large or, as is often the case, it becomes infected, surgical treatment is indicated. Such infections can be extremely painful and the gland, normally tiny, can grow to the size of a lemon. Treatment usually involves oral antibiotics, applying hot compresses, and surgical incision and drainage. Among the organisms responsible for such infection is gonococcus, so a GONORRHOEA culture is also necessary. Bartholin cysts tend to recur because scarring from one infection often creates new blockage of the gland's secretions. Then either the entire cyst has to be removed (*cystectomy*) or even the entire gland. Occasionally this can be avoided by *marsupialization*, in which, after the cyst is removed, the gland is so cut and stitched that a permanent opening (pouch) is created.

4 **Nabothian cyst** Also *cervical cyst*. A cyst formed when one of the many mucus-producing glands that line the cervix becomes blocked. Nabothian cysts may occur singly or in groups, and occur most often on the surface of the cervix. In size they usually grow no bigger than a small pea; they look like small, white pimple-like bumps on the surface of the cervix. Unless such cysts are associated with other irritation of the cervix they usually cause no problem and require no treatment, but if they occur in conjunction with CERVICITIS they are treated in the same way, by cauterization or cryosurgery.

5 **Chocolate cyst** Also *endometrical cyst*. See under ENDOMETRIOSIS.

6 **Ovarian cyst** A cyst that develops on the ovary. Ovarian cysts may occur at any age, singly or in numbers, on one or both ovaries. The cyst consists of a thin, transparent outer wall enclosing a centre of clear fluids or jelly-like material. Such cysts range in size from that of a raisin to that of a large orange. They may cause a feeling of fullness in the abdominal area, or pain on vaginal intercourse. Often, however, there are no symptoms at all, and the cyst is discovered only during a gynaecological examination, when the doctor finds one ovary is considerably enlarged. At that point it is important to rule out malignancy (See CANCER, OVARIAN), since ovarian cancers in their early stages also have no warning symptoms and can occur at any age.

Many ovarian cysts – some authorities say more than half – are *functional*, that is, they arise out of the normal functions of the ovary during the MENSTRUAL CYCLE. A cyst can form when a follicle has grown in preparation for ovulation but fails to rupture and release an egg; this type is called a *follicle cyst* or *follicular cyst*. Sometimes the structure formed from the follicle after ovulation, the CORPUS LUTEUM, fails to shrink and forms a cyst; this is called a *corpus luteum cyst*. If there is no severe pain or swelling, a doctor may decide to wait for one or two more menstrual cycles to be completed, during the course of which such functional cysts frequently disappear of their own accord. Sometimes this process is hastened by administering oral contraceptives for several months, which establishes a very regular menstrual cycle. (Women already taking oral contraceptives rarely develop ovarian cysts.)

A different kind of ovarian cyst found most often in younger women is a *dermoid cyst*, which contains particles of teeth, hair, or calcium-containing tissue that are thought to be an embryologic remnant; such cysts do not usually cause menstrual irregularity.

Ovarian cysts cause problems when they become very large, when they rupture and cause severe internal bleeding, or when their pedicle (a tail-like appendage) suddenly twists and cuts off its blood supply, creating severe pain. In these cases surgical treatment is indicated, preferably a *cystectomy*, which means removal of the cyst only and preservation of as much of the normal ovarian tissue as possible. Sometimes, with a very large cyst, the ovary cannot be saved and must be removed.

The diagnosis of an ovarian cyst is determined by the patient's age, medical and family history, symptoms, and size of the enlarged ovary. In women under thirty, doctors will usually recommend waiting through one or two menstrual cycles to see if the ovary will return to its normal size. If it does not and pregnancy has been ruled out, an abdominal X-ray and/or sonograph (see ULTRA-SOUND, definition 1) can determine the exact size of the ovaries and distinguish between a cyst and a solid tumour. In older women (over forty) X-ray and sonograph may be done sooner and, if uncertainty still exists, the doctor may recommend LAPAROSCOPY to look at the ovaries through a small incision, or a larger incision and a biopsy. See also STEIN-LEVENTHAL SYNDROME.

7 Breast cyst See CYSTIC DISEASE, BREAST.

Cyst, breast See CYSTIC DISEASE, BREAST.

Cyst, cervical See CYST, definition 4.

Cyst, ovarian See CYST, definition 6.

Cystic disease, breast Also *fibrocystic disease*, (*chronic*) *cystic mastitis*, *mammary dysplasia*. The most common benign (noncancerous) disorder of the breast, characterized by the formation of cysts in one or both breasts. Cysts, which are small, fluid-filled sacs, occur most often in the breasts of women between the ages of thirty-five and fifty-five, when levels of oestrogen and progesterone are relatively high. Indeed, it is estimated that between 15 and 30 per cent of all women have cystic disease during those years. Unlike cancerous growths, cysts are movable, spherically shaped, fairly soft, and subject to rapid changes in size. Often they are associated with nodules or lumps of the breast; they usually occur multiply (not singly) and in both breasts. Some cysts are painful, and others are not.

The formation of cysts appears to be directly related to oestrogen. Not only do cysts rarely appear after menopause, when oestrogen levels are much lower, but they often become firmer and more tender just before a menstrual period, when oestrogen levels are high. Some women find temporary relief by lowering their salt intake during the premenstrual days or by taking a mild diuretic. Although a cyst is, strictly speaking, harmless, a large one is usually subjected to *needle aspiration*, that is, drainage with a needle syringe or, if it refills after such drainage, it is surgically excised. The fluid and tissue withdrawn are always examined by a pathologist in order to rule out malignancy. Because women with cystic disease have a considerably greater chance of developing breast cancer (some studies say three times greater) than women who do not, and the presence of numerous cysts could conceal the presence of a cancerous growth, many doctors advise that women at 'high risk' for developing breast cancer have cysts removed surgically (for a detailed description see under CANCER, BREAST). Others, however, minimize the dangers in a woman with multiple cysts that repeatedly prove to be benign. Cysts do not appear as 'hot spots' on a thermogram but can usually be differentiated from solid tumours on a mammogram (see MAMMOGRAPHY; THERMOGRAPHY).

Treatment for cystic breast disease, which in some women causes considerable discomfort, has ranged from administering hormones, diuretics, and other medications to the very extreme measure of surgically removing all the breast tissue under the skin and replacing it with synthetic implants. Recent studies point to the possible effectiveness of much simpler remedies, among them eliminating all foods that contain methyl xanthines, the best known of which is caffeine; taking large doses of vitamin E, which, however, can be toxic and therefore requires close medical supervision; and administration of a synthetic male hormone, danazol for about six months, which appears to relieve tenderness and lumpiness in a majority of patients. See also CANCER, BREAST.

Cystic fibrosis A severe and chronic disease of the exocrine (externally secreting) glands that affects principally the pancreas, respiratory system, and sweat glands, causing them to overproduce normal secretions and/or produce abnormal secretions. It may also affect the intestines, causing malabsorption syndrome, that is, failure to absorb needed nutrients. It occurs primarily in persons of North European ancestry and is carried as a recessive trait (see under CHROMOSOME for explanation), so that if both parents are carriers, any of their children (of either sex) has a 25 per cent chance of inheriting the disease. If only one parent carries it, the disease is not passed on. Recent studies indicate that its presence in unborn babies might be detected by FOETOSCOPY.

Cystic fibrosis is usually recognized in infancy or early childhood, but in some patients few or no symptoms appear until late adolescence. The principal symptoms are respiratory problems and failure to grow despite normal appetite and vigour. No cure has yet been found, but health can be maintained by close attention to respiratory difficulties – young children, for example, may need regular suctioning of mucus several times a day – and prompt treatment of any infections so as to avoid involvement of the lungs. Treatment includes administering pancreatin, to make up for inadequate pancreatic functions, and careful attention to adequate diet – more calories than normal, especially in the form of fats – as well as treatment of specific manifestations of the disease when they occur.

Cystitis Also *bladder infection*. Infection of the bladder, which is usually caused by bacteria and may be triggered by mechanical irritation. A common trigger in women is frequent sexual intercourse; in fact, cystitis of this origin is called *honeymoon cystitis* because so many women used to be affected in the early weeks of marriage, when engaging in intercourse for the first time and/or very frequently. Intercourse, especially in the conventional position with the woman on her back and the man lying on top of her, directs the penis along the roof of the vagina and against the floor of the urethra and bladder. The pumpimg action of the penis irritates those structures and pushes bacteria normally resident on the external vulva into the urethra. The best way of preventing such infection is to empty the bladder before intercourse and again immediately afterward, and to drink considerably more water than usual, so as to dilute the urine and make it less hospitable to bacterial growth. A diaphragm can also irritate the urethra if the rim rubs against it during intercourse. Bubble baths and swimming pools with chemically treated water are occasionally responsible.

Sexual intercourse is by no means the only way of contracting cystitis for even young children can be afflicted. The causative bacteria are often such normal residents of the intestinal tract as *Escherichia coli*. They may move from the rectum into the vagina (as a result of wiping from back to front after a bowel movement, for example) and thence into the urinary tract; or they may be introduced by instruments used to withdraw urine (a catheter) or to examine the urinary tract (cystoscope). A CYSTOCELE (fallen bladder) may also contribute to infection by preventing the complete emptying of the bladder; the urine that remains is hospitable to bacteria. For a similar reason, cystitis is common during pregnancy, when the foetus is pressing on the bladder.

The symptoms of cystitis are urgency, frequency (needing to void much more often, but producing less urine at one time), and pain – usually a burning sensation – felt on urination. Some blood or pus may appear in the urine, and there may be a feeling of pressure just above the pubic bone. Diagnosis should include a urine culture and sensitivity test to determine what organisms are responsible and which drugs will be most effective against them. Treatment involves drinking six to eight glasses of water per day (in addition to other beverages) and taking appropriate medication – sulphonamides (sulpha drugs) or antibiotics to kill the bacteria, and perhaps also phenazopyridine hydrochloride (Pyridium) to soothe the mucous membranes in the area and relieve urinary frequency (this drug tends to turn the urine a bright orange and stains underwear). Drinking cranberry juice helps make the urine more acid, and therefore inhospitable to bacteria, and also enhances the effect of some drugs used against the infection (especially tetracycline but not the sulpha drugs); cranberry juice contains benzoic acid, a natural preservative used to prevent the growth of moulds, yeasts, and bacteria in foods. (If cranberry juice increases the burning sensation, drink lots of water with a teaspoon of sodium bicarbonate, or baking soda, per glass; however, omit the baking soda if you have high blood pressure or heart disease.) A follow-up urine test should be done after medication relieves the symptoms to make sure the infection has been completely eliminated.

Women who prefer HERBAL REMEDIES report relief from pain is provided by a tea made from cornsilk (*Zea mays*), buchu leaf (*Barosma betulina*), or pipsissewa (*Chimaphila umbellata*). For infections with bleeding they use a tea made from a combination of shepherd's purse (*Capsella bursa pastoris*), burdock root

(*Arctium lappa*), bearberry (*Arctostaphylos uva-ursi*), and echinacea root (*Echinacea augustfolia*).

Cystitis is one of the most common ailments affecting women; nearly every woman contracts it at some time during her life. (A woman's bladder is only about one inch from her urethra; in a man the distance is six or more inches, and therefore cystitis is much less common in men.) Although distressing, it is usually not serious. However, cystitis should be treated, for it tends to recur, and chronic bladder infection over a period of years can result in permanent kidney damage. See also URETHRITIS.

Cystocele   Also *dropped bladder, fallen bladder.* A bulging of the bladder into the vaginal canal, owing to pelvic relaxation, that is, impairment of the muscles that normally hold the bladder in place. It may occur alone or in conjunction with a PROLAPSED UTERUS and so is usually, like the latter, a result of childbirth (a long, difficult labour, very large babies, or many pregnancies). Cystocele usually gives rise to some symptoms, the most common of which is leaking of urine, especially when coughing, laughing, or sneezing (see STRESS INCONTINENCE). It often leads to repeated urinary infections, marked by frequency of urination, a burning sensation when voiding, and a feeling of incomplete voiding (see also CYSTITIS). The condition is readily diagnosed with a pelvic examination.

Treatment for minor cystocele may consist merely of KEGEL EXERCISES to strengthen the pelvic muscles. For more severe cases surgery is indicated, after other causes of chronic incontinence have been ruled out. In the standard repair procedure, the surgeon makes an incision along the front wall of the vagina, pushes the bladder upward, and sews it into normal position. This may be combined with repairing the back wall of the vagina (near the rectum) for better support (see also RECTOCELE). About four out of five patients find relief in this way. For the remaining 20 per cent, more complicated surgery, called a *Marshall-Marchetti procedure,* may be needed to eliminate incontinence. For this procedure the surgeon makes an incision in the abdomen and changes the angle of the bladder opening. See also URETHROCELE.

Cystosarcoma phyllodes   A rapidly growing but relatively uncommon tumour of the breast. It is usually benign (noncancerous) but is occasionally malignant; moreover, it is not easy to distinguish the benign form from the malignant, and therefore evaluation of the tumour tissue by at least two pathologists is recommended. Treatment consists of surgical removal; because this kind of tumour grows so fast, sometimes the entire breast must be removed to eliminate the whole tumour, even when it is benign.

Cytology   The study of cells, including their structure, function, origin, and pathology (diseases and other abnormalities). A PAP SMEAR is one of the most common cytological studies.

D

D and C Abbreviation for *dilatation and curettage*, or scraping of the uterine lining, currently one of the most frequently performed surgical procedures in Britain. It is estimated that each year 4 per cent of all British women undergo a D and C, and 90 to 95 per cent have one sometime during their lives. The operation consists of dilating (stretching) the cervix, or neck of the uterus, sufficiently to allow the insertion of a curet (currette), a small instrument that is used to scrape away part of the endometrium (uterine lining). Among the principal reasons for performing a D and C are to determine the cause of abnormal bleeding or staining; to stop heavy bleeding (see ENDOMETRIAL HYPERPLASIA); to remove bits of placental or other tissue remaining after childbirth, miscarriage, or abortion; to determine if ovulation has occurred in cases of infertility; to detect early uterine cancer or a FIBROID; and to remove endometrial POLYPS (see definition 3). Even when the principal purpose of a D and C is not for diagnosis, the tissue removed should always be examined in the laboratory to make sure no cancer cells are present.

Until about 1960 a D and C also was the principal method of performing an early abortion (during the first trimester of pregnancy), but since then VACUUM ASPIRATION has largely replaced it. Furthermore, for purposes of biopsy as well as to stop heavy bleeding, many doctors prefer to use the simpler vacuum procedure first, following it up with a surgical D and C only if necessary (see BIOPSY, definition 8).

A D and C requires either general or regional (epidural, spinal, or caudal) anaesthesia. Occasionally local anaesthesia, usually a paracervical block is used; in that case the patient will feel some cramps during the procedure. The patient is placed in the same position as for a pelvic examination. Next the surgeon inserts a speculum, holds the cervix steady with a special clamp, a *tenaculum*, and determines the angle of the cervical canal and depth of the uterus by inserting a narrow metal rod called a *sound* through the cervix to the top (fundus) of the uterus. The cervix is then gradually dilated by inserting a series of ever larger rods; the largest is about one-half inch (11 millimetres) in diameter. Sometimes LAMINARIA are used for this purpose, but they take about twenty-four hours to dilate the cervix and are generally reserved for procedures where considerable dilation is needed, more than for a diagnostic D and C. If there are polyps, they are located and removed, and a spoon-shaped curette is used to scrape shreds of tissue from all around the endometrium. The entire procedure takes fifteen to twenty minutes. The instruments are then removed and the procedure is finished; no sutures (stitches) are required.

Recovery from a D and C takes anywhere from a few hours to a couple of days. There may be some bleeding and staining for about two weeks, and mild cramps or backache for the first day or so. Fever, severe cramps or abdominal pain, heavy bleeding, or foul-smelling discharge all are signs of infection and should be promptly reported to the doctor. Such infections, which are the most common complication of a D and C, usually respond to antibiotic treatment but should never be ignored, because they can become serious. Most doctors advise patients to avoid vaginal intercourse, douching, and the use of tampons for two weeks, because the cervix takes time to return to its normal closed position and any of these activities is a potential source of infection. If a woman does wish to engage in vaginal intercourse, her partner should use a condom (to prevent entry of bacteria). After two weeks most doctors see patients for a postoperative check-up.

Complications after a D and C are rare. It is possible for the uterus to be punctured (perforated) by a surgical instrument, but even then no treatment may be needed, the injured tissue simply healing by itself. They can also be damage to bladder or bowel, both of which are adjacent to the uterus, but this rarely happens. Relatively safe as a D and C is, it still constitutes surgery and should be undertaken only if there is a genuine need for it. For irregular bleeding in young women, for example, many doctors prefer first to try hormone therapy for several months (see BREAKTHROUGH BLEEDING). In addition, not only is it essential that pregnancy be ruled out before performing a D and C – provided that the woman wishes to continue the pregnancy – but if there is any infection or inflammation of the uterus, tubes, or cervix, these conditions should, if possible, be cleared up before surgery. See also ASHERMAN'S SYNDROME.

D and E Abbreviation for *dilatation and evacuation*. A procedure that combines the traditional dilatation and curettage (or D AND C) with VACUUM ASPIRATION (definition 2) and is used chiefly to terminate pregnancies of thirteen to eighteen weeks, counting from the first day of the last menstrual period; technically it can be used up to twenty-four weeks, but in practice it is not usually done after eighteen weeks because the cervix would have to dilate too much in too short a time. It requires anaesthesia, either general or regional, and should be performed in a hospital or surgical clinic by a gynaecologist. The cervix must be dilated more than for a D and C; often this is done with the aid of LAMINARIA, beginning twelve to twenty-four hours before surgery. A vacuum curette (suction tube) of the kind used in vacuum aspiration but with a larger bore (because more tissue must be removed) is inserted through the dilated cervix and suction applied to remove foetal and placental material; then forceps are generally used to complete the procedure, as well as a surgical curette to make sure all the tissue has been removed. Following surgery (sometimes during the procedure, as well), most doctors administer oxytocin to promote uterine contractions, which limits blood loss and returns the uterus to its normal pre-pregnant size. Dilation and evacuation takes fifteen to forty-five minutes and does not always require overnight hospitalization. If regional anaesthesia is used, most patients experience sensations similar to those following vacuum aspiration, although the recovery period is somewhat longer, the patient usually being kept several hours for observation. See also ABORTION.

Decompression bubble Also *decompression suit, birthing bubble.* A device that reduces the atmospheric pressure surrounding the abdomen of a woman in labour in order to make her contractions more effective in expelling the baby. It consists of a large plastic shell, or 'bubble', that is fitted around the woman's abdominal area and is connected by a hose to a suction pump. When the pump is on, suction withdraws air from the bubble, causing the woman's abdomen to be lifted up and away from her uterus, so that the uterine muscles can work more efficiently. The woman can switch the pump off and on by herself. When she feels a contraction beginning, she switches it on, and a negative pressure is exerted – the exact amount can be adjusted by turning a dial – reducing the resistance offered the uterus by the abdominal walls. The decompression bubble is said to speed up labour and make it more comfortable as well. Invented in the late 1950s by a South African obstetrician. O. W. Heyns, the decompression bubble is widely used in that country.

Defloration Literally, 'deflowering', meaning a woman's first vaginal intercourse, when penile penetration breaks the HYMEN. See VIRGINITY.

Delayed puberty See under PUBERTY; also see AMENORRHOEA, definition 2.

Delivery The birth of a baby; childbirth. See LABOUR.

Demand feeding A programme of BREAST-FEEDING based on the infant's wish to nurse rather than on specific times.

Deodorant A class of COSMETICS that helps eliminate the odour of perspiration by killing some of the bacteria that cause it, or by adding a fragrance to mask it, or both. Deodorants are generally harmless when used on the armpits but should not be used in the pubic area. Occasionally they give rise to an allergic reaction, usually caused by their perfume component. Switching to another brand may solve the problem. A deodorant does not stop perspiration; if it does, it is classed as an *antiperspirant*, which contains a substance – usually aluminium salts – that temporarily closes the openings of the sweat glands and thus stops their secretions.

Depo-Provera See under PROGESTERONE.

Depression 1 Also *melancholia*. An emotional disorder that ranges in severity from unusually intense or long-lasting feelings of sadness, disappointment, and frustration, to chronic insomnia, inability to concentrate or perform ordinary tasks, and attempts at suicide. Depression is one of the most common afflictions of British adults, affecting an estimated 8 to 20 per cent of the entire population. It is at least twice as prevalent in women as in men; estimates range from a ratio of 4 or 5 depressed women to every man, down to only 1½ or 2 to 1 in the form known as MANIC-DEPRESSIVE ILLNESS. The symptoms of depression are very numerous indeed (see the accompanying chart), and some of them are experienced by practically every man, woman, or child

Symptoms of Depression*

blues
anhedonia (inability to feel pleasure)
loss of appetite
weight loss
constipation
sleep disturbances, insomnia
  (especially waking during the night or early in the morning)
diminished energy, fatigue, lethargy
restlessness, agitation
slowed-down speech, movement, thought
stooped posture, sad facial expression
decreased sex drive
loss of interest in work
feelings of worthlessness, self-reproach, guilt
diminished ability to think and concentrate
forgetfulness
indecisiveness
low self-esteem
feelings of helplessness, anxiety
pessimism, feelings of hopelessness
thoughts of death, suicide attempts
self-absorption, bodily complaints

* None alone is symptomatic of a clinical depression, but the persistent presence of six or more simultaneously may be suspicious.

at some time or anther. They constitute an illness – a so-called *clinical depression* – only when they are long-lasting or severe enough to interfere with normal functioning for a number of months or years.

Doctors frequently distinguish between a *reactive depression* (also called an *exogenous depression*), which begins as a natural reaction to a particular situation or event (such as death of a parent) but persists for more than a normal amount of time and seems more extreme than the situation that provoked it, and an *endogenous depression*, which has no discoverable cause. They further distinguish between *neurotic* and *psychotic* or *major* depressions. Some believe that the difference is largely one of degree, the psychotically depressed person being virtually incapable of functioning and more likely to attempt suicide, but others believe biological factors are definitely implicated in a major depression and less so or not not at all in a mild depression.

The more severe psychotic depressions respond better to drugs and electro-convulsive shock therapy than do milder ones (see ANTIDEPRESSANTS), supporting the view that psychotic depression has an organic basis. Some studies suggest that certain individuals may have a genetic predisposition for such illness. Others maintain that some persons lack, or have an excess of, some chemical that affects the activity of neurotransmitters in the brain or some other objective physical factor. Depression is known to be associated with certain physical illnesses; for example, mononucleosis and infectious hepatitis both are linked with mild depression, and arteriosclerosis with more severe depression. In addition, some researchers have linked clinical depression to the use of oral contraceptives.

There is no conclusive evidence yet concerning these hypotheses, but certain social and emotional aspects of depression have been long observed. Consequently therapists continue to treat depression with psychotherapy, ranging from psychoanalysis to various behaviour therapies, as well as with drugs and electroconvulsive shock treatment, with varying degrees of success. Many feminists maintain that depression is often at least in part, a normal response of women to a repressive sexist society. They tend, therefore, to endorse treatment that teaches women (in particular) to cope more effectively, principally by changing their behaviour so as to receive more positive reinforcement of their self-esteem. Such treatment may involve keeping records to discover the relationship between one's mood and one's expectation of reinforcement, consciousness-raising contacts with other women, assertiveness training to learn to express appropriate anger and to take independent action, and similar measures. See also FEMINIST THERAPY.

2 **Postpartum depression** Also *after-baby blues*. A form of depression experienced by many – perhaps most – women three to four days after giving birth. It is typically characterized by feelings of fear or apprehension about being able to take care of the baby, as well as a general let-down following the exhilaration of giving birth. Because it is so common, many authorities believe postpartum depression may be caused by physical changes, especially the marked drop in oestrogen levels following delivery (back to normal within twenty-four hours) and the drastic reduction in total blood volume (up to 30 per cent). The feelings generally last anywhere from a day or two to a week. If depression persists or is severe enough for a woman to withdrawn from her family, professional help may be indicated. However, contact with a support group of other new parents is often sufficient.

A few women – an estimated 1 in 600 – suffer from more severe (but also temporary) mental illness following childbirth. This condition comes on suddenly, within two weeks of delivery, and ends in about three months, with the woman fully recovering. Symptoms here are more marked than a mood of sadness or withdrawal, and include confusion and rambling speech. Some women become euphoric and hyperactive; others are incapable of caring for their babies and ask for help or supervision in even the simplest tasks. Most women with this condition, one study indicates, have particularly high levels of oestrogen and low levels of progesterone, as well as abnormal levels of other hormones, suggesting an endocrine imbalance.

DES See DIETHYLSTILBOESTROL.

Diabetes Also *diabetes mellitus, sugar diabetes*. A disorder characterized by failure of the pancreas to provide enough effective insulin, a hormone that removes excess sugar from the blood and stores it in the liver, or the inability of body cells to receive insulin. Its prevailing sign is the presence of increased quantities of glucose (sugar) in the blood (*hyperglycaemia*) and urine (*glycosuria*). Symptoms include urinary frequency, increased hunger and thirst, and weight loss. The cause is not known, although diabetes does appear to be connected with age, overweight, hereditary factors, virus infection, and possibly an autoimmune response. The condition cannot be cured, but it can usually be controlled, by diet alone or by oral medication or by administering insulin in various forms. Uncontrolled, diabetes may have serious complications, especially in the circulatory system, where in extreme cases it causes impairment leading to gangrene and the loss of limbs, and in the eye, where blindness may result. Diabetes is a leading cause of death in Britain, and over 500,000 people in Britain are diabetics. However, it is hoped that new methods whereby diabetics can regularly monitor their own blood levels of glucose – a far more accurate indicator than older urine tests – will enable many to control the disease better and avoid its worst complications.

Diabetes may begin in childhood, but then appears to be due to a defect in the pancreas itself, and is more apt to develop serious complications, and usually requires insulin therapy for life. This form is also known as *insulin-dependent, juvenile-onset,* or *Type 1 diabetes*. In adults the disease usually, but not always, attacks after the age of forty, and is slightly more common in women than in men. This form is called *non-insulin-dependent, maturity-onset,* or *Type II diabetes,* and some researchers believe the two forms

are separate diseases. Of the two, maturity-onset diabetes is often controlled simply by means of a strict diet (high in carbohydrates and fibre is recommended) and may not require the administration of insulin. It may occur during pregnancy, and sometimes – but not always – disappears after delivery; some authorities believe that in such cases pregnancy may 'unmask' an already existing disease. Diabetes has no effect on fertility but diabetic women are often advised to avoid oral contraceptives.

The disease poses a considerable problem in pregnancy, so that a pregnant woman with diabetes is usually classed as a HIGH-RISK PREGNANCY. Too much insulin causes a diabetic to go into shock; too little insulin causes another dangerous condition, ketoacidosis. The balance of insulin is a delicate one, and whenever the body goes through a major metabolic or hormonal change, as during the adolescent growth spurt (SEE PUBERTY) or during pregnancy, that balance is upset. Babies of diabetic mothers, for reasons that are not understood, tend to be very large, with oversize organs, but not well developed (mature) for their size. They tend to be born prematurely, and consequently are more likely to develop hypoglycaemia and respiratory distress syndrome. The diabetic mother has a much greater risk of developing pre-eclampsia and eclampsia (four times greater than the non-diabetic), as well as infections of various kinds during pregnancy. The larger size of the baby often makes for difficult delivery. The incidence of stillbirth is high, HYDRAMNIOS is common, and postpartum haemorrhage is frequently a threat.

Although fastidious antenatal care of the diabetic mother will usually safeguard her during the pregnancy, the outlook for her baby is less optimistic: perinatal mortality (before, during, or just after delivery) is estimated to be 10 to 15 per cent, and those babies who survive often have one or more disabling birth defects.

Because of the high risk and the tendency to have unusually large babies, some doctors insist that all their diabetic patients be delivered by Caesarean section by the 38th week, because the risk of foetal death is so much higher then and the cervix is often not ripe enough to induce labour. Many others, however, prefer a more conservative approach. Some recommend hospitalization from the 35th or 36th week of pregnancy on, depending on the severity of the diabetes. Others prefer to try INDUCTION OF LABOUR if the baby is not too large, the pelvis not too small, the cervix soft and somewhat effaced and dilated, and the baby is head first and fixed in the pelvis.

After delivery the mother's insulin dosage must be drastically lowered to meet her body's new needs and must continue to be carefully monitored. Some doctors feel that diabetic women who already have several children and who have circulatory or kidney impairment of any kind should seriously consider sterilization to avoid the hazards of another pregnancy.

Diaphragm 1 A muscle separating the abdominal and chest cavities.

2 A cup-shaped spring device that is inserted into the vagina along with spermicidal jelly or cream in order to prevent conception. It is *not* effective alone as a mechanical barrier to sperm, which can enter around its edges. Rather, it keeps sperm-killing material (see SPERMICIDE) in place over the cervix, so that sperm are killed before they can enter

there. (Sperm do not survive for more than eight hours in the vagina because of its acid secretions.) In theory, the diaphragm, which requires a doctor's prescription, is one of the most effective and safest means of BIRTH CONTROL; when it is used properly its success rate is allegedly about 98 per cent. However, it must be properly fitted, large enough to allow for expansion of the vagina during sexual excitement but not so tight that it is uncomfortable when the vagina returns to normal size. Furthermore, the fit should be checked yearly, as well as after childbirth, abortion, or a weight loss or gain of ten to fifteen pounds or more, since a woman's size can change. The diaphragm must be properly inserted each time, along with an adequate amount of active (not outdated) spermicide. It must be used for each act of intercourse and left in place for eight hours therafter; additional spermicide must be inserted with an applicator if intercourse is repeated before eight hours are up. Because spermicide is effective for only six to eight hours, the diaphragm should not be inserted more than two hours before intercourse. If more than two hours pass, it should be removed and fresh spermicide added before intercourse takes place. Given all these requirements, the actual effectiveness of a diaphragm in preventing unwanted pregnancy is far less than claimed, some studies saying only 84 per cent or so. The diaphragm itself consists of a flexible metal ring (spring) covered with rubber, taking the shape of a shallow dome. For insertion, spermicidal cream or jelly is placed inside the dome and all around the edges of the rim, about 1 tablespoon in all. Then, squeezing the diaphragm in one hand and spreading the vaginal lips with the other, the woman slides the

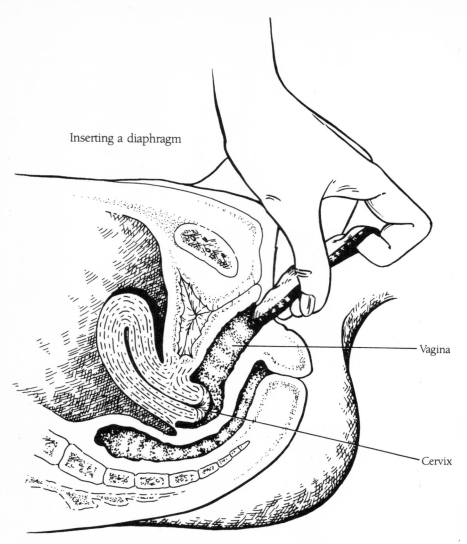

Inserting a diaphragm

Vagina

Cervix

diaphragm into the vagina, where it is held in place by spring tension. Its rim should rest behind the pubic bones, where it cannot be felt (except by touching) and the dome should cover the cervix. The diaphragm is easier to insert from a squatting position (or standing with one foot up on a chair). For women who have trouble inserting it, a plastic inserter, which looks somewhat like a crochet hook with a series of notches in it, is available for use with some kinds of diaphragm. The diaphragm is stretched onto the inserter, which is then put inside the vagina; once in, the diaphragm is released by giving the inserter a little twist, and it is withdrawn while the diaphragm remains in place. After removing the diaphragm (eight hours after the last intercourse) it should be washed with soap and water, rinsed, and dried (if desired, dusted with cornstarch), and stored in a container away from light. It should never be boiled and should regularly be checked for holes, either by holding it up to the light or by filling it with water and looking for leaks (especially near the rim). With regular care a diaphragm will last two years or so.

Diaphragms come in diameters of 50 to 105 millimetres (2 to 4 inches; most women require one between 70 and 90 millimetres), and with one of four types of rim: coil spring, flat spring, arcing spring, and bow bend spring (a coil with two rigid semicircles that form an arc shape when compressed). The coil spring fits women of average size and shape who have good vaginal muscle tone; the flat spring works best for women with a shallow pubic arch, with moderate descent of bladder or rectum (cystocele, rectocele), or with a uterus tilted forward more than average (anteverted). The arcing spring works best for women with poor vaginal muscle tone, a cervix that protrudes considerably, moderate descent of bladder or rectum, or extreme forward or backward tilt of the uterus (anteverted, retroverted). Very occasionally, however, women cannot be properly fitted, usually because they have a severely prolapsed uterus, or their vagina is either too tight (as in a virgin; it may take some months of regular intercourse for it to stretch) or too relaxed, or if the uterus is severely tipped. Occasionally a woman's partner is allergic to either the rubber or the spermicide; in the latter case a different brand may solve the problem. For oral sex, many find the spermicide tastes unpleasant.

A diaphragm can be used during menstruation, both for contraception and to collect the menstrual flow during intercourse. Occasionally the diaphragm may become displaced in intercourse, mostly in the position where the woman is on top of the man when his penis is withdrawn or when the penis is withdrawn and reinserted repeatedly. Occasionally women find that a diaphragm irritates their urethra and then contributes to infection (see URETHRITIS); such irritation usually occurs when the diaphragm rim presses on the urethra and may indicate that the diaphragm is somewhat too large.

Devices like diaphragms have been in use for centuries. In the 18th century women sometimes inserted half of a squeezed lemon in their vagina over the cervix; presumably the acidity of the lemon juice helped kill sperm. The modern diaphragm was developed in the late 19th century in Europe. It was widely recommended by birth control clinics in the first half of the 20th century and, although briefly replaced in popularity by oral contraceptives and intrauterine devices in the 1960s, begain to regain favour as women realized that is disadvantages and risk were considerably less than those of alternative methods of BIRTH CONTROL. See also CERVICAL CAP.

Diet   A regimen of food intake. A basic *normal diet* consists of a wide variety of foods that provide adequate amounts of all the essential nutrients; that is, a balance of carbohydrates, proteins, and fats, containing sufficient quantities of the essential vitamins, minerals, and trace elements. At certain times of life, notably during adolescence, pregnancy, and lactation, nutritional requirements are greater, both in terms of total food intake (usually measured in calories) and increased need for particular nutrients. Even then, individual requirements vary according to body build, height, and amount of daily exercise.

During the adolescent growth spurt (see PUBERTY) – for girls from ages ten or eleven to fifteen, for boys from twelve or thirteen to nineteen – calorie requirements rise for both sexes. During this period most adolescents acquire half of their final adult weight. The precise amount needed depends on physical activity, but adolescent boys require at least 2,750 calories per day while girls need at least 2,200; participation in active sports may raise those amounts by 1,500 or more calories per day. Adult men continue to require more calories than women simply because they are taller and have a heavier build.

During pregnancy the average woman needs 300 or so extra calories per day for proper nutrition. Protein in particular is important to nourish the growing foetus, and daily intake should be about 50 per cent higher than before, or about 80 grams a day. Although some doctors routinely prescribe vitamin supplements, a healthy pregnant woman eating a well-balanced diet composed of fruits, vegetables, meat, fish, eggs, whole grains, and dairy products probably does not need any. However, unless she gets the calcium equivalent of two pints of milk per day she may need a calcium supplement, and most authorities agree that she should iron and folic acid supplements as well (aiming for a haemoglobin level of 12 to 16 grams per 100 cc. of blood). Adequate liquid intake also is important, but alcoholic beverages in large amounts can be harmful to the baby and so should be limited to two drinks a day (for more detail, see under ALCOHOL USE).

During lactation a woman may need 500 extra calories a day above her pre-pregnant level, mostly in the form of protein. The diet of the breast-feeding woman should also be high in calcium and the B vitamins, with adequate fluids to replace what is lost through her milk. Some women find that if they eat certain foods their babies have more gas pains and colic; among the offenders often named are vegetables of the cabbage family (cauliflower, Brussels sprouts, broccoli, cabbage), onions, garlic, and chocolate. Others maintain they can eat anything without ill effect on their babies.

With age, food requirements lessen; actually the total calories intake needed to maintain weight declines by a small amount every year after the age of twenty, by an estimated 5 to 10 per cent each decade. By menopause only two-thirds as many calories are required to maintain weight, and after menopause, with the reproductive system no longer active, still fewer are needed. However, the need for calcium, vitamin D, and the B vitamins continues to be great (some believe it is greater, since there is no longer much oestrogen to help absorption of essential nutrients), and if the average woman must limit her total calories to 1,800 or so a day she may need supplements of these nutrients to ensure adequate intake. The suggested level is 1 gram of calcium per day, along with 400 to 500 units of vitamin D (but no more, since higher amounts are toxic), along with a single B-complex supplement. Some women have found that vitamin E helps control HOT FLUSHES but there still is no conclusive evidence concerning its role, and it should not be used by women with hypertension (high blood pressure). Finally, certain substances should be restricted after the age of 50, notably cholesterol (found chiefly in animal fats), which appears to contribute to atherosclerosis, and salt (no more than 1.5 grams per day), which may call for a drastic reduction since the average Briton

Daily Eating Plan

	Milk and milk products	Meat and meat substitutes	Fruit and vegetables	Bread and cereals
Adolescent Women	4+ servings (8 oz. milk or yogurt, or 1½ oz hard cheese, = 1 serving)	3+ servings (2 to 3 oz. meat, fish, or poultry, or 4 tb. peanut butter, or 1 cup cooked legumes, or 1 egg = 1 serving)	4+ servings (½ cup or 3½ oz. = 1 serving), including 1 citrus fruit daily and 1 dark green or yellow vegetable 4 times a week	4+ servings, preferably whole grain (1 slice bread, 1 oz. dry cereal, ⅔ cup cooked cereal, rice, or pasta = 1 serving)
Adult Women	2+ servings	2+ servings	4+ servings	4+ servings
Pregnant* and Lactating Women	3 servings first trimester; 4 servings last six months	3 servings + 1 egg first trimester; 4 servings + 1 to 2 eggs last six months	4 to 5 servings, including 1 citrus and 1 dark green or yellow vegetable daily	3 servings first trimester; 4 to 5 servings last six months
Postmenopausal Women**	2+ servings	2+ servings	2+ servings	2+ servings

* Supplements of iron (30 to 60 milligrams per day) and folic acid are usually prescribed
** A general multivitamin and mineral supplement may be prescribed

consumes up to twenty times that amount, which contributes to high blood pressure. (See also under MENOPAUSE; OBESITY.)

During old age good nutrition becomes still more difficult to achieve. The elderly often are lonely and depressed, which diminishes their appetite and interest in taking care of themselves. They may have difficulty in shopping for food and preparing it; lose interest in preparing meals for themselves; lack teeth or have poorly fitting dentures, making it hard to chew healthy foods; and live on a fixed income that limits their buying power. Consequently many older persons so not get enough protein, calcium, iron, vitamins, fibre, or even total calories. Some gain weight on a diet high in carbohydrates but are still malnourished in terms of the proper nutrients. Many doctors now recommend routine vitamin and mineral supplements for all elderly patients, on the assumption that they cannot get sufficient amounts of them without consuming far too many calories. Furthermore, they suggest drastically lowering consumption of salt, refined sugars and starches, as well as fats, in order to help prevent diabetes, hypertension, and arteriosclerosis.

Diethylstilboestrol   Also *DES*. A form of synthetic oestrogen developed in 1938 and widely used until about 1955 to prevent miscarriage. Although by then its effectiveness for this purpose was seriously questioned, it continued to be used for almost twenty years longer. The daughters of women who were given DES during pregnancy have shown a significant incidence of clear-cell ADENOCARCINOMA (see definition 2), a rare form of vaginal cancer, as well as ADENOSIS (see definition 1) and other abnormalities of the reproductive tract.

In addition, some studies indicate that in their own pregnancies DES daughters have higher rates of miscarriage and premature birth. Sons of DES mothers have shown a higher than normal incidence of genital and urinary abnormalities, and the mothers themselves are suspected of having a higher incidence of cancer of the breast and pelvic regions. DES is still officially approved for use in a variety of other conditions, notably for treating certain advanced breast and prostate cancers, as OESTROGEN REPLACEMENT THERAPY for postmenopausal women and for 'oestrogen deficiency' in younger women, to suppress lactation in women not wishing to breast-feed, and in the MORNING-AFTER PILL for birth control.

Because of the potential dangers to children born of DES mothers and the fact that anyone who gave birth after 1940 or was born after that date may unknowingly have been exposed to DES, certain guidelines have been developed. Firstly, women suspecting that they may have received DES during pregnancy are urged to try to obtain their past medical records. Secondly, daughters of women who did receive DES are advised to have pelvic examinations every year beginning after their first menstrual period (or by the age of fourteen, whichever comes first), and also to have a check-up whenever they see unusual spotting, bleeding, or heavy discharge. The examination should include a complete history, careful observation and palpation of the vagina and cervix, a Pap smear, and COLPOSCOPY of the vagina and cervix, including examination with an iodine stain (see SCHILLER TEST). Furthermore, DES mothers are advised to perform monthly BREAST SELF-EXAMINATION and undergo annual breast exams by doctors, as well as annual pelvic examinations (including a bimanual examination and a Pap smear). Both DES mothers and daughters are advised to avoid when possible the use of oestrogens for other purposes, such as oral contraceptives, menopausal oestrogen replacement, and the like. Finally, DES sons are advised to visit a urologist immediately following puberty to be screened for genital abnormalities that have been found in other DES sons, notably urinary problems, cysts, undescended testes (cryptorchidism) or underdeveloped testes, low sperm count, abnormally shaped sperm, or absence of sperm.

Dilatation and curettage   See D AND C.

Dilatation and evacuation   See D AND E.

Discharge, vaginal   Also *leukorrhoea*. The normal secretions of the endocervical glands (located in the cervical canal) and Bartholin's glands, mixed with dead vaginal cells and bacteria normally residing in the vagina. These secretions are either clear or whitish (leukorrhoea means 'white discharge'), and with exposure to air often turn light yellow. After puberty higher oestrogen levels, especially during ovulation and pregnancy, serve to increase the amount of these secretions, as do emotional stress and sexual excitement. The secretions normally are slightly acid, owing to lactic acid produced by the action of the döderlein bacilli.

The consistency of the cervical mucus changes during the menstrual cycle and therefore can be an indication of when ovulation takes place (see CERVICAL MUCUS METHOD). Normal vaginal discharge has practically no odour and does not cause itching, burning, or other irritation. If such irritation occurs or if the discharge is smelly, copious, yellow greyish-green, cheesy, or blood-specked, it usually signals the presence of an infection (see CERVICITIS; VAGINITIS).

Discrete Separate and distinct, a term used to describe lesions that are separated from one another.

Diuretc Also *water pill*. A drug that acts on the kidneys to produce an increased output of sodium (salt) and water into the urine. It is used to treat disorders of the heart, circulatory system, kidneys, or liver that result in excess fluid retention (oedema, formerly called 'dropsy'), especially hypertension (high blood pressure). The principal diuretcs are: (1) thiazides and related drugs, such as chlorothiazide; (2) ethacrynic acid (Edecrin) and frusemide (Lasix), which are more powerful; and (3) carbonic anhydrase inhibitors,

mild drugs used to treat glaucoma (acetazolamide, or Diamox).

Some thiazides, particularly chlorothiazide, developed in 1958, were for a time widely used for pregnant women to counter excess fluid retention, but in 1973 studies showed that they can damage both mother and foetus, and have many adverse side effects (loss of appetite, stomach irritation, diarrhoea, constipation, cramping, jaundice, pancreatitis, hypertension and others).

Women who prefer HERBAL REMEDIES use infusions made from yarrow leaves (*Achillea millefolium*) or hibiscus flowers (*Hisbiscus*), which are said to have diuretic properties. See also the accompanying chart.

Douching Rinsing the vagina with water or some other solution. As a

---

Herbal Diuretics*

SIMMER 1 TABLESPOON OF HERB PER CUP OF WATER FOR 20 MINUTES

Asparagus (*Asparagus officinalis*)**
Celery (*Apium graviolens*)**
Cleavers, or bedstraw, or goosegrass (*Galium aparine*)
Cucumber (*Cucumis sativus*)**
Dandelion root and leaf (*Taraxacum officinale*)
Ground ivy (*Glechoma hederacea* or *Nepata glecoma*)
Hydrangea leaves or root (*Hydrangea*)
Juniper berries (*Juniperus communis*)
Parsley (*Petroselinum crispum*)**
Shepherd's purse (*Capsella bursa pastoris*)
Slippery elm (*Ulmus fulva*)
Wintergreen, or partridgeberry (*Gaultheria procumbens*)

* Herbs, like man-made drugs, have chemical constituents whose particular properties are what makes them effective. However, like other drugs, they may contain allergens, and a person who is allergic to a particular substance can have an allergic reaction. Therefore herbs should be used with care.
** Eat as a vegetable

method of preventing pregnancy (douching after intercourse), it is considered less than 60 per cent reliable (some authorities say 0 per cent). Sperm can quickly move through the cervical opening into the cervical canal, beyond the reach of the douche solution, within a minute or two of ejaculation, and can reach the Fallopian tubes in as little as ten minutes. Moreover, the pressure of the douching liquid may speed the sperm's progress. As a method of hygiene, comparable to bathing other parts of the body, douching is rarely necessary, and indeed by changing the relative acidity of the vagina it can encourage the growth of infection-causing organisms (see VAGINITIS), as well as help spread infection from the vagina up into the uterus and Fallopian tubes. Women who feel unclean unless they douche are advised to do so no more than once a week, with only very gentle pressure (with a drainage bag at shoulder height or lower), using either plain warm water or 1 tablespoon white vinegar per quart of water. Douching should be avoided if pregnancy is suspected, after a D and C or abortion (for two weeks), after childbirth (for four to six weeks), and for three days prior to any gynaecological examination (because it may flush out organisms before they can be detected by the doctor).

Vaginal hygiene sprays sold over the counter often cause uncomfortable irritation and should be avoided; there is no clinical reason whatever for their use. Douching with antibacterial agents and home or over-the-counter remedies such as boric acid solution or vinegar and water is effective against some vaginal infections, but it is better to find out what organism is responsible for the condition before embarking on a course of douches.

Dowager's hump See also SCOLIOSIS. Also *kyphosis*. Curvature of the upper vertebrae of the spine, giving a humped-back appearance. It is so called because it appears mostly in postmenopausal women, as a result of OSTEOPOROSIS.

Down's syndrome Also *mongolism*. A BIRTH DEFECT that is usually caused by the presence of an extra chromosome and is characterized by such abnormalities as mental retardation, retarded growth, poor muscle tone, a small, flat nose and slanting eyes (accounting for the older name, 'mongoloid'), a protruding lower lip, and small, broad hands and feet. In 80 per cent of cases the extra chromosome comes from the mother, from whom the embryo thus gets twenty-four chromosomes that pair up with twenty-three from the father (see under CHROMOSOME for further explanation). Most Down's babies have three chromosomes in what would normally be a pair identified as number 21, so the disorder is also called *Trisomy 21*. About 3 per cent of cases, however, are caused by translocation (genes out of order) and are hereditary, a defect that can be detected by KARYOTYPING.

Down's syndrome is thought to be the most common form of mental retardation. It occurs in about one in every six hundred babies born and is responsible for almost three-tenths of all cases of severe retardation in the Western world. Many Down's syndrome babies suffer from serious heart defects as well and, until recently, most died before reaching adulthood; those who did survive were generally institutionalized. Today, it is recognized that Down's syndrome children vary in intelligence level and that many, if their physical defects permit survival, can be educated sufficient to manage adult life in some kind of supervised setting.

The cause of Down's syndrome is not known, but, because the frequency of Trisomy 21 increases in direct proportion to the age of the mother (see the accompanying chart), it is strongly suspected that ageing adversely affects the ova (eggs) in some way, a fact that has been demonstrated in other species of animal even though there is no direct evidence for human ova. Fortunately, the extra chromosome can be detected by AMNIOCENTESIS, so that women whose choose not to bear a baby with this defect may have the option of abortion. See also AGE, CHILDBEARING.

Age of mother	Incidence of Down's syndrome
Under 20	1 in 2,500
20-29	1 in 1,500
30-34	1 in 850
35-39	1 in 280
40-44	1 in 100
Over 44	1 in 40

Dropping See LIGHTENING.

Drug use and pregnancy Practically all substances ingested by a pregnant woman – including tobacco smoke, alcoholic beverages, prescription drugs, illegal drugs, and over-the-counter remedies such as aspirin and laxatives – have some effect on the baby she is carrying. The placenta transports almost every substance the mother takes in to the unborn child. Therefore most authorities agree that no drug should be used during any stage of pregnancy (or of BREASTFEEDING) unless it is absolutely needed, and then only in the smallest dose and

for the shortest time possible. Habit-forming drugs such as *opiates* (opium, heroin, morphine, codeine, methadone) all can cause drug-dependency in the baby, which will be born addicted and immediately begin to experience withdrawal symptoms. Tranquillizers and antidepressants have not been fully evaluated in terms of their effect on the foetus (except for a few, among them the disastrously damaging THALIDOMIDE). The phenothiazines, major tranquillizers such as Larqactil, Stelazine, Depixol, and Mellaril, have caused infant death in test animals, and at least one has been connected with the development of jaundice in human babies. Librium and Valium, the two most commonly prescribed minor TRANQUILLIZERS have both caused skeletal abnormalities in animal foetuses and babies.

Other mind-altering drugs—LSD, mescaline, marijuana, PCP or 'angel dust', hashish—as well as the amphetamines ('speed', diet pills, 'uppers') and barbiturates (Seconal, Amital, sleeping pills) also reach the foetus, with varie effects. Even such a seemingly harmless remedy as aspirin can, especially when used in large doses in late pregnancy, disrupt the blood-clotting mechanism of both baby and mother, causing danger at delivery; it also should be avoided during the first trimester if possible. Frequent use of laxatives can interfere with the absorption of nutrients. Antibiotics can also damage the foetus; tetracycline is known to cause permanent discoloration of the baby's teeth and also may affect bone growth. Some sulpha drugs taken in late pregnancy can disturb the baby's liver function. Caffeine, present in coffee, tea, cola drinks, and some pain relievers (usually together with aspirin), also may be implicated in birth defects and should not be taken in large quantities.

To avoid possible damage, a woman who discovers she is pregnant should fully discuss any prescription medications and over-the-counter remedies she might use at her first antenatal care visit. Throughout her pregnancy she should be careful to remind other doctors she may consult (including her dentist) that she is pregnant. On balance, use of an occasional aspirin or laxative is unlikely to cause any damage, but beyond such minimal use any drug taken during pregnancy should always be evaluated as to its risks versus its benefits.

Dry labour Labour that occurs after the breaking of the membranes, that is, the spontaneous rupture of the AMNIOTIC SAC and release of the amniotic fluid. In most cases the sac does not rupture of its own accord until late in the first stage of LABOUR, but occasionally it occurs very early in labour or prior to it. Sometimes it is broken by the doctor as part of INDUCTION OF LABOUR or to strengthen uterine contractions. Actually, subsequent labour is not truly dry, since the cells lining the amniotic sac continue to secrete large amounts of fluid.

Dryness, vaginal See VAGINAL ATROPHY.

Ductal papilloma Also *intraductal papilloma*. A benign (noncancerous) tumour in the breast's system of ducts, which may produce both a mass (lump) in the breast and a serous (clear) or bloody discharge from the nipple. The serum secreted by papillomas tends to dam up in the duct and may become infected, leading to inflammation of the duct and surrounding tissue. Because such a tumour is hard to distinguish from a cancerous growth, it is nearly always surgically removed.

Duke's test A blood test to discover if a woman has developed antibodies against her partner's sperm and therefore cannot become pregnant. See SPERM.

Dysfunctional bleeding, vaginal Also *functional bleeding*. Heavy bleeding from the vagina with no discoverable cause, as opposed to bleeding that has a definite cause such as a fibroid or some other lesion. Some authorities restrict the term 'dysfunctional' to exceptionally heavy menstrual flow; others use it for any abnormal bleeding, either during a period or between periods (BREAKTHROUGH BLEEDING). See also ANOVULATORY BLEEDING; ENDOMETRIAL HYPERPLASIA.

Dysmenorrhoea 1 Any physical or emotional discomfort associated with menstrual periods.

2 **Primary dysmenorrhoea** Dysmenorrhoea associated directly with menstrual periods rather than some underlying disorder.

3 **Secondary dysmenorrhoea** Dysmenorrhoea usually spasmodic (see definition 4 below), that results from a specific condition or disorder, such as endometriosis, uterine fibroids, pelvic inflammatory disease, or the presence of an intrauterine device (IUD).

4 **Spasmodic dysmenorrhoea** Also *menstrual cramps*. Painful cramps – spasms of dull and/or acute lower abdominal discomfort – that occur on the first day of menstrual flow but sometimes some hours before the flow begins and/or on the second or subsequent days as well. The pain normally involves only the lower abdominal and genital area, but sometimes it is felt in the lower back, on

the inner thighs, and throughout the pelvis. Along with pain, some women experience nausea, vomiting, dizziness, and fainting. Such cramps usually do not occur during the first year or two of menstrual cycles, appearing (if at all) only after ovulation becomes established. Possibly the shedding of endometrial tissue after ovulation causes stronger uterine contractions that, along with spasms of small arteries in the uterine walls, are the source of the pain. Cramps tend to lessen in severity after the age of thirty. However, some women never (or hardly ever) experience spasmodic dysmenorrhoea, and never enough to disable them even temporarily, whereas others continue to suffer from it monthly until menopause. In 5 per cent or so of women the condition is severe enough to interfere significantly with their lives.

For some years doctors prescribed hormones, especially oestrogens, to alleviate severe cramps, but more recent evidence indicates that the principal purpose served by such treatment, which is not without risk, was to eliminate ovulation; indeed, women taking oral contraceptives for birth control often find they no longer have menstrual cramps. More recently, increased levels of hormones called *prostaglandins*, which cause uterine contractions, have been suspected to be the underlying cause of most spasmodic dysmenorrhoea, and treatment with anti-prostaglandins or prostaglandin inhibitors – among them fenoprofen, ibuprofen, naproxen, and mefenamic acid – has met with considerable success. Since these drugs are also commonly used as pain relievers, the results are not wholly conclusive. Furthermore, they cannot be used by women with a history of ulcers or of asthma, which these drugs might aggravate, or if there is a possibility of pregnancy (they pass through to the foetus).

Women have long used a variety of home remedies for cramps; Heat tends to relax the spasms, and relief is often afforded by use of a heating pad or hot-water bottle applied to the lower abdomen, or deep-heating oil (such as tiger balm) rubbed into the affected area. Avoiding long periods of standing also helps. A hot bath (but not so hot as to provoke nausea or fainting) may ease the discomfort, along with drinks of warm herbal teas (see below) or broth. Some women find a strong alcoholic drink helpful for relaxing uterine muscles. The deep breathing and back massage used in some methods of prepared childbirth may help, as do muscle-relaxing exercises such as the cobra, bow, and pelvic rock of yoga. There is no need to avoid ordinary exercise, and some women actually find jogging or a game of tennis helpful. Orgasm also affords relief, probably by increasing blood circulation to the pelvis.

Good nutrition is important, and some women are helped by balanced supplements of calcium and magnesium in a 2 to 1 ratio (500 mg. calcium, 250 mg. magnesium), taken for a week before each period. Vitamins A, C, and D are needed for good calcium absorption. a high-fibre diet (rich in whole grain, raw fruit and vegetables), with its natural laxative effect, may help relieve the constipation that often is associated with both spasmodic and congestive dysmenorrhoea (see definition 5 below).

Among HERBAL REMEDIES used by women for cramps are: for mild cramps, an infusion of red raspberry leaves (*Rubus idaeus*), alone or with squaw vine or partridgeberry (*Mitchella repens*); for moderate cramps, capsules of cramp bark (*Viburnum opulus*) taken with red raspberry tea (see above). Also used are infusions made from sweet or lemon balm (*Melissa officinalis*), chamomile or camomile (*Matricaria chamomilla* or *Anthemis nobilis*), mugwort (*Artemisia vulgaris*), or motherwort (*Leonurus cardiaca*).

If severe cramps do not respond to simpler remedies and there is no underlying disease causing them (see definition 3 above), a prescription for a stronger analgesic such as codeine, or for anti-prostaglandins, may be needed.

5 Congestive dysmenorrhoea Also *premenstrual tension, premenstrual syndrome.* A series of one or more symptoms that occur, alone or at times together, before the onset of a menstrual period, usually during the preceding week. The most common of them are oedema (fluid retention, with bloating or swelling in the abdomen, breasts, fingers, and ankles, and accompanying weight gain), a dull ache in the lower abdomen, headache, backache, joint and muscle pains, skin lesions (especially acne), irritability, depression, and fatigue. The occurrence of these symptoms more or less regularly before each (or nearly each) menstrual period, and relief from them soon after menstrual flow begins are what pinpoint diagnosis.

The term 'premenstrual tension' was coined in 1931 by Dr. Robert T. Frank. It is thought to occur to some degree in at least half (some say three quarters) of all women of child-bearing age; in about 10 per cent it seriously affects their lives, requiring time off from work or school. The underlying cause of most of the symptoms may be the influence of oestrogen on the body's salt and water exchange, with higher oestrogen levels toward the end of the MENSTRUAL CYCLE inhibiting the normal flushing of sodium and water through the kidneys. The extra water is then redistributed into the body tissues, with resultant oedema. Some researchers believe the adrenal hormone ALDOSTERONE may be responsible for fluid retention. As for the mood changes associated with congestive dysmenorrhoea, which are as characteristic of the condition as fluid retention, some believe they are largely the result of negative attitudes toward menstruation, but others blame biochemical factors. Like spasmodic dysmenorrhoea (see definition 4 above), congestive dysmenorrhoea is often relieved by oral contraceptives that stop ovulation, and some studies report good results from administering progesterone alone. Thus, although the precise mechanisms of cause and effect are not understood, it is generally agreed that the changes triggered by ovulation play an important role in both kinds of dysmenorrhoea.

A number of simple remedies may be helpful. Fluid retention may be minimized by reducing sodium intake (avoid table salt, carbonated drinks, soy sauce, very salty foods such as most cheeses and smoked meats and fish) and increasing intake of potassium (found in ripe bananas, orange juice, peanuts and peanut butter) and calcium (milk and milk products). A high-fibre diet (whole grains, raw fruits and vegetables) helps counter the constipation often associated with the syndrome, thought to be caused by the shift of fluid from the bowel to the intestinal walls, or by the effects of hormones on the muscles of the bowel. Prescription diuretic drugs, formerly widely recommended, may decrease fluid retention but do not seem to afford relief of other symptoms, and tranquillizers, while having a general calming effect, do not deal with the specific symptoms. Some HERBAL REMEDIES used are infusions made from camomile (*Matricaria chamomilla* or *Anthemis nobilis*), catnip (*Nepeta cataria*), hops (*Humulus lupulus*), motherwort (*Leonurus cardiaca*), mugwort (*Artemisia vulgaris*), skullcap (*Scutellaria lateriflora*), spearmint (*Mentha spicata*), sweet balm or lemon balm (*Melissa officinalis*), or valerian (*Vaeriana officinalis*).

Dyspareunia Painful vaginal intercourse. Pain in the vagina itself may be caused by a local disorder, such as irritation from a spermicide, a vaginal deodorant spray, or the rubber of a diaphragm or condom, which is subsequently aggravated by the movement of the penis inside the vagina, or by an infection such as a yeast infection or trichomonas. If a woman has had little sexual experience, entrance into the vagina may be uncomfortable owing to an insufficiently stretched hymen, or tension, or inadequate foreplay (sexual stimulation before actual penetration, which causes the vaginal walls to secrete lubricating fluids). Occasionally even considerable stimulation will not create enough fluid for lubrication. This is particularly common after menopause (see VAGINAL ATROPHY) and during breast-feeding, and can be relieved by using saliva, a water-soluble jelly such as K-Y jelly, or a spermicidal cream, or jelly, or foam. If the pain is deep in the pelvis, the cause may be a pelvic infection (such as pelvic inflammatory disease), endometriosis, ovarian tumours or cysts, or some other conditions that should be investigated and treated by a doctor. However, some women who have no such disorder always experience pain when the penis hits the cervix; this can be avoided only by less deep penetration, which may be effected by a change in the woman's or the couple's position for intercourse.

Dysplasia Mild to moderate abnormalities in the surface cells of the uterus (endometrium) and cervix. It is not certain whether or when such abnormalities are PRECANCEROUS LESIONS, and opinion differs as to whether they should be left alone (since some disappear spontaneously), or treated conservatively, or treated by surgery.

The surface, or epithelium, of the cervix is made up of several cell layers, and there is constant growth and development within the cervical epithelium. New cells are produced at the bottom layer, mature, and move to the top, replacing old cells that are shed from the top. When precancerous cell changes occur, the maturation process is upset and there are more immature cells on the surface, along with unusually large or malformed cells. It is these cells that are picked up by a PAP SMEAR. With mild dysplasia, a significant number of young (immature) cells appear in the top layers of the epithelium (constituting a Grade II Pap smear), and with moderate dysplasia (Grade III smear) there is an even higher proportion of such cells. When there are few mature cells on the surface, the condition is usually called CANCER IN SITU; that is, a localized cancer without invasive (into neighbouring tissue) propensities. With cervical cancer there are no mature cells on the top layer, which is now made up entirely of immature cells (see also CANCER, CERVICAL).

Dysplasia can result from infection, or from oral contraceptives or other hormone therapy, environmental pollutants, radiation, profound emotional stress, or any combination of these factors. In dysplasia the cervix may have a red bumpy ('mosaic') appearance, or leuko-plakia ('white patches'), or it may show no overt signs at all. There is rarely any pain.

Dystocia Difficult labour or childbirth. It usually is due to three factors, either alone or, more often, in combination: ABNORMAL PRESENTATION (position) of the baby; too small a passage in the pelvis (see PELVIMETRY); and uterine dysfunc-tion (see under PROLONGED LABOUR).

Dysuria Pain on urination, usually caused by a bladder or kidney infection. See CYSTITIS; PYELONEPHRITIS.

E

Early pregnancy test Strictly speaking, any PREGNANCY TEST made within a few days of the first missed period (or even before that). However, the term is usually reserved for various kinds of do-it-yourself pregnancy-test kits, which are available in chemist shops, without prescription and at nominal cost. All of the kits currently available are urine tests that yield results in two hours. Positive results could be obtained as early as nine days after a missed period. However, the incidence of false negative results (that is, indicating no pregnancy when there really is one) is higher than with the same kinds of test performed in a laboratory, probably because of a greater chance of error in reading the results, the use of too dilute urine, or similar factors. For this reason some of the kits instruct a woman who gets a negative result to repeat the test a week later (if her period has not begun in the meantime) and then, if the result is still negative and her periods do not resume, to consult a doctor.

Eclampsia Also *metabolic toxaemia of (late) pregnancy, toxaemia.* An acute illness occurring after twenty-four weeks of pregnancy or just after childbirth that is characterized by severe convulsions and loss of consciousness, followed by coma. It may be fatal. The condition is nearly always preceded by PREECLAMPSIA, which can often be controlled, so that eclampsia can usually be prevented. Eclampsia occurs three times as often in women carrying a first child as in women who have borne other children. Approximately half of all cases develop before delivery (nearly always in the last trimester), one quarter during labour, and one quarter after delivery (usually within twenty-four hours). Eclampsia occurs four times more often in multiple pregnancies than in single ones. It is also associated with ECTOPIC PREGNANCY and HYDATIDIFORM MOLE. Women whose mothers had eclampsia are also more likely to develop it.

Eclampsia is readily diagnosed by the onset of convulsions and coma. A convulsion can occur at any time, sometimes when the patient is sleeping, and is followed by coma of varying duration. Other signs are oliguria (decreased urinary output), high pulse rate, elevated blood pressure and temperature, proteinuria (protein in the urine), oedema (fluid retention), and hyper-reflexia (exaggerated reflexes). When eclampsia occurs during labour or after delivery, there may be only a single convulsion. More often, however, the first is followed by more convulsions, ranging from one or two in mild cases to as many as one hundred in severe ones. The patient may recover consciousness between convulsions but sometimes does not, and in severe cases may die before awakening. If convulsions occur before delivery, labour generally begins soon afterward and progresses very quickly to completion, sometimes before anyone is even aware that the patient is having contractions. If convulsions occur during labour, the contractions rapidly become more frequent and much stronger, shortening the duration of labour. After delivery the condition usually improves with a day or so, although occasionally the convulsions resume and the second attack may be more severe or even fatal.

As with preeclampsia, the cause of eclampsia is not known, although many theories have been advanced. Prevention consists of treating preeclampsia. When eclampsia does develop, treatment is directed at stopping the convulsions with sedatives. The patient is hospitalized immediately and given medication to lower her blood pressure and increase urinary output. Although the delivery in itself may cure the mother, it is usually delayed (if possible) until she is free of convulsions and coma; nevertheless, some women can go into labour spontaneously.

The risk of eclampsia for babies is high. Many succumb for lack of oxygen, from the heavy sedation required to control convulsions, from injury during too rapid a delivery, and from prematurity. A woman who has once had eclampsia is more likely to develop it with subsequent pregnancies. Eclampsia may also predispose a woman to the development of hypertension (high blood pressure) later in life (or it may simply signal the fact that she is already predisposed to develop it). Both these factors should be considered when another pregnancy is contemplated.

Ectasia See MAMMARY DUCT ECTASIA.

Ectopic pregnancy Also *tubal pregnancy*. The implantation and growth of a fertilized egg in some organ other than the uterus, usually in one of the Fallopian tubes but occasionally (although quite rarely) in the ovaries, peritoneum, or cervical canal. The condition is usually caused by distortion or damage of the Fallopian tubes resulting from endometriosis, gonorrhoea, pelvic inflammatory disease, or some other disorder, or past or present use of an IUD. Because of scar tissue, the fertilized egg cannot move down to the uterus, as it normally would, and remains in the tube, generally growing there for a period of two to three months. When the tube can no longer accommodate the enlarging embryo it ruptures, which may result in haemorrhage, a true medical emergency. Or, if the embryo is near the upper end of the tube, the muscular actions of the tube may push it into the pelvic cavity; if this occurs at an early stage of pregnancy, the embryo will generally be absorbed, giving rise to no further symptoms.

Diagnosing an ecotopic pregnancy can be difficult. There may or may not be pain. There may or may not be a positive pregnancy test. Usually there will be at least one missed menstrual period, and then some slight bleeding and pain. Some women continue to have periods, however, and experience no other symptoms of early pregnancy—morning sickness, enlarged or tender breasts, fatigue. Therefore the diagnosis of ectopic pregnancy is often not made until the tube ruptures. Danger signals are sudden sharp pain or persistent one-sided pain in the lower abdomen, shoulder pain, irregular bleeding or staining, and abdominal pain following a very light period or a late period; these warrant seeking emergency treatment at once. If tubal pregnancy is suspected, LAPARO-SCOPY and/or CULDOCENTESIS can establish the diagnosis.

Treatment depends on the extent of the damage, the presence of infection in the area, and the patient's age (whether she wishes to bear subsequent children), but a decision must be made quickly because of the danger of haemorrhage. The affected Fallopian tube must usually be removed, but if possible it is preferable to spare the adjacent ovary. When, however, the pregnancy has occurred in the only remaining tube (usually because the other was already removed for an earlier ecotopic pregnancy) and this tube cannot be saved, hysterectomy (removal of the uterus) may be considered since no subsequent pregnancy is possible.

The occurrence of one ectopic pregnancy greatly increases the likelihood of another, since the underlying cause may still be present. Other predisposing factors are tubal surgery (see TUBERO-PLASTY), gonorrhoeal infection, conception while an intrauterine (IUD) is in place, and conception while taking oral contraceptives.

Egg See OVUM.

Ejaculation 1 Also *coming* (slang). The release of seminal fluid from the PENIS, which is caused by a complex spinal reflex involving the contraction of the bulbar muscles at ORGASM. (See also SEXUAL RESPONSE; SPERM). Approximately 2 to 5 cc. (millilitres), or about 1 teaspoon, of seminal fluid are released in each ejaculation; the fluid is also called *ejaculate.*

2 **Premature ejaculation** A problem experienced by couples when man can rarely or never delay ejaculation sufficiently for his partner to become fully aroused. The term actually is quite im-precise, because what may be too quick for one partner may be fine for another. In some cases, however, ejaculation occurs within a minute or two of achieving erection, which would be too fast for most partners.

Learning how to delay ejaculation can be accomplished by means of a simple manoeuvre called the *squeeze technique,* usually executed by the woman. As the man approaches ejaculation, he signals to his partner, who then grasps his penis between the fingers, with the thumb on the underside of the glans and the first and second fingers held together on top, right at the coronal ridge (see under PENIS for an illustration); pressing the thumb and fingers firmly together for a few seconds causes loss of the desire to ejaculate (although the erection remains). By practicing this manoeuvre a number of times most men can learn to control ejaculation themselves. Use of a CONDOM also may help prevent premature ejaculation in men who find that it sufficiently lessens the exquisite sensitivity of the glans.

3 **Retarded ejaculation** Inability to ejaculate while the penis is inside the vagina. For couples desiring children, this can be a cause of infertility. Most often the cause is psychological and requires SEX THERAPY or other counselling to be corrected.

4 **Retrograde ejaculation** A condition in which the seminal fluid flows backward into the bladder instead of out through the penis during ejaculation. It eventually is eliminated in the urine. Retrograde ejaculation may occur after prostate surgery and causes no harm to the man; it does however, lessen or eliminate the chances for impregnating a woman since few or no sperm reach her vagina.

5 Split ejaculation See under OLIGOSPERMIA.

Electrocautery See CAUTERIZATION.

Embolism The blockage of an artery by an *embolus*, which may be a blood clot (see THROMBUS), air bubble, or some other material that has been transported through the circulatory system from elsewhere in the body. An air bubble (*air embolism*) can enter the bloodstream in the course of an intravenous infusion, or by exposure to increased air pressure, as in deep-sea diving. A *fat embolus* sometimes forms following the fracture of a large bone, such as the hip. Among the most dangerous kinds of embolism is a *pulmonary embolism* (also called *thromboembolism*), in which a blood clot, usually originating in one of the deep veins of the leg or pelvis, lodges in an artery serving the lungs (pulmonary artery). A pulmonary embolism may be fatal, depending on the extent of the blockage and the person's general condition. It is a major complication of PHLEBITIS, whose treatment is directed primarily at preventing it. A *systemic embolism* arises within the heart or an artery and is transported through arteries to the legs or elsewhere. If it cuts off the blood supply to an essential part of the brain – a *cerebral embolism* – it may cause permanent damage there. See also ARTERIOSCLEROSIS.

Embryo A fertilized egg, or ZYGOTE, that has begun to increase in size by cell division. Some authorities call the human fertilized egg an embryo as soon as the process of cell division has begun; others continue to call it an 'egg' or 'ovum' until four weeks after fertilization, when organ development begins. Still others call it an 'ovum' for about two weeks after conception, until it has become implanted in the uterine wall, and thereafter use the term 'embryo'. After the age of about six weeks (following fertilization), it is called a FOETUS.

Emmenagogue A drug, herb, or other chemical agent administered to bring on a delayed menstrual period. Very strong emmenagogues may also bring on uterine contractions and, if a woman is pregnant, result in abortion (see under ABORTIFACIENT). Menstrual periods are often delayed in non-pregnant women, however, by illness or malnutrition or stress. To hasten the onset of a period when there is doubt about possible pregnancy, or to eliminate premenstrual discomfort, or simply for the sake of convenience, women have long resorted to a large variety of agents, principally herbs. Literally dozens of HERBAL REMEDIES have been used for this purpose, among them infusions made from a mixture of blue cohosh (*Caulophyllum thalictroides*), pennyroyal or squaw mint (*Mentha pulegium*; use the plant only, for the oil is dangerous), rue (*Ruta gravelolens*), and yarrow (*Achillea millefolium*); or a mixture of black cohosh (*Cimicifuga racemosa*; avoid in presence of low blood pressure), common tansy blossoms (*Tanacetum vulgare*), and motherwort (*Leonurus cardiaca*).

Endocervical Inside the cervical canal; see under CERVIX. For endocervical curettage, see BIOPSY, definition 7.

Endocervicitis Inflammation of the cervix that affects the cervical canal, or endocervix. It is treated with locally applied antibiotics. If these are ineffective, cauterization (burning) or cryosurgery (freezing) may be necessary. See CERVICITIS.

Endocrine Also *ductless*. Literally, 'internally secreting', referring to glands that secrete hormones and other chemical substances important for the maintenance of basic body functions directly into the bloodstream rather than through special ducts (as certain other glands do). The principal *endocrine glands* are the pancreas, the pituitary, thyroid, parathyroid, and adrenal glands, the hypothalamus and the pineal body, and the gonads (or sex glands, that is, ovaries and testes) and placenta. There is a separate entry for each of them.

Together the endocrine glands make up the *endocrine system*, whose study, the field of *endocrinology*, is one of the newest branches of medicine, dating from the beginning of the 20th century. As a group, the endocrine glands are critically influenced by one another, both for their secretory ability and their control of many body functions, including the human reproductive cycle. Indeed, it is these interdependent relationships that account for changes in endocrine activity during a lifetime, governing puberty, conception, pregnancy, childbearing, and menopause. See also HORMONE.

Endometrial aspiration See VACUUM ASPIRATION.

Endometrial cancer See CANCER, ENDOMETRIAL.

Endometrial cyst See under ENDOMETRIOSIS.

Endometrial hyperplasia A thickening of the lining of the uterus (endometrium), which during a woman's men-

struating years is normally thin, about half its thickness being lost each month in the menstrual flow. If the thickening occurs in one spot only, it forms a growth called a *uterine polyp* (see POLYP, definition 3); if it occurs throughout it is called *hyperplasia*. In the monthly cycle, first oestrogen and then progesterone cause the endometrium to thicken in preparation for implantation of a fertilized egg. If no egg is implanted, the thickened layer is sloughed off. In menstruation without ovulation, called ANOVULATORY BLEEDING, no progesterone is produced and the mechanism triggering the regular sloughing-off process is disturbed. Anovulatory cycles occur principally at menarche and menopause (when, in effect, the endocrine system is gearing up for reproduction and winding down for non-reproduction). At menarche, however, anovulation is usually too short-lived for endometrial build-up to progress to hyperplasia, which therefore is found chiefly in women of forty-five or older. It may also occur in organs other than the ovaries (a process not fully understood). In all these instances, the underlying cause is persistent stimulation of the endometrium by oestrogen in the absence of progesterone.

The main symptom of endometrial hyperplasia is heavy, prolonged bleeding; there is no pain. Diagnosis is by VACUUM ASPIRATION or D AND C, which in many cases also cures the condition by simply removing a sufficient quantity of endometrial tissue. If bleeding persists, in young women the administration of oral contraceptives containing both oestrogen and progesterone, or, in women of any age, of progesterone alone may correct the condition. However, while in younger women endometrial build-up is always benign (noncancerous), in menopausal and postmenopausal women the condition can be precancerous (see PRECANCEROUS LESIONS). Therefore, if the condition recurs following a D and C and the subsequent administration of progesterone does not correct it, many doctors recommend a prophylactic (preventive) hysterectomy (surgical removal of the uterus) to eliminate the risk of cancer entirely.

Endometrial polyp See POLYP, definition 3.

Endometriosis The appearance of tissue from the endometrium (lining of the uterus) outside the uterus, in such locations as on the ovaries or surface of the Fallopian tubes, on the outer back wall of the uterus, or in the pelvic space between the uterus and rectum. About three out of four cases of endometriosis appear between the ages of twenty-five and forty-five, most often in women in their thirties. The principal symptoms are menstrual disturbances, most commonly extremely painful periods, and may progress to persistent pain. Some women also suffer pain, sometimes very severe, during vaginal sexual intercourse. There is, however, no true correlation between the severity of the pain and the extent of the disease.

The cause of endometriosis – why endometrial tissue should migrate out of the uterus – is not known, although its course is understood. Endometrial tissue outside the uterus is just as responsive to hormone stimulation as that inside the uterus. During menstruation, when the uterine lining, which was built up in preparation for pregnancy, is shed, the endometrial tissue outside the uterus responds in the same way, breaking down and bleeding. This blood is trapped in the pelvic cavity, and eventually a blood-filled cyst—an *endometrial cyst* or *chocolate cyst* (so-called because it is filled with old, dark, chocolate-coloured blood)—can form.

At first the pelvic pain is felt only during menstruation. In time, however, as adhesions (scar tissue) form and endometrial tissue presses against them, pain may precede menstrual flow by as much as two weeks. Because the symptoms of endometriosis are similar to those of pelvic infection, degenerating fibroid tumours, and other disorders, the only certain diagnosis is by LAPAROSCOPY or exploratory surgery.

Following menopause, endometriosis nearly always subsides. However, women with a diagnosis of endometriosis who can conceive and intend to bear children are urged to do so without delay, since until menopause the condition tends to be progressive (gradually worsen) and, even after conservative surgery, may recur. See also ADENOMYOSIS.

Endometritis An inflammation of the endometrium, or lining of the uterus. The main symptoms are pelvic or lower abdominal pain, a tender uterus (when a pelvic examination is performed), and a thick, foul-smelling, yellowish cervical discharge. Endometritis may result from irritation by an intrauterine device (IUD), or as a complication of an early (first-trimester) abortion. It nearly always responds to antibiotic treatment.

Endometrium The lining of the UTERUS, a thin, pinkish, velvety mucous membrane. It consists of several layers: surface epithelium; glands that secrete a thin alkaline fluid which keeps the uterine cavity moist; blood vessels; and tissue spaces. In thickness it varies during each menstrual cycle from 0.5 mm. (milli-metres) to 3 to 5 mm., gradually being built up in preparation for pregnancy and, in the absence of fertilization, much of it being shed in the menstrual flow with some blood. After MENOPAUSE the entire endometrium atrophies, its epi-thelial tissue flattening, its glands gradually disappering, and the gland tissue becoming fibrous.

The endometrium is subject to a number of disorders and diseases, the most serious of which is cancer (see CANCER, ENDOMETRIAL). A common benign growth is endometrial POLYPS (see definition 3). Occasionally endome-trial tissue begins to grow outside the uterus, a condition that can cause severe menstrual pain (see ENDOMETRIOSIS). Menstrual irregularities may lead to an over-build-up of endometrial tissue called ENDOMETRIAL HYPERPLASIA, which can often be corrected simply by removing some of the extra tissue by suction (see VACUUM ASPIRATION) or scraping (see D AND C). Both of these procedures are also used to diagnose endometrial cancer and other cell changes as well as to terminate a pregnancy.

Engagement In childbirth, the descent of the baby's head so that its widest portion has passed through the *pelvic inlet* (see under PELVIMETRY). Engagement may not occur until the second stage of LABOUR, that is, until the cervix has been fully dilated, or it may occur during the last few weeks of pregnancy, before labour begins. The latter happens in 90 per cent of women pregnant for the first time. One way to tell whether or not the head is engaged is to locate its lowermost part in relation to the *ischial spines* (part of the woman's hipbones), which the doctor or midwife can feel in either vaginal or rectal

examination, or even by palpating the abdomen. Engagement demonstrates that the pelvic inlet is definitely large enough for the baby, but lack of engagement before labour begins does not necessarily indicate that the pelvis is too small. Engagement is the first of a series of movements made by the baby's head (provided the head is the presenting part, as it is in 95 per cent of all deliveries) in the process of labour.

Engorgement, breast See under LACTATION.

Epidural anaesthesia Also *lumbar epidural block*. A kind of REGIONAL ANAESTHESIA that is administered during the second half of labour. It involves injecting a local anaesthesia into a space between the ligaments of the bony verte-brae and the dural sac (which encases the spinal fluid and spinal column), thereby deadening pain from this level and lower but retaining motor function so that uterine contractions can continue although they will be slowed down. It can be given fairly early in labour, when the cervix is 4 centimetres dilated (of the total 10 centimetres required) and can be maintained throughout the remainder of labour and delivery by means of a catheter, through which additional anaes-thetic is injected as needed. If continued through the second stage of labour (expulsion of the baby), the urge to push will not be felt, making pushing less effective and often necessitating the use of FORCEPS.

Epidural anaesthesia has definite dis-advantages. It is difficult to perform, need-ing a highly skilled anaesthetist to find just the right space for injection. It may not work correctly, some nerves being blocked (all the nerves on one side, for example) and others not. If the needle is not in exactly the right position, some anaesthetic may escape into the spinal fluid, which may cause a precipitous drop in the mother's blood pressure, dangerous to both her and the baby. Because of potential problems, an anaesthetist must watch her constantly. Because she feels no sensation whatever from the lumbar area down, she must be carefully directed to bear down for each contraction in expelling the baby. Finally, EPISIOTOMY and forceps are necessary more frequently when an epidural anaesthetic is used.

Epidural anaesthesia is also sometimes used for abdominal TUBAL LIGATION and CAESAREAN SECTION.

Episiotomy A surgical opening of the perineum made during the second stage of LABOUR, when the baby is being pushed through the vagina, in order to avoid tearing of the delicate perineal tissues. An incision is made in the bottom of the vagina at the time the baby's head is actually being delivered; if the woman is awake at the time, a local anaesthetic is usually injected into the site to be cut, which extends from the vagina toward the anus. After delivery the cut is repaired with sutures (stitches) – either the kind that are absorbed or a kind that fall our within two or three weeks. The site of the incision may be painful for a week or more until it heals.

Critics contend that episiotomies are performed too often. There is great variation in episiotomy rates between different countries; one study indicated they were done in 70 per cent of all deliveries in America and in only 6 per cent of deliveries in Sweden. Perineal tearing, it is said, may often be avoided by performing perineal massage (rubbing the area). Such massage, done daily for several weeks before the baby is due, as well as during labour and while the baby's head is crowning (begins to appear in the vagina), often allows the surface perineal tissue to stretch without tearing, although it cannot help the underlying muscle that also determines perineal elasticity. More important, tears can often be avoided by the birth attendant's gently controlling the advancing head and allowing it to emerge only between contractions (not during one).

Erection The condition of tissue that has become stiff and elevated in response to stimulation. Such tissue, called *erectile tissue*, contains numerous small arteries that dilate in response to sexual or other stimulation, causing engorgement (swelling). The swelling in turn blocks the flow of blood from the veins, thereby causing more engorgement. Engorgement causes the tissue to darken in colour, increase in size, and stiffen. In women, the prime areas of erectile tissue sensitive to sexual stimulation are the nipples, clitoris, inner labia, and vaginal opening; in men, the penis, especially near its tip (the glans), is the most sensitive, but the nipples are also erectile. Although other areas of the body respond to sexual stimulation, they do not become erect. Some erection of the penis is necessary for *intromission* (insertion of the penis into the vagina); inability to have or maintain an erection is called IMPOTENCE. See also SEXUAL RESPONSE.

Ergot A fungus that grows on rye and some other grains, and for centuries has been known to produce uterine contractions. In its pure form it is toxic, causing severe pain, convulsions, gangrene, and death. However, an alkaloid isolated from ergot—ergonovine—can be used after childbirth to help the uterus contract and return to its normal size. Other ergo alkaloids have been used in mental illness, particularly for poor memory and confusion in the elderly, and ergotamine is useful in treating MIGRAINE.

Erosion, cervical See CERVICITIS.

Erythroblastosis Also *erythroblastosis fetalis, RH disease.* Haemolytic anaemia of the foetus or the newborn baby, usually caused by Rh incompatibility. See RH FACTOR.

Excise To cut out, to remove by surgery. Any such procedure is called an *excision.*

Exercise Physical exertion that is undertaken deliberately to promote and maintain good health, as well as for recreation. Regular exercise is important for men and women throughout life, from infancy on. It improves blood circulation and muscle tone (including the muscle tone of the diaphragm and heart), enlarges lung capacity, benefits the digestive system and aids bowel function, contributes to good posture and a more vigorous appearance, lowers body weight, and promotes relaxation and good sleep patterns.

Women in particular are apt to neglect exercise at certain times of their life when it can be most beneficial. One such time is during pregnancy and following childbirth, when fatigue, fear of harming the unborn baby, and preoccupation and lack of sleep from caring for a newborn infant may prevent normal patterns of exercise. However, a programme of simple exercises during and after pregnancy can greatly improve muscle tone, aid delivery, and prevent some of the problems that can develop with normal weight gain and loss involved in childbearing. Another time when women are tempted to avoid or curtail exercise is during and after the menopausal years. It is precisely then that regular exercise – which need be nothing more complicated than regular brisk walks – can be of great benefit in maintaining cardiac (heart) function and delaying or offsetting the problems of bone loss (see OSTEOPOROSIS).

Before embarking on a specific exercise programme (other than brisk walking or swimming), women with any chronic condition, such as high blood pressure, as well as all women over the age of forty-five who have been leading largely sedentary lives, are usually advised to have a general physical examination. Further, if they are considering a formal or strenuous exercise programme, the doctor may advise a *stress test*, which measures pulse and blood pressure (sometimes also heart function by means of an attached electrocardiograph machine) during and/or immediately after increased levels of exertion. As a rule, all exercise programmes should be started slowly and gradually increased in length and difficulty.

Exercise is also useful for those who wish to lose weight, both in using up some extra calories (although not as many as most people tend to believe) and in firming muscles after some body fat has been lost. It is estimated that brisk walking (a mile in fifteen minutes) uses only about five calories a minute, bicycling about eight calories a minute, and swimming, eleven calories a minute. See also ATHLETIC ABILITY; KEGEL EXERCISES.

F

Face presentation In childbirth, the position of the baby when its face is presenting or leading part as it descends into the birth canal. In this posture the baby's neck is sharply extended so that the top of its head virtually touches its back. Face presentation occurs about one in every 400 to 500 deliveries. If the mother's pelvis is normal in size and shape and the baby's chin is not extended too much, a vaginal delivery—either spontaneous or with some help from low FORCEPS—is possible in most cases. If the chin is severely extended, however, the baby's head becomes caught under the pubic bone (*symphysis pubis*) and cannot be delivered. The doctor may try to flex the face or it may flex spontaneously during the course of labour, but in stubborn cases a Caesarean section (surgical delivery) may be necessary.

Fallen bladder See CYSTOCELE.

Fallen uterus See PROLAPSED UTERUS.

Fallopian tubes Also *oviducts*. A pair of narrow passages that are attached high on either side of the uterus and transport eggs to it from each OVARY. Each tube is 4 to 5 inches (10 to 12½ centimetres) long. It is quite narrow in the central portion—the outside about the diameter of a drinking straw, the inside that of a hair bristle—and flared at the trumpet-shaped open end near the ovary. This end is lined with *fimbria*, tiny fingerlike projections that are constantly in motion. After ovulation (the monthly release of an egg from an ovary) their movement draws the egg from the ovary's surface into the tube, and the muscles in the tube walls then contract, moving the egg down and the tube toward the uterus. This action is further assisted by the waving motion of tiny hairs called *cilia*, which line the inside surface of the tube. If fertilization (the union of the egg with a sperm) takes place, it happens when the egg is about one-third of the way down the tube, a journey that must be made within twenty-four hours of its release from the ovary; thereafter the egg is no longer viable. Whether fertilization took place or not, the muscular contractions of the tube continue to move the egg into the uterus, which takes four to five days.

The principal functions of the Fallopian tubes are to provide a hospitable environment for both sperm and eggs, and to move eggs into the uterus. Occasionally the latter function fails (or is blocked) and a fertilized egg becomes implanted in the tubal walls and begins to grow there, a dangerous condition called tubal or ECTOPIC PREGNANCY. Without properly functioning Fallopian tubes, conception cannot take place. Some women are infertile because their tubes are blocked by scar tissue or some other condition (see also TUBEROPLASTY). Indeed, scarring of the Fallopian tubes is the single most common cause of infertility in young women. Women who do not want to bear children may have their tubes 'tied', or closed off, so as to prevent conception (see TUBAL LIGATION). One surgical technique for sterilization is *fimbriectomy*, the removal of the fimbria, without whose action an egg cannot enter the tube.

The principal disease affecting the Fallopian tubes is *salpingitis*, or inflammation and infection of the tubes, which may be caused by GONORRHOEA, PELVIC INFLAMMATORY DISEASE, pelvic tuberculosis, or as the result of an abortion, childbirth, or intrauterine device. Cancer that originates in the Fallopian tubes is rare, although it can spread there from the uterus or ovaries. Surgical removal of the Fallopian tubes is called *salpingectomy*, and may be done in conjunction with HYSTERECTOMY or removal of an ectopic pregnancy.

False labour The irregular contractions of the uterus that occur throughout pregnancy and can be mistaken, near term, for true labour. (See BRAXTON-HICKS CONTRACTIONS.) False labour may be perceived three or four weeks before actual labour begins, but it is differentiated from true labour because the contractions are relatively painless and intermittent, rather than increasing in intensity and regular. Also, they are felt chiefly in the lower abdomen, they do not become more frequent (the intervals between contractions remain long, rather than becoming shorter and shorter), they are not intensified by walking, and discomfort is relieved by mild sedation. In true labour, on the other hand, contractions occur with increasing frequency at regular intervals and are intensified by walking. They are felt in the lower back and abdomen and are not affected at all by mild sedation. However, the only way to distinguish false and true labour with certainty is to examine the cervix, which after some hours of true labour shows progressive dilation (widening). See also CONTRACTIONS, UTERINE; LABOUR.

False pregnancy The appearance of some of the signs of pregnancy in a woman who is not pregnant. Among them are weight gain, breast enlargement, amenorrhoea (cessation of menstruation), morning sickness (nausea), and, sometimes, sensation of foetal movements. However, the pelvic organs when examined are normal, and the uterus is unchanged in size from its non-pregnant state. Since such symptoms occasionally are associated with ECTOPIC PREGNANCY, a CORPUS LUTEUM cyst, or a missed abortion (see MISCARRIAGE, definition 5), these conditions must first be ruled out. In their absence, false pregnancy is nearly always the result of a woman's desperate wish to conceive – although very occasionally it results from the opposite, that is, extreme fear of pregnancy – and can often be managed with careful counselling on INFERTILITY and, if desired, treatment for infertility.

Family planning Planning for or preventing a pregnancy. In Britain family planning services are provided free by family doctors or family planning clinics run by the health authority. Referral to a gynaecologist for sterilization or abortion, or to a genitourinary clinic for venereal disease can be arranged by the family doctor or a family planning clinic.

Fatigue A feeling of excessive weariness that is both unrelated to an underlying illness and seems out of proportion to the amount of physical exertion and sleep a person has had. Fatigue is one of the most common complaints brought to doctors, and its cause is often very difficult to find. It can be, of course, the symptom of numerous underlying disorders, ranging from low-grade minor infections to diabetes and cancer. Moreover, it is often symptomatic of an emotional problem of some kind, such as depression or anxiety. In women fatigue is sometimes related to fluctuation in hormone levels. Many women regularly experience intense fatigue at some point during their menstrual cycle, most often premenstrually, that is, just before the onset of a period and/or during the first day or two of menstrual flow. Fatigue is a classic symptom of the early months of pregnancy, as well as of menopause (particularly for women whose sleep is disturbed by hot flushes and night sweats). It is also a classic symptom of iron-deficiency ANAEMIA.

Even though serious illness is relatively seldom the cause of prolonged fatigue, it cannot be overlooked, and anyone who feels drained of energy for weeks on end should have a thorough physical check-up. If no physical problem is found, it is very possible that too much stress is responsible. If stressful situations cannot be pinpointed or changed, professional counselling of some kind should be considered. Meanwhile, a well-balanced diet, regular physical exercise, and adequate sleep (the amount needed varies greatly among individuals, and also in the same person at different times) are indicated. Treatment with sleeping pills, tranquilizers, strong stimulants (caffeine, alcohol, and other drugs) should be avoided; in the long run they are more likely to compound the original problem, and

they can never eliminate its basic cause. See also INSOMNIA.

Fellatio   Also (slang) *blowing, blow job, going down*. A form of oral sexual intercourse in which the man's partner uses his or her mouth (lips, tongue) to stimulate his genitals. See also CUNNILINGUS; ORAL SEX.

Feminine hygiene   See HYGIENE.

Feminist health clinic   See under SELF-HELP.

Feminist therapy   Psychotherapy performed by a mental health specialist who incorporates the basic beliefs of feminism in her approach to treatment. In theory feminist therapists can be either male of female, but in practice nearly all are women. They do not use any special therapeutic method; rather, each uses whatever method of psychotherapy she prefers that also is compatible with feminist thinking. Although there is a wide range of opinions and ideas among feminists, they share a number of fundamental beliefs, which underlie feminist therapy. Chief among them is the idea that the traditional role of women as passive and powerless, subordinate to and dependent on men (economically and emotionally), must be replaced so that they are (and feel they are) active, equal, and autonomous. The feminist therapist therefore tries to help women understand the connection between their social conditioning as women and their present psychological situation. Unlike traditional psychotherapists, who usually focus on internal conflicts as the primary (or only) source of emotional distress, feminist therapists believe that social factors are largely if not entirely responsible for many women's emotional problems. Another central belief is that a therapist should not behave as a powerful authority figure who dominates or intimidates her client. Rather, she should help the client overcome the feelings of helplessness and dependency associated with traditional female roles, and encourage her assertiveness and independence. To this end, feminist therapists may use such techniques as avoiding technical jargon, giving the client access to her own records and files, and generally establishing a sense of equality between therapist and client. The client is encouraged to establish her own goals for therapy, rather than having the therapist set goals and standards for her. The use of group therapy, often recommended, also helps reduce a client's feelings of dependency on the therapist and at the same time helps her see what she has in common with other women in the group and elsewhere.

Feminist therapy grew out of the women's movement of the 1960s, and represents a reaction against the influence of Sigmund Freud and his followers. The Freudians believe, among other things, that normal women are sexually less desirous or active than men, that they fulfil themselves best by childbearing (especially male children), and that a woman's emotional problems can often be traced to unresolved childhood conflicts such as unconscious envy of men for having a penis or the repressed desire to marry their fathers. Even though few male psychotherapists today wholeheartedly accept these ideas, their influence continues to be felt in culturally assigned sex roles, to which a woman is traditionally expected to adjust (or else be considered maladjusted, abnormal, or 'sick').

One organization which offers feminist therapy is the Women's Therapy Centre.

Fern test   See under CERVICAL MUCUS METHOD.

Fertility   In women, the ability to become pregnant and carry a child to term. Fertility reaches its peak during a woman's mid-twenties and then begins to decline, slowly in the thirties and more rapidly in the forties. It ends completely with MENOPAUSE. In men, fertility is the ability to impregnate a woman. It reaches its peak in a man's early twenties and begins to fall off after the mid-twenties, but the decline remains very gradual, and men in their seventies have been known to father children. An estimated 15 per cent of all British couples have trouble conceiving. See also AGE, CHILDBEARING; INFERTILITY; STERILITY.

Fertility pill   One of several compounds that either induce ovulation or replace hormones in women who, for lack of them, cannot become pregnant. One of them, *clomiphene citrate,* or *Clomid,* is a synthetic compound that causes the hypothalamus to be stimulated so that it, in turn, stimulates the pituitary to release more FSH and LH in order to induce ovulation (see MENSTRUAL CYCLE for an explanation of this process). It succeeds in establishing ovulation in about 70 per cent of the women treated with it. It has been used also to regulate highly irregular menstrual cycles and to correct progesterone deficiency that leads to ANOVULATORY BLEEDING, as well as to stimulate sperm production in men (see STERILITY). If Clomid does not establish ovulation, a stronger preparation, made from *human menopausal gonadotrophin* (HMG) extracted from the urine of postmenopausal women, may be used. Sold under the trade name Pergonal, it is similar to human chorionic gonadotrophin ˙(HCG), found in the urine of pregnant women which also is used for this purpose. Both are chemically similar to LH. However, they can be used only under close medical supervision because they tend to overstimulate the ovaries, sometimes resulting in the formation of large ovarian cysts. Both are more expensive than Clomid, and they tend to produce MULTIPLE PREGNANCY – not only twins but triplets, quadruplets, and quintuplets, who have a much poorer chance of survival than single births. HMG has been used in men suffering from a pituitary deficiency that makes them infertile; in men, however, it appears to have no connection with multiple births or to produce any other side effects. See also INFERTILITY.

Fertility in Women*	
Age	Chance of Conception
under 25	73%
26 to 30	74%
31 to 35	61.5%
36 to 40	53.6%

* Based on data from a large-scale study of women in artificial insemination clinic, in which each woman's fertility is calculated over a one-year period.

Fertilization Also *conception*. The mating of a sperm with an egg, involving the fusion of the nuclei, which results in a fertilized egg, or ZYGOTE. In human beings fertilization takes place inside the FALLOPIAN TUBES. For an explanation of how both the mother's and father's characteristics are transmitted to their offspring, see under CHROMOSOME.

Fibroadenoma Also *adenofibroma*. A benign (noncancerous) breast tumour, consisting of a firm, well-defined, movable, slow-growing, painless mass. It occurs most in women between the ages of fifteen and thirty-five, in black women more than in white. Fibroadenomas are easily recognized on a mammogram (see MAMMOGRAPHY) but because they resemble breast cancer they can be definitely diagnosed only by biopsy and examination by a pathologist. Fibroadenomas are made up of connective tissue, duct and gland cells, which have multiplied faster than normal. Some authorities believe these tumours as a rule should be removed, but in teenagers they feel it may be advisable to wait until the breasts are fully developed before undertaking surgery. Others are more conservative and believe they should simply be left alone. See also CYSTIC DISEASE, BREAST.

Fibrocystic disease of breasts See CYSTIC DISEASE, BREAST.

Fibroid Also *fibromyoma, leiomyoma, myoma*. A benign (noncancerous) growth of the uterine wall that occurs only after puberty. It may occur singly or, often, in numbers. Fibroids are extremely common. Some 20 per cent of all women over thirty-five have at least one fibroid, and they are more common in black women than in white. Their growth is apparently stimulated by oestrogen, and consequently they shrink and even disappear entirely after menopause.

Fibroids range in size from a small bean to a large grapefruit or larger; a larger

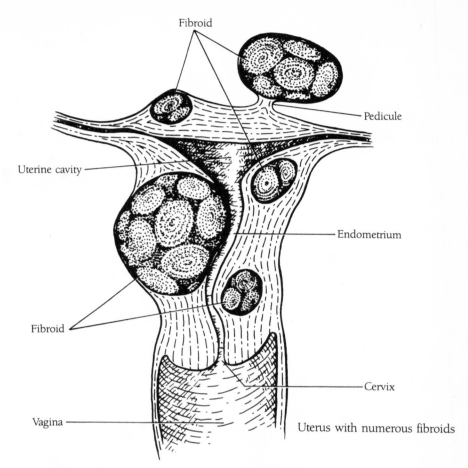

Fibroid

Pedicule

Uterine cavity

Endometrium

Fibroid

Cervix

Vagina

Uterus with numerous fibroids

fibroid can weigh twenty pounds or more. The symptoms of a fibroid include a palpable lump in the abdomen, heavy and prolonged menstrual periods (but, usually, no bleeding between periods), and a feeling of fullness. Sometimes there is urinary frequency owing to pressure on the bladder. Usually there is no pain, but sometimes, if fibroids press on the ureters or rectum, there may be quite severe pain, and severe pain also occurs if a tumour degenerates, that is, twists and cuts off its own blood supply.

Diagnosis is based on pelvic examination, but because a fibroid may be difficult to distinguish from an ovarian cyst (see CYST, definition 6) it may be necessary to perform a D AND C; a submucous fibroid cannot usually be detected by examination alone (the uterus simply feels enlarged) but must be verified by a D AND C or ultrasound. In the removal of a fibroid, called *myomectomy*, the surgeon usually tries to leave the uterus intact, especially in women who still want to bear children. In the case of a very large fibroid, however, the uterus may have to be removed in order to .remove the tumour, a procedure defended on the grounds that the very size of the fibroid so distorts the uterus that pregnancy is highly unlikely. Severe bleeding from fibroids can give rise to ANAEMIA, which must be treated with iron supplements.

If already present before conception, fibroids tend to grow during pregnancy, when oestrogen levels are high. Despite such growth, which can be very rapid during the early months (sometimes the tumour fills the entire pelvis), they rarely interfere with the pregnancy, because they usually move out of the pelvis (most often up into the abdomen). When this occurs a normal vaginal delivery is quite feasible. When fibroids remain in the pelvis, however, the baby may have to be delivered by Caesarean section. Also, a fibroid may interfere with the placenta, and the closer it is to the placenta, the greater the chance of its causing bleeding during the pregnancy.

For another benign uterine growth, see POLYP, definition 3.

Fibromyoma See FIBROID.

Fibrosis, cystic See CYSTIC FIBROSIS.

Fimbria, fimbriectomy See under FALLOPIAN TUBES.

Fissure See ANAL FISSURE.

Fistula An abnormal narrow pathway between some body cavity and the outside skin or another body cavity. A *vaginal fistula* may connect the vagina and bladder (*vesicovaginal fistula*) or the vagina and rectum (*rectovaginal fistula*). The principal symptom of the former is leakage of urine from the vagina; for the latter it is leakage of gas or faecal matter (or both) from the vagina. Most vaginal fistulas are caused by injury of some kind, frequently inflicted during Caesarean section, hysterectomy, or some other surgical procedure. Small vaginal fistulas may close spontaneously. If they do not, they require surgical repair.

An *anal fistula* usually leads from the anal canal to an opening in the skin near the anus, from which faecal matter may leak. Anal fistulas rarely heal by themselves and nearly always require surgical repair.

See also MAMMARY DUCT FISTULA.

Fluid retention See OEDEMA.

Foam, contraceptive See under SPERMICIDE.

Foetal alcohol syndrome See under ALCOHOL USE.

Foetal monitoring Assessing the physical condition of a baby before and during labour and delivery. The oldest and simplest form of foetal monitoring is listening to the baby's heartbeat, which can first be detected about halfway through the pregnancy (between sixteen and twenty weeks). It can be heard with the ear alone but it sounds much clearer through a stethoscope, particuarly a special obstetrical stethoscope with a metal headband that further amplifies the sound through bone conduction. It can also be detected by means of an ultrasound device called a Doppler as early as eleven to fourteen weeks. The foetal heartbeat is a double beat like the tick of a watch and has a normal rate of 120 to 160 beats per minute. If, during pregnancy or labour, the heart rate slows down markedly and/or becomes irregular, it is a definite sign that something may be wrong with the baby.

The amniotic fluid also provides means of foetal monitoring; AMNIOCENTESIS is performed to discover severe genetic defects in mid-pregnancy. A simpler investigation can be made just before the onset of labour. Normally the fluid at this time is quite clear; if it is brownish-green, it signals the presence of meconium (the baby's stool), which is passed when the baby is in distress. The amniotic fluid can be observed just before labour by passing a small viewing instrument through the cervix and observing whether it is cloudy or clear.

Most often, however, the term 'foetal monitoring' refers to electronic devices used during labour and delivery to keep track of both the baby's heartbeat and the mother's uterine contractions. These devices augment or replace the older practice of listening to the heart through a stethoscope and manually feeling the abdomen during a contraction. Developing in the late 1950s, electronic foetal monitoring originally was used only in potentially abnormal births, when the mother had diabetes, severe heart or kidney disease, Rh-factor incompatibility, or some other disorder associated with severe distress in a baby. When the monitor showed *foetal distress*, that is, a slowdown in heart rate, a Caesarean section would be performed. Today electronic foetal monitoring is used much more widely, in some hospitals for as many as 75 per cent of all births.

In *internal foetal monitoring*, two electronic catheters are inserted into the vagina and through the cervix. One is attached to the baby's scalp and relays its heart rate, while the other lies between the foetus and the wall of the uterus and measures the rate and pressure of uterine contractions; the latter is rarely used, however, except for research. In *external foetal monitoring* two straps are placed around the mother's abdomen. One,

around the upper abdomen, contains a pressure gauge to record contractions; the other, around the lower abdomen, contains a device to measure the foetal heart rate. Both kinds of monitor are connected to a machine that records the findings on a roll of paper. Not only can these devices show changes in the ordinary course of labour, but they can show how the baby's heart rate responds to artificially stimulated contractions. In the *oxytocin challenge test*, the hormone oxytocin is administered to the mother by intravenous infusion, and the monitor attached to her (or to the baby) shows how her uterus and the baby's heartbeat respond. If the contractions cause the heart rate to slow down, it is a sign that the baby is in distress and should be delivered at once.

The oxytocin challenge test has in some centres been replaced by the *Non-Stress Test* (NST), which uses the external foetal monitor to detect at least two foetal movements during a twenty-minute period, each accompanied by a rise of fifteen beats per minutes in the baby's heart rate. Studies show that a baby responding in this fashion is in good condition and is likely to remain so for another seven days, provided there is no change in the mother's condition. If the test is nonreactive, that is, shows no foetal movement or no accompanying increase in foetal heart rate, then an oxytocin challenge test is performed.

Supporters of foetal monitoring claim that the different patterns in the foetal heart rate cannot be discerned simply by a stethoscope and counting. Foetal monitoring provides a continuous record, and its simultaneous record of the pressure of contractions (with their possible effect on the foetal blood supply) permits more accurate correlation of these events.

Moreover, if an interal foetal monitor indicates possible distress, it also permits taking a blood sample from the baby's scalp to determine whether it is being deprived of oxygen or not, and whether labour should be allowed to continue or a Caesarean section should be performed. Supporters also hold that many babies have been saved from brain and other damage that would have resulted if a difficult labour had been allowed to continue.

Critics counter that foetal monitoring not only makes the mother uncomfortable but may compress the *vena cava* (a large vein) and thus compromise the uterine blood flow, interfere with efficient contractions, and slow down labour. In addition, internal monitoring may require artificial rupture of the membranes and cause injuries to the baby's scalp, the most common complication. For both internal and external monitoring, moreover, much of the information recorded may be misleading or be misinterpreted (for example, the mother's abdominal noises are often picked up as well), leading to unnecessary interference with a normal delivery. Certainly the increasing use of foetal monitoring in all births has been partly responsible for the increase in the performance of CAESAREAN SECTION. Opponents of monitoring say there has been no difference in outcome for infants, but there has been a higher rate of post-partum infection, presumably from the insertion of a foreign object into the uterus. Consequently some authorities suggest that *internal* foetal monitoring should be limited to high-risk births or instances where complications develop in the course of labour, and no kind of monitoring – external or internal – should be used merely as a matter or routine.

Foetoscopy A procedure in which an instrument called an *endoscope* is inserted inside the AMNIOTIC SAC in order to see parts of a foetus, withdraw skin or blood samples from it, and determine whether or not it has certain disorders or defects. An exceptionally delicate operation that is still considered experimental, it is performed under local anaesthetic some fifteen to twenty weeks into a pregnancy. Usually ULTRASOUND (see definition 1) is used first to locate the foetus, placenta, and umbilical cord. Then a small incision is made into the uterus through the abdomen and a narrow tube, as thin as a pencil lead, containing an endoscope is inserted into the amniotic sac. To obtain a blood or tissue sample, a tiny needle or forceps is inserted through the endoscope into the placenta.

Foetoscopy is much riskier for the foetus than AMNIOCENTESIS – it induces miscarriage in about 5 per cent of cases, as well as ABRUPTIO PLACENTAE – and therefore is performed only when there is a considerable risk of bearing a defective child. It enables not only discernment of gross visible defects in the limbs, eyes, ears, mouth, and genitals, but diagnosis of blood disorders such as haemophilia and thalassaema, as well as the 40 per cent or so of cases of SICKLE CELL DISEASE that are missed by amniocentesis. With further refinement, it is expected to detect such disorders as albinism, muscular dystrophy, and foetal levels of toxic substances to which the mother was exposed, as well as to permit administering medication directly to the foetus and performing minor surgery on the foetus.

Foetus A name for a developing EMBRYO that is used either from six weeks after FERTILIZATION on or from eight weeks on, depending on which authority one follows. By the end of the second month of development the foetus is about 1 inch (2.5 centimetres) long and weighs $\frac{1}{30}$ ounce (slightly more than 1 gram). At this point centres of ossification (bone formation) appear throughout the skeleton, especially in the skull and long bones; the features of the head, which is quite large compared to the trunk, are well developed; the fingers and toes are present; and the ears form definite bumps on each side of the head. For subsequent foetal development, see under GESTATION.

Follicle-stimulating hormone See FSH.

Forceps Also *obstetrical forceps*. A two-bladed instrument, resembling a pair of tongs, that is used to extract a baby. The blades are inserted into the vagina separately and articulated after being placed in position to grasp the baby's head. The most important function of forceps is traction (pulling), but they also can be used for version (turning), especially if the baby is in POSTERIOR PRESENTATION.

Forceps procedures are classified according to where the baby's head lies at the time the blades are applied. *Low forceps* are applied after the head has reached the perineal floor; *midforceps* are applied sooner but after ENGAGEMENT has taken place; *high forceps* are applied before engagement. Today high forceps are practically never used, and even mid-forceps are becoming rare, a Caesarean section usually being regarded as safer.

Forceps were invented in the late 16th or early 17th century to hasten a slow labour. They were kept secret by four generations of a family of Huguenot surgeons in England, but finally came into general use in the 18th century. Today

their use is largely restricted to life-threatening conditions that will be relieved by quicker delivery, such as ECLAMPSIA, heart disease, acute pulmonary OEDOEMA, PLACENTA PRAEVIA, prolapse of the umbilical cord, pressure on the baby's head, or problems in the foetal heart rate. However, they can be used only during the second stage of LABOUR and when there is room enough to apply them. See also VACUUM EXTRACTOR.

Foreskin See PREPUCE.

Fraternal twins See under MULTIPLE PREGNANCY.

Frequency, urinary An urgent desire to void more often than usual, with no increase in the amount of urine voided. It is a common symptom of pregnancy, especially in the early months (until the tenth or twelfth week) and again during the weeks preceding delivery. It can be particularly annoying at night (*nocturia*), since it may require two or three trips to the bathroom each night. In early pregnancy frequency is usually caused by anteversion of the uterus (a kind of forward tilt), which irritates the bladder; in the late stages it is caused by pressure of the enlarged uterus and presenting part of the baby on the bladder.

Urinary frequency may also be caused by pressure from a FIBROID, it is the chief symptom of urinary and kidney disorders (see URETHRITIS; CYSTITIS), and it may be aggravated by a fallen bladder (see CYSTOCELE). See also STRESS INCONTINENCE.

FRH Abbreviation for *follicle-releasing hormone*, also called *follicle-stimulating hormone release factor* (FSH-RF). See under LRH; also under MENSTRUAL CYCLE.

Frigidity An older name for female SEXUAL DYSFUNCTION, specifically the inability to achieve orgasm. Until the mid-20th century little or nothing was done for this condition, but today an estimated 90 per cent of women who seek treatment are helped. Present-day sex therapists believe that the term 'frigidity' implies a permanent condition and so prefer the terms 'pre-orgasmia' or 'dysfunction'. See also SEX THERAPY; VAGINISMUS.

Frozen section See BIOPSY, definition 1.

FSH Abbreviation for *follicle-stimulating hormone*, a hormone produced by the pituitary gland. In women it stimulates growth of the follicles in the ovaries (see FOLLICLE) and in part is responsible for the explusion of a mature egg (see OVULATION) and the manufacture of oestrogen in the ovaries. In men FSH contributes to the maturation of sperm cells. See also MENSTRUAL CYCLE.

Functional bleeding See DYSFUNCTIONAL BLEEDING, VAGINAL.

Fundus See under UTERUS.

G

Galactocele Also *milk cyst*. A CYST in the breast that is caused by blockage of one of the lactiferous (milk-secreting) glands.

Galactorrhoea The spontaneous flow of breast milk in a woman who has not recently given birth. See also under LACTATION; POLYGALACTIA; PROLACTIN.

Gall bladder A pear-shaped sac in the rear upper quadrant of the abdomen, underneath the liver, whose main function is the collection of bile. Bile, which is secreted by the liver and assists in various digestive processes, is transported from the gall bladder through bile ducts to the duodenum, part of the small intestine. The gall bladder is subject to a very common disorder, the development of *gallstones*, which occur in 10 per cent of all British adults (20 per cent over the age of forty and five times more often in women than in men). Gallstones are abnormal concretions made up of crystals that precipitate out of bile. Both obesity and pregnancy are believed to contribute to their formation, but it is not known exactly how; possibily high levels of oestrogen are involved. Gallstones, technically called *biliary calculi*, may give rise to no symptoms at all, but they usually cause upper abdominal discomfort, bloating, belching, and intolerance to certain foods (especially fatty foods).

The pain usually takes the form of an 'attack', that is, a fairly sudden episode of acute discomfort, generally after a fatty meal or at night. Many individuals with gallstones experience no attacks, or only a single one; others suffer repeated episodes. Because gallstones can lead to serious complications, severe or repeated attacks call for prompt treatment. If the stones cannot be dissolved by oral medications, surgical removal of the gall bladder, called *cholecystectomy*, may be indicated.

Gallstones See under GALL BLADDER.

Gardnerella vaginalis See HAEMO-PHILLIS VAGINALIS.

Gaucher's disease An incurable and hereditary disease that, like TAY-SACHS DISEASE, is characterized by the lack of an enzyme enabling the body to break down and eliminate the accumulation of certain fats in the cells. Also like Tay-Sachs disease, it is a recessive-gene disorder (see under BIRTH DEFECTS) and is most common in Jews of European ethnic origin, among whom an estimated 4 per cent are carriers. If both parents are carriers, a fact that can be determined only by a culture of cells taken from a skin biopsy, there is a 25 per cent risk that any child of theirs will have the disease. However, its presence in a foetus can be detected by AMNIOCENTESIS.

The disease is named after Philippe Gaucher, a French physician who discovered it in 1882. Unlike Tay-Sachs, it is not invariably fatal. Fatty substances tend to accumulate in the liver, spleen, and bone marrow, causing gross enlargements of the affected organs, painful swelling of the joints, and brittleness of the bones. However, its course varies from patient to patient. If the disease appears in infancy, it tends to be more severe and survival is often limited to a year or two. If it appears later in life, it is generally less acute and patients may survive for many years. In 1987 no specific treatment was yet known, although enzyme replacement therapy was showing encouraging improvement in some adult patients.

Gender identity 1 A person's physical identification with a particular sex. For most individuals there is never any question about which sex they belong to, but in persons with a congenital abnormality, such as TURNER'S SYNDROME or KLINEFELTER'S SYNDROME, characteristics of both sexes are present, and a decision must be made as to whether the child should be brought up as a boy or a girl. See also TRANSSEXUAL.

2 A person's emotional identification with a particular sex, leading him or her to seek out sexual partners of the same of the opposite sex, or sometimes both. See BISEXUAL; HETEROSEXUAL; HOMOSEXUAL.

Gene See under CHROMOSOME.

General practitioner unit (GPU)
This is usually a small hospital where the woman's family doctor can admit women for labour and delivery under his/her care, although like other hospitals fully

trained midwives are in attendance. These units tend to be less formal and regimented than the larger hospitals where consultant obstetricians work. Before being booked for delivery in a GPU women are carefully checked to ensure that they do not represent a HIGH-RISK PREGNANCY or indicate in any way that they may have a complicated birth. Some GPUs are in close proximity to a consultant unit so that a transfer can be effected quickly in the event of any difficulty in labour. After delivery the mother and child are often able to go home within two days.

Genetic counselling Professional advice concerning the probability and implications of transmitting a hereditary disorder within a family, and the alternatives available. The process usually begins with determining the reason for seeking such advice. Some couples already have a child with a birth defect. Others known they have a potential problem (as shown by a blood test, for example) or have a family member who is affected. Women over the age of thirty-five may wish advice concerning the chances of giving birth to a child with a chromosomal defect (see also AGE, CHILDBEARING). Others may be concerned about the effects of their exposure to environmental hazards, and still others may have a history of HABITUAL MISCARRIAGE.

The first step in genetic counselling is formulating a complete family history and personal medical history for both parents, which systematically reviews all past and present medical problems. The individual's (and couple's) age, nationality or ethnic background, habits, diet, hobbies, education, and vocation all are included, as well as information about former marriages, family illnesses, and abortions. Possible exposure to infection and hazards such as X-rays, drugs, and toxic chemicals is investigated. This careful review is followed by a detailed physical examination; if needed, specialists of various kinds are consulted. Specific laboratory tests, including biochemical and cytogenetic studies, may be performed. Among these are *metabolic screening*, with an amino acid chromatogram; *urinary screening* if there is more than one retarded child in the family; and *chromosome analysis* based on a simple blood test. (See also KARYOTYPING.) Sometimes physical examination and laboratory tests may be carried out on close relatives as well.

When all the relevant information has been gathered, the counsellor tries to determine if there is a genetic problem or one caused by a known environmental factor; if it is the former, he or she tries to establish the mode of inheritance. The conclusions then are reviewed with the concerned individual or couple, the mode of inheritance and recurrence risks are fully explained, and various options (ARTIFICIAL INSEMINATION, AMNIOCENTESIS, and others) are considered.

Genetic counselling, which is available principally at major hospitals is time-consuming and expensive. However, many couples who are at risk find it less costly than bringing into the world a child who cannot survive or perhaps may never function as a self-sufficient adult.

An estimated 2 million people in Britain carry traits due wholly or partly to defective genes or chromosomes, and although some defects, such as colour blindness, are a very minor handicap, others are exceedingly serious. Some 40 per cent of all infants who die do so because of hereditary disorders; of all surviving newborn babies, 15 per cent have one or another genetic disorder. Indeed, it is estimated that every individual carries five to eight genes for genetic defects, and each couple has a 3 per cent risk of bearing a child with a birth defect, which may be as minor as a birth mark or very major. When a serious condition is suspected, genetic counselling may prevent at least some of the tragedy. See also BIRTH DEFECTS; CHROMOSOME.

Genetic disorders See under BIRTH DEFECTS.

Genitals Also *genitalia*. The external reproductive organs. In women the principal external organs also are called the pudenda or VULVA; in men they include the PENIS and SCROTUM.

Genital warts See CONDYLOMA ACUMINATA.

German measles See RUBELLA.

Gestation Also *term*. The period of development of human beings and other animals whose young grow inside the mother's body from conception until birth. For the mother this period is called PREGNANCY. The average duration of gestation of the human foetus is nine months. However, since most women cannot tell exactly which act of intercourse was responsible for a given pregnancy (and, even if they could, there is some variation in the length of gestation from individual to individual), gestation is calculated in terms of menstrual age; that is, counting from the *last menstrual period* (LMP), even though that may precede conception by two weeks or more. Thus the average gestation is $9\frac{1}{3}$ months, or 40 weeks, or 280 days, and the date of delivery is calculated by adding exactly 9 months and 7 days to the first day of the LMP. A baby born close to this time is described as *full-term*; a baby born before about 36 weeks gestation is usually PREMATURE, and one born after 42 weeks gestation is usually POSTMATURE.

Although the exact time for each stage of development also varies among individuals, and the size of foetuses varies considerably, the general sequence is roughly the same, and is as follows:

WEEK 4   Implantation has occurred; egg barely visible to naked eye (see IMPLANTATION).

END OF WEEK 8   Embryo measures 22 to 24 millimetres long, weighs 1 gram (.07 ounce); fingers and toes appear; ear buds seen on head.

END OF WEEK 12   Fingers and toes fully formed, have nails; external genitals appear; foetus measures 7 to 9 centimetres (3½ inches) long, weighs about 14 grams (½ ounce). In another week or two risk of miscarriage becomes very small.

END OF WEEK 16   Foetus is 13 to 17 centimetres long (6 inches), weighs about 100 grams (3½ ounces).

END OF WEEK 20   Downy hair (lanugo) covers body; foetal movements have been felt for several weeks; heartbeat sometimes heard; foetus weighs more than 300 grams (10 ounces).

WEEK 24   Foetus weighs about 600 grams (20 ounces); skin wrinkled; if born, may try to breathe but cannot live more than a few minutes.

WEEK 28   Length 37 centimetres (14 inches), weighs more than 1,000 grams (2.2 pounds); skin is red, covered with *vernix caseosa*, a white cheesy substance.

WEEK 32   Weighs 1,700 grams (3½ pounds), length 42 centimetres (16 inches); if born, with special care has chance of survival.

WEEK 36   47 centimetres (18 inches) long, 2,500 grams (5½ pounds). Has good chance of survival if born.

WEEK 40   Fully developed newborn baby. Average length, 50 centimetres (20 inches), weighs 3,100 to 3,400 grams (7 pounds); smooth skin still covered with *vernix caseosa*; (black babies are dusky bluish-red, not yet dark-skinned).

Ginseng   Also *American ginseng, man root, flower of life, fountain of youth root*. A herb, *Panax quinquefolium*, the root of which has been used in many primitive cultures, as well as in ancient and modern China and in the Soviet Union, as a general tonic, to help the body adapt to heat stress and reduce sweating, to prevent numerous infectious diseases, and to treat impotence. Most recently it has been suggested as a remedy for the HOT FLUSHES of menopause. As of 1986 there were still no reliable controlled studies showing that ginseng was effective or how it works. Nevertheless, it is widely available in chemist shops, both the root itself and an assortment of powders, instant teas, capsules, and liquid concentrates made from it. American ginseng and Oriental ginseng are slightly different plants, distinguished as *Panax quinquefolium* and *Panax schinseng* or *chinensis*; another close relative is Siberian ginseng, *Eleutherococcus senticosus*. Still another related plant is *dong kwai* (*Angelica sinensis*). As with all HERBAL REMEDIES, it is important to remember that, while some may be just as effective as inorganic drugs, they can also give rise to allergic reactions and undesirable side effects. Moreover, since information about herbs is based largely on hearsay and the experience of others, it is more difficult to determine proper dosages for effectiveness and non-toxicity.

Goitre See under THYROID.

Gonad Sex gland. In the human female the gonads are the ovaries, in the male, the testes. See OVARY; TESTES.

Gonadotrophin A hormone that controls the functions of a sex gland, or gonad. Two such hormones are produced by the pituitary gland, follicle-stimulating hormone (FSH) and luteinizing hormone (LH), whose production in turn is controlled by the hypothalamus. (See under MENSTRUAL CYCLE for an explanation of their effect.) Another pituitary hormone, prolactin, inhibits production of the gonadotrophins and so is sometimes called an *antigonadotrophin*.

Gonorrhoea Also *GC*, (slang) *clap, dose, drip, strain*. The most common reportable VENEREAL DISEASE in Britain today, usually transmitted by sexual intercourse (vaginal, anal, or oral). It is caused by a bacterium, the gram-negative gonococcus *Neisseria gonorrhoeae*. Outside the body the gonococcus dies within seconds, so the disease cannot be spread by towels, toilet seats, or other objects touched by an infected person. It thrives only in mucous membrane, the moist lining of the mouth, throat, urethra, and cervix. Symptoms appear one to fourteen days (usually three to seven days) after the sexual contact, but *no* symptoms whatever occur in about 80 per cent of infected women and perhaps 20 per cent

of infected men. If symptoms do appear, in women they tend to consist of a greenish or yellow-green vaginal discharge and very occasionally irritation of the vulva; in men they consist of painful urination and a urethral discharge, usually white, but sometimes yellow or yellow-green. Both men and women may have a sore throat if infection is by oral sex, as well as tender enlarged lymph glands in the groin. Anal gonorrhoea (infecting the anus) rarely gives rise to any symptoms. Gonorrhoea can also affect the eyes, in adults usually from contact with the urethral discharge of an infected man and in newborn babies while the baby is passing through the infected mother's birth canal. The principal complication of gonorrhoea in both men and women is sterility.

Diagnosis of gonorrhoea requires examination and testing of mucus from the cervix, penis, and, if oral or anal contact are possibilities, the mouth, throat, and anus. (In women the anus always should be checked because infection may spread there from the vagina.) With speculum inserted in the vagina, the doctor takes a sample of cervical secretions, since the cervix is usually the first site of infection. A bimanual pelvic examination should also be performed, to make sure the Fallopian tubes are not infected. The kind of laboratory test performed on the mucus is important as well. The commonly used Gram stain, which shows up many kinds of bacterium fails to reveal the gonococcus in 40 to 60 per cent of women; a bacteriological culture, in which the bacteria are allowed to grow and multiply in a nutrient jelly, is far more accurate.

Treatment of gonorrhoea consists of a very large dose of penicillin, which must be injected, plus an anti-gout drug called probenecid, given by mouth, which prevents the otherwise rapid excretion of the penicillin by the kidneys. Other forms of penicillin (aluminum monostearate penicillin or benzathine penicillin), which are absorbed slowly into the bloodstream and excreted slowly by the kidneys, are *ineffective* against gonorrhoea (although very effective against syphilis) and therefore should not be used. An alternative to penicillin by injection is ampicillin by mouth, also taken with probenecid. For those who are allergic to penicillin (an estimated 5 per cent of people), the treatment of choice is tetracycline (by mouth), which, however, should not be taken by pregnant women. If a woman with gonorrhoea is both allergic to penicillin and pregnant, erythromycin is considered the best drug, although a newer antibiotic, spectinomycin hydrochloride, seems to be quite effective, especially against penicillin-resistant strains. Contraindicated for gonorrhoea are streptomycin, kanamycin, chloramphenicol, and hetacillin.

After treatment, three follow-up tests are required to make sure the disease has really been eradicated. The first test should be performed within one week following treatment, and the second and third can be performed the following week. All sexual contact – vaginal, oral, anal – should be avoided until three consecutive cultures are negative. If they are not, treatment with a higher dose of the same antibiotic or with another medication may be required. Some authorities believe that oral contraceptives give rise to an ideal environment for gonococcal growth and therefore must be avoided while an infection is being treated; others disagree. An IUD (intrauterine device) must always be removed once gonorrhoea is diagnosed.

Untreated gonorrohoea in women may lead to infection of the Fallopian tubes (salpingitis) or generalized PELVIC INFLAMMATORY DISEASE, which develops in half of all women not treated for eight to ten weeks. These infections in turn can produce scar tissue that causes sterility and also increases the risk of ECTOPIC PREGNANCY. Symptoms of *gonorrhoeal salpingitis* may begin with a menstrual period that is longer and/or more painful than usual, with pain developing on one or both sides of the lower abdomen within a few days. In acute cases the pain becomes severe, the temperature rises to about 102°F., and there may be headache, nausea, and vomiting. In some women the infection is less acute, marked only by dull aching in the lower abdomen, pain during or after intercourse or pelvic examination, backache, and low fever (99°F.) Other possible complications are *gonococcal ophthalmia* (eye infection), usually only in babies born of infected mothers, which requires very prompt treatment with silver nitrate or penicillin eye drops to prevent blindness, and *septicaemia* (blood poisoning), which may give rise to an *arthritis-dermatitis syndrome.* Septicaemia occurs more commonly in woman and homosexual men who have had gonorrhoea for months without any other symptoms. Spread of the bacteria in the bloodstream causes fever (100° to 104°F.), chills, loss of appetite, general malaise, and stiffness or pain in several joints. In about 3 per cent of cases of *gonococcal arthritis* may develop, affecting the knees, wrists, fingers and hands, ankles, and elbows. In about half of such cases a characteristic and painful skin rash (dermatitis) develops also, usually on the arms, hands, legs, and feet, and especially around the affected joints. Though the rash may heal by itself in a few days, new joint pains tend to develop. Intravenous antibiotic treatment must be given without delay to avoid permanent joint damage.

In pregnant women gonorrhoea may lead to miscarriage or tubal infection in the early months. After the third month the infection is usually confined to the lower genital tract, but, as noted, the baby may become infected during delivery.

Gonorrhoea has been known since ancient times. The symptoms are described in the Old Testament book of Leviticus, dating from about 1500 B.C., and were known to Hippocrates (400 B.C.) and Galen (200 A.D.). The mode of its transmission was not recognized until the late Middle ages. The slang name 'clap' (from *clapoir*, 'bubo') was introduced by the French in the 14th century. The gonococcus was identified in 1879. Gonorrhoea has always been far more common in wartime, presumably passed on to soldiers by prostitutes. Prostitutes run a very high risk of catching the disease because of the large numbers of men with whom they have sexual contact, and, once infected, they can unknowingly pass the disease on to many others. The first significant worldwide gonorrhoea epidemic occurred during and after World War I. Incidence fell between wars but rose drastically again during World War II, and dropped again after the war when penicillin came into widespread use. In the early 1960s incidence again began to climb. During the 1960s strains of gonococcus resistant to penicillin began to develop, so that the disease became much more difficult to cure. By the late 1970s gonorrohoea was considered virtually epidemic in many developed countries. More than half of those affected were under the age of twenty-five, and more than half lived in large cities. Also, penicillin-resistant forms of the disease were increasing; a new strain of the gonococcus produces a penicillin-destroying enzyme called penicillinase. This form of gonorrhoea is called PPNG (for *penicillinase-producing Neisseria gonorrhoea*).

Gossypol See under MALE CONTRACEPTIVE.

Graafian follicle The one ovarian FOLLICLE (sometimes, but rarely, there are two) that develops to maturity during each ovulatory menstrual cycle and eventually breaks through the wall of the ovary and releases a mature egg cell (ovulation). It is named after Reinier de Graaf, who discovered it in 1672. Before ovulation takes place, this one follicle may occupy as much as one quarter of the entire volume of the ovary and measure up to 1.5 centimetres (½ inch) in diameter. Since at puberty there are an estimated 75,000 immature egg cells in each ovary, it is obvious that the Graafian follicle grows many times larger than the others.

The Graafian follicle consists of two primary layers of cells, the *granulosa*, which surround the mature egg in the centre, and the *theca interna*, which surround the granulosa and are the prime repository and producer of the hormone oestrogen. After the egg ruptures through the ovarian wall, the Graafian follicle in effect collapses in on itself. The space left by the egg is filled with blood, and a new structure, the CORPUS LUTEUM, is formed.

Gram stain A special staining method used on tissue samples to help identify certain organisms under the microscope. It is used to detect GONORRHOEA, for which it is not very reliable, and TRICHOMONAS.

Gravida A woman who is pregnant.

Growth and development The progressive increase in size (height and weight) and the maturation of certain organs and physiological functions that mark the changes from infancy to adulthood. The rate of these changes, and their total extent, vary enormously among individuals and depend on numerous factors: hereditary, diet, general health, and others. Despite such variation, broad guidelines have been developed to differentiate normal growth and development from that influenced by diseases and deficiencies. Standardized growth charts represent one such guideline. Another is the progressive development of the foetus (see under GESTATION; FOETUS). During adolescence the development of certain secondary sex characteristics, notably the growth of the breasts and of pubic hair, tends to occur in certain stages, which are used for similar guidelines to assess normal development. See also PUBERTY.

Growth spurt See under PUBERTY.

Gynaecological examination A physical check-up that includes special attention to the pelvic area and breasts in order to detect any abnormalities at an early stage and/or treat an existing disorder. It may be performed by a GYNAECOLOGIST, or a family doctor (general practitioner, family practitioner). It is highly desirable for all women to have such check-ups at regular intervals, but there is some disagreement concerning how often. Most authorities agree that the first check-up should take place between the ages of sixteen and nineteen, but earlier if a girl is sexually active before sixteen, or is about to become sexually active, or has not yet begun to menstruate. Thereafter, some procedures should be carried out once a year whereas others need to be performed only every two or three years, until the age of forty, when the guidelines change again.

A thorough gynaecological examination includes: (1) taking of history; (2) the physical examination itself; (3) certain tests; and (4) a discussion with the doctor concerning his or her findings and recommendations for the future. *History-taking* consists of a discussion with the doctor of a complete history of the patient's health and that of her immediate family. Among the topics covered are age, number of pregnancies and their outcomes, chief complaint and present illness (if any), menstrual history, contraceptives used (past and present), previous gynaecological problems, general medical history (including certain illnesses in parents, grandparents, and siblings), hospitalizations and surgery, medications currently used (including alcohol, smoking, drug use), any previous adverse reactions to drugs, and any past use of DES (diethylstilboestrol) by the patient or her mother.

The *physical examination* should include measuring height, weight, temperature, pulse, and blood pressure. Many doctors also listen to the heart and lungs with a stethoscope, check the inside of the throat and mouth, and examine the neck for tender lymph nodes and thyroid enlargement. (For women using or planning to use oral contraceptives, heart and lung examinations are mandatory.) The breasts should be examined for lumps, tenderness, nipple discharge, dimpling or puckering, and any other signs of a possible tumour (see BREAST SELF-EXAMINATION).

The *pelvic examination*, includes both

external and internal pelvic organs. The external genital area is checked first, including the labia, pubic area, clitoris, anus, and urethra, for lumps, sores, growths, discolouring, discharges, or lice. Both BARTHOLIN'S GLANDS and SKENE'S GLANDS are palpated to detect lumps. It is followed by an *internal examination* (before which the patient should empty her bladder). A metal or plastic SPECU-LUM is inserted in the vagina so that the vaginal walls and cervix can be inspected for redness, swelling, unusual discharge, or irritation. At this time specimens for laboratory tests are collected, the doctor simply inserting a swab or spatula through the speculum to remove tissue shreds for a PAP SMEAR, gonorrhoea culture, or wet smear (see the discussion of tests below). After removing the speculum (or before inserting it – the exact order of procedures varies with different doctors) the doctor performs a *bimanual examination* inserting two fingers of one hand into the vagina and placing the other hand on the abdomen. In this way he or she can check the position, size, firmness, and mobility of the uterus, locate the Fallopian tubes and ovaries (and feel any lumps there), and inspect the entire abdominal area for tenderness and lumps. Some doctors ask the patient to bear down (as for a bowel movement) to check for relaxed muscles or a pro-lapsed uterus. Next comes a *rectovaginal examination* in which the doctor keeps one finger in the vagina and inserts another into the rectum, both to check the wall between rectum and vagina and to feel the pelvic organs from this angle. Finally, there should be a *rectal examin-ation*, in which one finger is inserted in the rectum only to check for growths or other abnormal conditions there.

The pelvic examination is usually not painful although it can be uncomfortable. Urinating immediately beforehand helps, but douching should be avoided during the preceding twenty-four hours (or longer), so as not to hide discharges or other symptoms. The speculum is much easier to insert if the woman's muscles are relaxed; open-mouth deep breathing helps many women to relax more. If insertion still seems quite painful, the doctor should be asked if a smaller speculum is available or if the one being used can be adjusted. Most women can be examined quite readily, even if they have never had vaginal intercourse or even never used tampons. (The doctor cannot tell from an examination whether a woman has had sexual experience.) Women who find pelvic examination agonizingly embarrassing or are unsure about a new doctor's attitude may find it helpful to ask a friend to accompany them on their visit.

Among the *laboratory tests* generally performed are: *urine test* for protein, sugar, blood, and diabetes (recommended annually); a *Pap smear* for cervical cancer (formerly recommended annually for all women, now recommended once every three years for women who have had two negative tests in successive years but more often in high-risk women; see PAP SMEAR); a *gonorrhoea culture* (some doctors do it routinely, others only when exposure is suspected); *blood count for anaemia* (some do it routinely once a year, others not). Other tests, usually per-formed only when they are specifically indicated, include: syphilis test; tests for vaginal infection (usually only in the presence of symptoms); urinalysis or urine culture (if infection is suspected); stool test (for blood); BLOOD TESTS for cholesterol, triglycerides, and other substances.

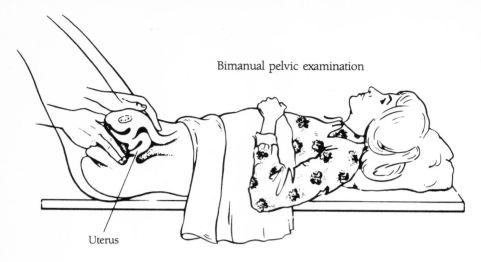

Bimanual pelvic examination

Uterus

After completing the physical examination and tests, most doctors sit down with the patient to discuss their findings, prescribe medication and/or contraceptives (if needed), answer questions, and plan future visits is necessary and/or the next check-up. See also ANTENATAL CARE.

Gynaecologist A doctor who specializes in women's health problems. This speciality is frequently combined with *obstetrics*, which includes all aspects of childbirth (antenatal care, delivery and postpartum care); such a specialist is called an *obstetrician-gynaecologist* (or *ob-gyn*). A consultant gynaecologist has had at least six years of specialist training and has passed special examinations. In Britain in 1985 approximately 88 per cent of consultant gynaecologists were men.

Although gynaecologists have studied general medicine as well, like other specialists they tend to focus on the particular areas they know best. Therefore a woman who uses a gynaecologist for routine private health care, such as physical check-ups, should make sure that her examinations include regular measurements of blood pressure and blood and urine tests, and not only pelvic and breast examinations. Routine gynaecological care may also be performed by general practitioners (GPs). They are able to perform standard breast and pelvic examinations but are both less experienced in and less highly trained for more specialized gynaecological care. Some authorities believe that routine or primary care if best carried out by a practitioner who is not specifically trained as a surgeon (as most gynaecologists are). See also SURGERY, UNNECESSARY.

H

Habitual miscarriage Also *habitual abortion*. The spontaneous loss of three consecutive pregnancies by MISCAR-RIAGE. The causes lie either in the foetus, which may have some genetic abnormality or other defect, or in the mother or father. Conditions affecting the mother include endocrine abnormalities (in the thyroid or adrenal glands, progesterone deficiency, or diabetes, for example), a structural abnormality in the UTERUS, such as an INCOMPETENT CERVIX, or genital HERPES INFECTION or some other infection. Women whose mothers were given the hormone DIETHYLSTILBOE-STROL while pregnant with them may be more likely to miscarry than untreated women, but this theory has not been satisfactorily verified. In some women the cause may lie in an immunological reaction that makes their body reject a foetus as foreign tissue. A newer field of investigation is abnormalities in sperm caused by environmental factors, such as exposure to toxic substances, which are also linked with a high risk of miscarriage.

The duration of pregnancy at the time of miscarriage is often a clue to the cause. Up to about twelve weeks it tends to be a genetic or hormonal abnormality; thereafter it tends to be a structural one. For repeated miscarriage during the first thirteen weeks, tests should include CHROMOSOME studies of both parents, a thyroid-function test, an endometrial biopsy (see BIOPSY, definition 8) timed so as to investigate hormone deficiency after ovulation, and, if the results of all these studies are negative, a hysterosalpingogram (special X-ray of uterus and tubes). Habitual miscarriage later in pregnancy calls for careful examination of the uterus and cervix by X-ray and other techniques.

Until recently it was commonly believed that women who miscarry three consecutive times will almost inevitably miscarry again. More recent studies indicate that the risk of a fourth miscarriage is only about 25 per cent; that is, there is a 70 to 80 per cent chance that the fourth will be a perfectly normal pregnancy. Such spontaneous cures of whatever condition caused the previous miscarriages are not fully understood, but it is suspected that they result from the self-correction of some delicate hormonal feedback mechanism that had gone amiss.

Haematuria The presence of blood in the urine, usually symptomatic of a urinary infection (most often urethritis or cystitis) but sometimes of a more serious condition, such as a tumour of the bladder or kidney, kidney stones, cysts, or sickle cell disease. The urine is reddish or brownish, depending on how much blood is present and on the chemical make-up (especially the acidity) of the urine itself. Because it may signal a serious problem haematuria always calls for careful diagnosis to identify the underlying cause.

Haemophilia A hereditary bleeding disorder that is due to a lack of or abnormality of some of the chemical factors that make blood coagulate (clot). It is a sex-linked recessive gene disorder (see under BIRTH DEFECTS and CHROMOSOME for further explanation) passed on by mothers to their sons. Depending on which clotting factor is defective, there are various kinds of haemophilia, the most common of which are haemophilia A (abnormal Factor VIII) and haemophilia B (abnormal Factor IX). The former accounts for more than four-fifths of all cases. The disease is usually detected early in life, when symptoms such as haematomas (internal blood clots) and haematuria (bloody urine) appear. In some cases superficial cuts and wounds heal slowly, but in others serious haemorrhages develop from trivial injuries or mild exercise, and haemarthrosis (bleeding into the joints) develops. There is no cure for the disease, but it can be controlled by administering the missing clotting factor. Factor VIII is present only in quite fresh plasma and has a short shelf life. However, it can be precipitated from plasma by freezing and can be stored frozen in blood banks. Therapy depends on the severity of the bleeding; internal haemorrhage into a large area, for example, may require transfusion at least twice a day for several days. In recent years arrangements have been made whereby the missing factor can be self-administered by the patient at home or injected by a family member.

Haemophilus vaginalis Also *HV*, *Corynebacterium vaginale, Gardnerella vaginalis*. An organism that causes VAGINITIS, marked by a greyish-white, foul-smelling vaginal discharge and intense itching. Its prinipal mode of transmission is sexual intercourse, so it is regarded as a VENEREAL DISEASE. It is diagnosed by means of a WET SMEAR and is treated with antibiotic suppositories or creams applied to the vagina, or with oral antibiotics.

Haemorrhage, vaginal Heavy uncontrollable blood flow from the vagina, frequently but not always originating in the uterus. Unlike heavy MENSTRUAL FLOW, it tends to come in spurts, irregularly, rather than at a steady rate. The most common causes in adult women are MISCARRIAGE or an ECTOPIC PREGNANCY. Following childbirth, a POSTPARTUM HAEMORRHAGE may occur when the uterus does not contract sufficiently after delivery or a portion of the placenta or foetal tissue is retained. It may also occur, for similar reasons, following abortion. During labour, haemorrhage can be caused by either ABRUPTIO PLACENTAE or by PLACENTA PRAEVIA.

Like uncontrolled bleeding elsewhere, vaginal haemorrhage constitutes a medical emergency and must be dealt with promptly, by stopping the bleeding, restoring blood volume (by blood transfusion), and combatting shock.

Haemorrhoid Also *piles*. A VARICOSE VEIN in the anus or lower rectum. It is caused, like other varicosities, by increased pressure that weakens the wall of a vein, destroying the valves that keep blood moving back to the heart and ultimately causing blood to pool in places. The causes of such increased pressure include constipation (leading to straining to defaecate), prolonged coughing or sneezing, obesity, pregnancy, and abdominal tumours. The principal symptom is bleeding, usually noticed after a bowel movement. Haemorrhoids may occur inside or outside the anus. *External haemorrhoids* are small, soft, purplish skin-covered mounds that become more prominent with straining at stool. They are rarely painful unless they thrombose, that is, a clot forms. The haemorrhoid then may become inflamed, break down, bleed profusely, and be extremely tender, especially during defaecation. After a few days the clot is absorbed and the swelling subsides. *Internal haemorrhoids* generally occur in clusters, and are covered by a thin layer of mucous membrane. Passage of a hard stool may cause them to ulcerate and bleed; frequently they also cause itching and leakage of mucus from the anus.

Small haemorrhoids that cause only slight occasional bleeding and otherwise are not troublesome need no treatment other than identifying and removing the underlying cause; those that appear during pregnancy often disappear after delivery. Constipation can often be relieved by a high-fibre diet and increased intake of liquids. For internal haemorrhoids that cause pain on defaecation, use of a stool softener may help. Also, the anal area should always be cleaned very gently to avoid irritating it further. Sitz baths often help relieve discomfort. The use of suppositories and any local manipulation of the affected area should be avoided. More troublesome haemorrhoids can often be treated by injection of phenol which causes shrinkage of the haemorrhoid. This can be carried out in a surgical outpatient clinic or a doctor's surgery. If these measures fail and the bleeding is sufficient to cause ANAEMIA, the pain is disabling,

or the itching intolerable, surgical removal (called *haemorrhoidectomy*) may be considered. However, the recovery period following surgery is quite uncomfortable for a week or so; also, haemorrhoids may recur after surgery. HERBAL REMEDIES for haemorrhoids include infusions made of dandelion root (*Taraxacum officinale*), chicory root (*Cichorium endiva*), cascara sagrada (*Rhamnus purshiana*), Oregon grape root (*Berberis aquifolium*), or liquorice (*Glycyrrhiza glabra*), which all are drunk as a tea, or direct insertion into the rectum of an infusion of witch hazel leaves (*Haemamelis virginiana*), bayberry bark (*Myrica cerifera*), and goldenseal (*Hydrastis canadensis*).

Hair loss Also *alopecia*. The thinning or falling out of scalp hair, which is affected to some extent by hormonal changes that are not completely understood. Some women experience loss of scalp hair when they take oral contraceptives. Since a common cause of such hair loss is an underactive thyroid gland (hypothyroidism), this condition should first be ruled out. Thereafter, switching to another kind of oral contraceptive may solve the problem. Other women experience hair loss when they stop taking oral contraceptives; usually this is a temporary condition, probably caused simply by the change in hormone levels, and is self-correcting within a few months. Pregnancy sometimes affects hair growth and also hair texture. Also, many women experience considerable thinning of scalp hair after delivery; again, it usually is a temporary condition that is self-correcting. After menopause, most women experience some thinning of both scalp and pubic hair, and sometimes an increase in facial hair. These changes are most likely to be caused by a relative increase in androgen levels (the male hormone produced by the adrenal glands) compared to oestrogen levels, which are lowered. Still another possible cause of hair loss is anaemia, which should be ruled out by means of a simple blood test.

Halsted radical mastectomy See MASTECTOMY, definition 2.

Headache A general term for moderate to severe pain in the head, which can be a symptom of numerous disorders but does not generally require medical attention unless it occurs often enough to be considered chronic and/or is severe enough to be disabling. The headache accompanying a cold or other infectious disease normally subsides when the disease does, and usually responds to aspirin or other over-the-counter remedies. Severe and recurrent headache, however, may be caused by a tumour or other brain lesion, by a serious infection such as meningitis or encephalitis, by infections of the eye, ear, nose, mouth, sinuses, or teeth, or by allergy. The most common kinds of recurrent headache, whose causes often are very difficult to determine, are those caused by various vascular disturbances, that is, disturbances of the blood flow to the head. Among these are the *cluster headache*, found twenty times as frequently in men as in women; the *tension headache*, in which tense muscles of the head, face, and neck cause blood vessels to constrict spasmodically; *toxic metabolic headache*, caused by a toxic state (overindulgence in alcohol – the typical 'hangover' headache – as well as lead, arsenic, morphine, or carbon monoxide poisoning); *hypertension headache*, caused by complications from high blood pressure;

and MIGRAINE, caused by arterial spasm. Headache also may be a side effect of ORAL CONTRACEPTIVES or other medication. A change to a different kind of oral contraceptive may help, but if the headache is of the migraine variety the oral contraceptives should be discontinued at once and another form of birth control substituted.

Numerous drugs, both prescription and over-the-counter, as well as psychotherapy have been used to fight chronic headache, with mixed success. One promising approach is *biofeedback*, in which patients are taught to increase the blood flow to the head. Another approach is learning relaxation exercises, which can be used whenever a stressful situation arises. Some researchers believe poor nutrition can cause sufficient physical stress to produce chronic tension headache, and suggest that eating foods rich in calcium and the B vitamins may be helpful. Another form of self-treatment is acupressure, which consists of pressing an index finger firmly on certain pressure points of the body and slowly rotating the finger for 20 to 30 seconds; this may relieve the headache within a minute or so. Many HERBAL REMEDIES have been used for headache, among them teas made from dried rosemary (*Rosmarinus officinalis*), skullcap (*Scutellaria laterifolia*), hops (*Humulus lupulus*), passion flower (*Passiflora incarnata*), peppermint (*Mentha piperita*), or valerian (*Valeriana officinalis*), or massaging the forehead and temples with peppermint oil.

Hegar's sign An early physical change of the reproductive tract in pregnancy, and therefore a useful presumptive sign in its diagnosis. Just above the cervix at the bottom of the corpus (body) of the uterus is a tiny area called the *isthmus*.

In early pregnancy this area, just a few millimetres long, feels softer than either the cervix or corpus. This softness, called Hegar's sign, is readily detected by the doctor during bimanual pelvic examination, because the area is readily compressed between the two hands.

Herbal remedies   Also *herbalism*. The use of plants to relieve or cure a variety of disorders, a practice that is thousands of years old. Herbal medicine was and is practised in virtually every part of the world, and became the basis of early European pharmacology. The ancient Greek physician Hippocrates left a valuable description of herbs in use in his time, some of which are still popular today, and Dioscorides (1st century A.D.) wrote a *materia medica* listing more than five hundred plants. Printed herbals appeared soon after printing was invented, and their circulations enabled anyone who wished (and could read) to medicate him or herself. Unlike other kinds of treatment, herbal remedies require no special skills or costly apparatus. As medicine became a formal profession, surgery (including blood-letting) and the use of chemical substances (such as arsenic and mercury) began to replace the use of plants in medicine. Nevertheless, the practice of herbalism survived, mostly passed down by word of mouth. By the mid-20th century, however, herbal medicine had fallen into disrepute. Drug companies manufactured more and allegedly better chemical remedies, often synthesizing some of the organic compounds (in effect, copying nature in the laboratory). In recent years interest in herbalism has increased, in part due to the women's movement, with its emphasis on women's right to control their own bodies, and in part to the advocates of vegetarianism and 'natural' foods. Actually, herbal medicines are more 'natural' only in that their preparation is simpler and their ingredients are wholly organic. Chemically they can be identical with, and just as toxic as, man-made inorganic compounds.

Herbs can be extremely effective medications. The leaves of the foxglove plant were used to treat heart disease long before their active ingredient, digitalin, was isolated, and digitalis is still an accepted remedy for heart patients. Herbs act on the body in the same ways as manufactured medications do, and potentially are just as dangerous – indeed, in some respects more dangerous, because potency and dosages are less exact (whereas the amount and quality of active ingredients in a pill or capsule are generally closely controlled). Herbal remedies can cause serious side effects or extreme allergic reactions. Consequently, it must be emphasized that **herbal remedies are not a substitute for professional medical attention for any acute illness or persistent ailment**. Because herbs may cause adverse reactions and do not work equally well for everyone, it is wise at first to use only one herb at a time (avoiding herbal teas that blend numerous plants) and in a small dose. Once it is fairly certain there will be no bad reaction, one can gradually increase dosage and add other herbs.

Like most plants, herbs have both common and scientific names. Because common names often vary, and sometimes the name is used for several different herbs, every herb mentioned in this book is identified with its scientific name. Herbs can be brought dried from herbalist suppliers, and the more common ones are also available in health-food shops, sometimes in the form of capsules. It is important to use a reliable supplier whose stock is adequately fresh. The best way to obtain fresh herbs is, if possible, to pick one's own; many grow wild in gardens, fields and industrial wasteland. They can then be dried, either by hanging in bunches in a well-ventilated place or by drying in a barely warm oven (but taking care the oven temperature is never higher than 35°C, or 94°F). They should not be dried in sunlight. Once dried, herbs may be stored in bags, jars, or tins, and can be expected to keep for about three years.

To prepare them for use, most herbs are made into an *infusion* or *tea*, usually one teaspoon of dried herb (three teaspoons of fresh) per cup of boiling water. Roots are usually simmered over low heat for fifteen minutes; with leaves or flowers the boiling water is poured over the herb, covered, and allowed to steep (brew) for ten to twenty minutes. For a remedy using both roots and leaves, simmer the roots first and then pour, with their water, over the leaves or flowers and let steep. All are strained before use. An infusion will keep for a day or two if stored in a cool, dark place.

Specific herbs used medicinally are mentioned in this book under the following entries: ABORTIFACIENT; ANALGESIC; ANAEMIA; BREAST-FEEDING; CERVICITIS; CYSTITIS; DYSMENORRHOEA; DYSPLASIA; EMMENAGOGUE; GINSENG; HEADACHE; HAEMORRHOID; HOT FLUSHES; HYPERTENSION; INSOMNIA; LACTATION; MASTITIS; MENOPAUSE; MENSTRUAL FLOW; PELVIC INFLAMMATORY DISEASE; SITZ BATHS; TRICHOMONAS; VAGINITIS; YEAST INFECTION;

Hereditary disease See under BIRTH DEFECTS.

Heredity See BIRTH DEFECTS; CHROMOSOME.

Hermaphroditism Also *pseudohermaphroditism*. A congenital condition that can affect both men and women, in which structural characteristics of both sexes appear in one person. The particular characteristics affected are those that ordinarily determine sex: chromosomal arrangement (see CHROMOSOME), external genitals, internal genitals, and gonads (sex glands). A *male hermaphrodite* may have testes but external genitals resembling a woman's vulva. A *female hermaphrodite* may have ovaries but the chromatin structure of a man. In *true hermaphroditism*, which is extremely rare (only a few hundred cases have ever been reported), both ovaries and testes are present.

All hermaphroditism results from defects in foetal development. One kind of female hermaphroditism is known to be caused by administering progesterone to the mother in order to prevent miscarriage. Treatment of hermaphroditism usually involves hormone administration and surgery to make both the external and internal sex organs conform to the sex with which a child can most closely identify. See also TRANSSEXUAL.

Hernia, umbilical An outward bulge of the naval that is caused by a weakness in the abdominal wall. Far more common in women than in men, such hernias often are associated with previous pregnancies, as well as with obesity. They usually have no effect on subsequent pregnancies. Umbilicial hernias also occur in newborn babies where, after the skin of the naval heals, there is usually still an opening in the deeper muscular layers of the abdomen. When the baby cries, a small portion of intestine is pushed through this hole, making the naval protrude more. Such hernias heal of their own accord, although when they are large it may take months or even several years. No treatment whatever is needed.

Herpes infection   Also *genital herpes, herpes genitalis, herpes simplex II*. A disease of the genital organs caused by the herpes simplex virus, also called *herpes virus hominis* (HVH). Unknown until the mid-20th century, it is now believed to be the third most common VENEREAL DISEASE (after GONORRHOEA) in Britain, especially in women, who contract it far more often than men. There are two closely related kinds of herpes virus: Type I and Type II. Type I usually causes 'cold sores' or 'fever blisters' on the lips and in the throat, and sometimes eruptions that affect the eyes (*herpes simplex keratitis*), stomach, or brain. Type II usually affects the genital area. How the virus infects the genitals is not completely understood. Since the virus cannot survive outside human cells, it is believed to be transmitted by vaginal, anal, and oral-genital sexual intercourse, but some persons whose sexual partner(s) are not infected somehow contract the infection anyway. Types I and II can be distinguished from one another by laboratory tests, but the symptoms of infection are the same for both, and occasionally Type I has been found in genital sores and Type II in mouth sores.

The principal symptom of infection is the appearance of one or several groups of small, painful, itchy blisters along the vulva and genital mucous membranes; the area most affected is the labia (vaginal lips), but the clitoris, outer part of the vagina, anal area, and cervix can also be involved. The blisters are moist and greyish in colour, with red edges. Men are most commonly affected on the glans or shaft of the penis and, in homosexual men, around the anus. The blisters soon rupture to form soft, extremely painful open sores on a reddish base, covered by a greyish-yellow secretion. (On the cervix, however, the sores are painless.) In women the sores can spread so as to involve the entire surface of the labia. There may also be inflammation and swelling around the urethra (and consequent pain when urinating), and irritation and ulceration of the cervix, causing a vaginal discharge and staining. In addition to these local symptoms, there is usually a low fever, general malaise, and swollen tender lymph nodes in the groin.

Untreated, the outbreak usually clears up by itself in two to three weeks. However, it frequently recurs, because the virus remains dormant in the body (most likely in the nerve cells) and consequently the body's immune system cannot dispose of it. It may remain permanently dormant or give rise to infection again and again. When infection does recur, subsequent attacks are usually milder and shorter-lived than the first one, probably because some antibodies have been built up. There appears to be more risk of recurrence during menstruation, ovulation, and pregnancy (all involving higher hormone levels), as well as with gonorrhoea, heat, emotional stress, tension, fever, or a general rundown physical condition. Recurrence may also be limited to certain triggering factors, notably trauma to the skin that can occur through kissing, rubbing, sunburn, shaving, dental work, smoking, and contact with particular foods.

Herpes infection is more uncomfortable than dangerous except for two factors. First, it appears to be somehow linked with the development of cervical cancer. This relationship is not understood, but women who have had herpes infections are thought to be more susceptible to cervical cancer and therefore are urged to have a PAP SMEAR every six months. It may also be associated with precancerous lesions on the vulva. Secondly, a baby may become infected while passing through the birth canal of an infected mother, and some babies may become infected before labour begins, while still in the uterus. Premature babies seem to be especially susceptible to such infection, which can quickly spread to the brain, leading to brain damage, blindness, and even death. A primary (first-time) infection in the mother during pregnacy appears to be more dangerous to the baby than a second or subsequent attack. To prevent infection of their babies, pregnant women with herpes infection may be advised to have a CAESAREAN SECTION, so that the baby does not pass through the birth canal. Of course, if infection has already spread through the placenta before labour begins, or the membranes have been ruptured for more than two hours, such surgery is useless. A baby usually shows signs of infection within four to seven days, although in severe cases it may be evident immediately. Treatment for such infants is difficult, since the only drugs effective – primarily anti-viral drugs or experimental drugs – may have toxic side effects.

Diagnosis of herpes is often missed because the sores resemble those of two other venereal diseases, SYPHILIS and CHANCROID. In all cases of multiple genital sores, therefore, herpes should be suspected. To test for the virus, a smear of secretions from the sores is put on a slide and fixed as for a Pap smear; in the presence of herpes virus, characteristic changes in the nucleus of cells are usually seen. This is the cheapest and among the most accurate tests for herpes for both men and women but can detect it only when sores are actually present. Viral cultures, where the virus from a sore is grown in a laboratory, are less accurate and costlier. Blood tests measuring antibody titres are also available. They require two samples, one taken during the first attack of herpes and the second two to four weeks later, or after symptoms have subsided. Blood tests are not accurate if they are performed *after* (rather than during) an initial attack because the results are unclear. None of these tests detects the difference between Herpes I and II virus, but the site of infection often indicates which is responsible.

No permanent cure for herpes has yet been found, but acyclovir (Zovirax) ointment is effective if used very early in a first attack of herpes, and intravenous and oral forms of the drug are also used in severe attacks. Other researchers are working to develop a vaccine to build up antibodies. Current treatment is aimed largely at relieving discomfort. Sulpha cream applied directly to the sores is used to kill other bacteria that might otherwise enter them. Wet dressings of cool water may help relieve itching and pain, along with oral analgesics such as aspirin and codeine. Cool sitz baths, with or without baking soda added, and local applications of soothing substances – such as cold milk, acidophilus milk, yoghurt, baking soda, milk of magnesia, cornstarch, witch hazel, wheat germ oil, vitamin E oil, and ointments containing either camphor or zinc oxide – have been recommended. For an anaesthetic effect, products containing benzocaine may afford relief. Because the mucous membranes affected by herpes are highly sensitive – far more so than skin – caution is advised in applying any topical agent lest it prove even more irritating; patients are advised to use only a tiny amount in one place and wait for a possbile adverse reaction before proceeding to more widespread application. Among the HERBAL REMEDIES for herpes are compresses with an infusion of cloves, black tea bags soaked in hot water, peppermint oil, and clove oil. Cotton underwear (or no underpants) and loose clothing promote healing, as does keeping the genital area clean and dry with normal bathing. Some authorities believe a diet rich in certain nutrients – especially vitamins C, B-complex, and B_6, along with zinc and calcium – and the daily use of kelp powder (1 capsule a day) and sunflower seed oil (1 tablespoon a day), help prevent recurrence.

Heterosexual Also *straight* (slang). Describing a male-female sexual relationship, or a person who prefers a sexual partner of the opposite sex. See also HOMOSEXUAL.

High-risk pregnancy A term used for pregnant women who have a chronic disease or some other condition that makes pregnancy more dangerous for them and/or their babies. Among the chronic diseases associated with such a risk are DIABETES, HYPERTENSION (high blood pressure), heart disease, kidney or lung disease, liver disease, SICKLE CELL DISEASE or related blood disorders, any form of CANCER, alcoholism (see ALCOHOL USE), and drug addiction (see DRUG USE). In addition, certain infections in the mother can have serious effects on her baby, especially RUBELLA, genital HERPES INFECTION, SYPHILIS, and GONOR-

RHOEA. Blood incompatibility (see RH FACTOR) represents a risk. Finally, there is increased risk to the baby if the mother is either over thirty-five or in her early teens (see AGE, CHILDBEARING), has had difficulty with previous deliveries, is known to have a small pelvis, is obese, or is known to be carrying more than one foetus (see MULTIPLE PREGNANCY). In all these instances ANTENATAL CARE must be more frequent and more cautious.

During pregnancy, hypertension, common especially among obese women, older women, and black women, can compromise the flow of blood through the placenta, resulting in smaller babies. Also, hypertension carries the risk of kidney damage, which can be life-threatening to both mother and child. The normal heart and kidneys must work considerably harder during pregnancy; for disease-damaged organs the overload may be too great. Pregnancy itself can induce hypertension in women whose blood pressure was previously normal (see PREECLAMPSIA). Cancer anywhere in the pelvic or abdominal area is particularly dangerous; CANCER IN SITU of the cervix can be treated conservatively during pregnancy, as can breast cancer, although extra efforts must be made to shield the foetus from damaging radiation exposure during either diagnosis or treatment. Marked OBESITY is dangerous to both mother and baby. The majority of obese women develop some obstetric complication, especially hypertension, diabetes, kidney disease, wound complications, and thromboembolism (blood clots). Women who smoke heavily are more likely to bear undersized and premature babies than women who do not, and their risk of MISCARRIAGE, PLACENTA PRAEVIA, and ABRUPTIO PLACENTAE also is higher.

Hirtsutism In women, excess body hair distributed as it is normally found in men, especially on the face, chest, and abdomen below the navel. Occasionally a hereditary trait, hirsutism more often is caused by excess production of androgens (male hormones) by the adrenal glands (ADRENOGENITAL SYNDROME), a tumour of the adrenals, CUSHING'S SYNDROME, or an abnormality in the ovaries, such as the STEIN-LEVENTHAL SYNDROME. Depending on the cause, hirsutism is treated with hormone therapy and/or electrolysis (for permanent hair removal). Occasionally, use of oral contraceptives causes hirsutism, which can usually be corrected by changing to a different blend of medication (although it may take months for the extra hair already produced to fall out). Other women experience hirsutism, along with acne and weight gain, after stopping oral contraceptives; here it is believed to result from a sudden but temporary increase in androgens, again secreted by the adrenal glands. See also HAIR LOSS.

Holiday pill An ORAL CONTRACEPTIVE taken only once a month, or for a few days whenever sexual intercourse is anticipated. It began to be used in China in the late 1970s, but little information has become available in the West about its effectiveness and other important details.

Home birth Also *home delivery.* Delivering a baby at home, rather than in a hospital. Such deliveries were the norm until about 1900, when the use of anaesthesia for childbirth and hospitalization became the accepted practice in most advanced countries. By 1967 75 per cent of births in Britain were in hospital and by the 1980s this had risen to 95 per cent. A woman has the right to choose to have her baby at home but this is not always easy to arrange. A woman is entitled to the services of a community midwife and it is especially important that good antenatal care is provided for a home birth. A family doctor who carries out maternity care must be notified of the expected home birth. Some hospitals have a 'Flying Squad' which is a team from the Obstetric department that will attend to the woman at home should an unexpected emergency occur during birth or soon afterwards. A 'confinement pack' containing sterile towels and other materials for the birth is provided by the health authority.

Home birth has both risks and benefits. For the 5 per cent of births that are not normal – that is, where complications of some kind arise – they clearly represent a greater risk than would be involved in a hospital. Among the most common complications are ABNORMAL PRESENTATION of various kinds, a disproportionately large baby (relative to the size of the mother's pelvis), haemorrhage from PLACENTA PRAEVIA or ABRUPTIO PLACENTAE, PROLONGED LABOUR and foetal distress from a PROLAPSED CORD or other causes that is not detected because of inadequate FOETAL MONITORING. Some of these complications are unpredictable beforehand.

Although there is conflict between those who oppose home birth for any woman and those who feel it is the only natural (and therefore desirable) way to have a baby, most knowledgeable supporters agree that no woman characterized as a HIGH-RISK PREGNANCY (representing 10 to 15 per cent of all women) should deliberately seek home birth. In addition, critics maintain that even low-risk pregnancies can without warning become high-risk during labour, since this is the most stressful time for the baby. Advocates of home birth, on the other hand, point out that most births are normal, and at home the parents can remain in control of the delivery, friends and family (including siblings) can be present and become intimately involved with the new family member from the start, and in a relaxed, familiar atmosphere labour tends to progress faster and medication of various kinds may be avoided. See also MIDWIFE; PREPARED CHILDBIRTH.

Homosexual Also *gay* (slang). Describing a sexual relationship in which both partners are of the same sex, or a person who prefers a sexual partner of the same sex. See also HETEROSEXUAL; LESBIAN.

Honeymoon cystitis See under CYSTITIS.

Hormone In human beings, a chemical substance produced by a gland that serves to stimulate and control vital bodily functions. Acting as a kind of chemical messenger, hormones are carried to various organs and tissues by the bloodstream. The most important hormones regulate growth, sexual development and reproduction, the composition of the blood, metabolism, the transmission of messages in the nervous system, and the production of other hormones, as well as still other functions not yet completely understood. Some hormones, such as insulin, are necessary to maintain life.

The discovery of hormones and their functions is quite recent. The word 'hormone' was coined in 1902, when the first hormone was identified. As hormones began to be synthesized in the laboratory, they came into increasing use to treat disorders associated with their lack, as in DIABETES and OESTROGEN REPLACEMENT THERAPY, as well as to prevent pregnancy (see ORAL CONTRACEPTIVES) and to treat some diseases not directly related to hormone deficiency, such as the use of cortisone to treat arthritis.

Most hormones are produced by ENDOCRINE glands, and sometimes all hormones are classified according to where they were produced – pituitary hormones, ovarian hormones, adrenal hormones, and so on. Another way of classifying hormones is by the functions they affect, as sex hormones, gonadotrophins (sex-gland-stimulating hormones), metabolic hormones, and so on. Still another way of classifying hormones is according to their chemical make-up, which for a few of them is still not known. Chemically there are two basic kinds of hormone: the *steroids*, which are derived from cholesterol and include the sex hormones and hormones produced by the adrenal cortex, or corticosteroids; and those based on single amino acids or strings of amino acids, called *protein* or *polypeptide hormones*, which include insulin and thyroxine. The chief steroid hormones are the androgens (principally testosterone and androsterone), oestrogens, and progesterone. Although androgens are usually produced by the testes, oestrogen and progesterone by the ovaries, and the corticosteroids by the adrenals, these same organs can make any kind of steroid hormone, and sometimes do. The principal protein hormones are human chorionic gonadotrophin (HCG), produced by the placenta during pregnancy, and follicle-stimulating hormone (FSH), luteinizing hormone (LH), prolactin, oxytocin, and somatotrophin (growth hormone), all released by the pituitary gland. Prolactin and oxytocin normally do not occur in men, although in certain diseases they may do so. The so-called gonadotrophic (gonad-stimulating) hormones function in both sexes; in men FSH stimulates sperm production and LH stimulates testosterone production.

Most of the body's hormones are intimately interconnected. For example, FSH and LH stimulate a woman's ovaries to produce oestrogen; the anterior pituitary gland in turn is stimulated to produce FSH and LH by release factors, which are hormones produced by the hypothalamus. When oestrogen levels drop, the hypothalamus is stimulated to produce release factors to stimulate the pituitary to produce FSH and LH to stimulate the ovaries, and so on. A similar feedback system is involved in the production of many other hormones. There are separate entries for the most important hormones; see also HYPOTHALAMUS; MENSTRUAL CYCLE; PITUITARY GLAND.

Hormone cream   See under VAGINAL ATROPHY.

Hospice   A facility or system of medical care for dying patients. In Europe, especially in Britain, the hospice is often a residential facility in a pastoral setting where the terminally ill may live out their days in peaceful surroundings. Such hospices are based on the medieval 'hospitality houses' from which the term is derived, shelters maintained by religious orders that took in strangers, travellers, and the indigent sick.

In Britain many hospices have a religious non-denominational foundation or are funded by charities such as the National Society for Cancer Relief.

Sometimes the hospices are able to give advice and help in care of a dying person at home avoiding the need for residential care.

Medical care for the dying is palliative, directed at making a person as comfortable as possible, and often including the use of alcohol and addictive drugs to ease pain. Essentially, hospice care provides an alternative to impersonal high-technology intensive care in a hospital, where patients may be kept alive by means of machinery even when there is no hope for recovery. In contrast, the hospice concept emphasizes the quality of life at the expense, perhaps, of duration.

Hot flushes   Also *hot flashes, vasomotor instability.* A sudden sensation of heat that passes over the upper body, usually from the chest up over the neck and face, which may actually become flushed and sweaty, and which is often followed by copious perspiration and chills. The single most common symptom of MENOPAUSE, hot flushes of varying frequency and severity occur in an estimated 60 to 80 per cent of women. A hot flush may last from a few seconds to several minutes, and may occur as seldom as once or twice a year or as often as fifteen or twenty times a day. Hot flushes occur at night as well, although often a woman is aware of them only after waking up soaking wet from the subsequent sweat (so-called *night sweats*).

Hot flushes are actually the rapid dilation of surface blood vessels, believed to be caused by a disturbance of the hypothalamus (which controls body temperature), in turn caused by hormone imbalance. After menopause, as the body adjusts gradually to lower oestrogen levels, hot flushes usually subside. Typically they begin to occur about the time that menstrual flow begins to wane and continue until after periods have ended (although a few women continue to experience them for a number of years after the last period). They also occur, often more suddenly and more severely, in women whose ovaries have been surgically removed (see OOPHORECTOMY).

Hot flushes can occur with or without obvious signs of their presence (red face, drops of perspiration). For a few women they are very severe indeed, sometimes accompanied by numbness of hands and feet, shortness of breath, a feeling of suffocation, palpitations, dizziness, and even fainting. They are greatly eased by OESTROGEN REPLACEMENT THERAPY, which, however, is associated with increased risk of cancer and therefore is considered a controversial treatment. Moreover, some authorities believe that oestrogen replacement simply staves off hot flushes for a time; when therapy is ended, the body reacts to the reduced oestrogen levels with a new set of hot flushes. And, for some women, oestrogen therapy is contraindicated anyway. However giving progesterone as well as oestrogen is thought to lessen the risk of cancer.

An alternative found effective by some women is clonidine, a drug used to treat high blood pressure, which works by causing vasoconstriction. Other approaches are vitamin therapy, especially supplements of vitamin E (either alone or combined with vitamin C and calcium supplements). However, vitamin E must be used very cautiously by women who have diabetes, rheumatic heart disease, or high blood pressure, and no one should take more than 600 International Units per day without medical supervision. Various HERBAL REMEDIES have been recommended for hot flushes, among them liquorice root (*Glycyrrhiza*

lepidota), which contains a substance chemically similar to oestrogen, and sarsaparilla (*Smilax officinalis*), which contains one similar to progesterone; ginseng root (*Panax quinquefolium*) and dong kwai (or tang kuei; *Angelica sinensis*), long used in China (see GINSENG); and red raspberry leaf (*Rubus idaeus*) tea. Also a simple but effective palliative at the time of a hot flush is a cold-water compress applied to the face. Another, still experimental, way of dealing with hot flushes is to alter the body's exposure to light (see under PINEAL BODY).

Hydatidiform mole   Also *hydatid mole.* An abnormal development of embryonic tissue (specifically the PLACENTA) resulting in the formation of a grapelike cluster instead of a foetus. It is distinguished from a normal pregnancy in that the uterus grows far more rapidly, there is vaginal bleeding in the third or fourth month (ranging from spotting to profuse haemorrhage), and no foetal heartbeat or movement can be discerned. Severe nausea and vomiting often occur, and eventually grapelike molar tissue is discharged through the vagina. Diagnosis can be confirmed by the presence of exceptionally high levels of human chorionic gonadotrophin (HCG) in the blood or urine at three and one-half months or so. Although 80 to 90 per cent of such moles are benign (noncancerous), they are considered potentially malignant because they occasionally give rise to a cancer called CHORIOCARCINOMA. Treatment is directed at expelling the mole, which often occurs spontaneously near the end of the fourth month. If it does not, a D AND C is performed, usually by means of suction (vacuum aspiration) followed by some scraping (curetting) to make sure all of the molar tissue has been removed. Usually chemotherapy, consisting of methotrexate, is administered. The patient is usually checked for HCG levels in the blood until there have been negative levels for one year. In addition, oral contraceptives are often prescribed for one year, provided there are no contra-indications for them, in order to prevent conception. After one year of negative HCG levels, it is safe to attempt another pregnancy.

Hydroalpinx A large, fluid-filled, club-shaped FALLOPIAN TUBE, closed at the fimbriated end (closest to the ovary), thus making it impossible for an egg from that ovary to enter the tube. It usually is the result of GONORRHOEA, which causes inflammation and infection of the tube. As the pus from the infection is absorbed, hydrosalpinx results. Often the condition is bilateral (affecting both tubes), making the woman infertile. Treatment is aimed at early detection by pelvic examination; confirmed by HYSTEROSALPINGOGRAPHY, it may then be surgically corrected.

Hygiene The science of health, and practices such as cleanliness, which help preserve it. Regular use of soap, water, and toothpaste generally suffice to keep the body clean. Body odour comes mostly from perspiration and can be controlled by daily bathing of those areas where it is most likely to be concentrated, chiefly the armpits and the pubic area. Hair removal on the underarms and legs is not related to health, but to appearance. Armpit hair does trap perspiration odours, and regular shaving minimizes that, but otherwise it is purely cosmetic. The use of underarm DEODORANTS Also helps, but they should not be used in the pubic area lest they irritate the very sensitive skin there.

The vagina does not ordinarily need to be washed or douched. Its normal secretions, menstrual flow, and seminal fluid all are alike in that they are not 'dirty'. Strong odours in the pubic area tend to be those trapped by the pubic hair, which simply requires regular washing. If a strong odour persists despite washing, it can be a sign of vaginal infection and should be investigated. Use of 'hygiene sprays' inside the vagina should be avoided; they frequently cause allergic reactions and, should a woman using them be pregnant, they can harm the baby. Wiping after a bowel movement should always be done from front to back, to avoid contaminating the vagina with faecal matter, which can contain bacteria harmful to it. See also DEODORANTS; DOUCHING.

Hymen Also *maidenhead*. A thin elastic membrane, about ⅛-inch thick, that partly covers the introitus, or vaginal opening. In most young girls and women who have never had vaginal intercourse, the hymen partly blocks the opening, allowing menstrual flow to pass through. The size and shape of the hymen vary enormously. It can be stretched by the use of tampons or with the fingers, as well as by physical exercise that causes stretching in that area, such as gymnastics, ballet, or horseback riding. Consequently it is not possible to tell, from examining the hymen, whether or not a woman has ever had vaginal intercourse. During the first vaginal intercourse the hymen may rupture, if it has not done so earlier, tearing at several points. The edges of the tears then heal, and the hymen may remain permanently divided into two or three sections. There may or may not be slight bleeding (occasionally severe bleeding) when it is ruptured; thus the presence or absence of such blood also does not signify virginity. Occasionally the hymen is very resistant to tearing and may require a small surgical incision (*hymenotomy*) or even removal (*hymenectomy*) before vaginal intercourse can take place. Even more rare is the condition called *imperforate hymen*, in which the membrane completely blocks the vagina so that menstrual flow cannot pass through; this condition requires minor surgery for correction.

Hyperemesis gravidarum See under MORNING SICKNESS.

Hypermenorrhoea Also *menorrhagia*. Exceptionally heavy bleeding during regular menstrual periods. See under MENSTRUAL FLOW.

Hyperplasia, endometrial See ENDOMETRIAL HYPERPLASIA.

Hypertension Also *high blood pressure*. Elevation of arterial systolic and/or diastolic blood pressure, occurring either alone (*primary* or *essential hypertension*) or as the byproduct of kidney disease or some other condition (*secondary hypertension*). It is just about equally common in women and men. As a whole it affects some 15 per cent of British adults. It tends to strike after middle age, but can occur at any age and is being recognized increasingly in young people.

There is usually no warning symptom of hypertension until a person suffers from one of its complications, most commonly a heart attack, stroke (cerebral vascular accident), or kidney disease. The only way to discover the disease is to measure the *blood pressure*; that is, the pressure of the blood on the walls of the arteries, which in turn depends on the energy of the heart action, the elasticity of the arterial walls (which decreases with advancing age), and the volume and viscosity (thickness) of the blood. There are two components to blood pressure. The first, the *maximum* or *systolic pressure*, is the pressure that occurs with the contraction of the left ventricle (the lower chamber of the left side of the heart, which pumps oxygenated blood out to the tissues of the body). The second, the *minimum* or *diastolic pressure*, is the pressure when the ventricle dilates and refills with blood (when the heart is at rest). Blood pressure is measured with a *sphygmomanometer*, an instrument containing a column of mercury, or a similar device.

There is no known cure for primary hypertension, but treatment can modify its course; secondary hypertension is treated by eliminating the underlying cause. Without treatment there is great risk of developing a serious, and possibly fatal, complication. The greatest dangers are congestive heart failure and stroke. The extra pumping needed may cause the left ventricle to fail entirely, or the increased pressure may cause some smaller blood vessel to burst (in the brain this releases blood that presses on and damages brain tissue, causing a cerebral haemorrhage or stroke; see CEREBRAL VASCULAR ACCIDENT). Another frequent complication is kidney damage.

General measures for treating hypertension include weight control (obesity definitely contributes to the disease, and, furthermore, creates a greater work load for the heart) and prudent physical exercise. Smoking should be avoided, and the intake of salt greatly reduced: These measures may be sufficient to control mild hypertension, provided there are no complications such as kidney disease or high-risk factors such as a strong family history of hypertension and heart disease. Antihypertensive drugs, when required, must usually be continued for life. Mild hypertension usually is treated with an oral DIURETIC drug, which stimulates the kidneys to increase elimination of salt and water and thereby reduces the blood volume; it also relaxes the walls of the smaller arteries, allowing them to expand and thus reducing the need for such high pressure to pump blood through them. Moderate and severe hypertension usually are treated with both an oral diuretic and a sympathetic nervous system depressant, which reduces the ability of the sympathetic nervous system to constrict blood vessels, and sometimes with a vasodilator. Since becoming available (in 1966), a class of drugs called *beta blockers* have been increasingly used to control hypertension. They include propanolol, timolol, and others. Herbalists say that the leaves and stem of hyssop (*Hyssopus officinalis*), brewed into a tea, has an antihypertensive effect.

With treatment most persons with uncomplicated hypertension can lead relatively normal lives. Women with hypertension should avoid using oral contraceptives, choosing another method of birth control. Women who desire to bear children must remember that hypertension makes pregnancy risky for both mother and child, but if the mother's blood pressure can be maintained within a normal range, by close antenatal supervision, restriction of sodium (salt) intake, and regular medication, the prognosis for both is quite good. For pregnancy-induced hypertension, see PREECLAMPSIA.

Hyperthyroidism See under THYROID.

Hypoglycaemia Also *low blood sugar.* A rare disease in which the body's regulatory system of the amount of glucose in the bloodstream is disturbed owing to a tumour of the pancreas, liver disease, or surgery on the gastrointestinal tract. Its symptoms usually involve the central nervous system and range from loss of alertness to coma and convulsions. Treatment involves eliminating the underlying cause. However, one form of hypoglycaemia, sometimes called *functional hypoglycaemia*, is more common. It develops two to four hours after eating, when too much insulin is released after a high-carbohydrate meal, giving rise to symptoms of faintness, weakness, tremors, palpitations, hunger pangs, and nervousness. Because these symptoms all are largely subjective (difficult to measure or otherwise demonstrate) and also may result from psychological problems, especially stress, anxiety, and depression, and because levels of blood sugar in healthy individuals are quite variable, the condition is difficult to diagnose. Treatment of functional hypoglycaemia consists of a fairly restrictive, high-protein, low-carbohydrate diet without concentrated sweets and with frequent small meals instead of three large ones per day, and psychotherapy if emotional problems are involved. Many patients find that their symptoms improve with this diet, possibly indicating that they actually were suffering from disturbances caused by too high an intake of sugar.

Hypomenorrhoea Exceptionally light bleeding during regular menstrual periods. See under MENSTRUAL FLOW.

Hypothalamus A part of the brain that is considered part of both the ENDO-

CRINE system and the central nervous system. Adjacent to the posterior pituitary gland, the hypothalamus produces two hormones that travel through the posterior pituitary and are released into the bloodstream as *oxytocin*, which influences labour (in childbirth) and milk production, and *vasopressin*, which constricts the blood vessels, raises blood pressure, and also influences the uterus and kidneys. The hypothalamus also controls the synthesis and release of hormones by the anterior pituitary gland.

Hysterectomy Surgical removal of the uterus. A *total hysterectomy* involves removal of the body of the uterus and the cervix; a *subtotal* or *partial hysterectomy* leaves the cervix intact, a procedure rarely performed today since the cervix alone has no function and carries the risk of developing cancer in the future. A hysterectomy as such does not involve removal of the Fallopian tubes or ovaries, and consequently does not bring on menopause since it does not stop ovulation or oestrogen production by the ovaries. It does, however, preclude childbearing, and it puts an end to menstruation. Surgical removal of the ovaries, or OOPHOREC-TOMY, and of the Fallopian tubes, or SALPINGECTOMY, can be and often is performed along with hysterectomy; in that case the operation is technically known as a *total abdominal hysterectomy and bilateral salpingo-oophorectomy* (abbreviated *TAH and BSO*) or, in lay terminology, a *complete hysterectomy*. 'Bilateral' means both ovaries and both tubes, 'unilateral' means only one; 'abdominal' refers to the fact that the incision is made through the lower abdomen, distinguishing it from a vaginal hysterectomy, where the uterus and cervix are removed through an incision

inside the vagina (see below).

Hysterectomy was first performed by Dr. Robert Battey in 1872. It became one of the most widely performed operations in developed countries by the 1970s, particularly the United States where critics claimed that perhaps 40 per cent of all hysterectomies were performed unnecessarily and that seeking a second opinion after hysterectomy was proposed resulted in greatly reducing the number of operations performed.

There are certain clear-cut indications for hysterectomy, when the operation may be necessary to save a woman's life: (1) to stop severe uncontrollable bleeding (haemorrhage); (2) as a last resort for severe infection, such as the bursting of an abscess secondary to PELVIC INFLAM-MATORY DISEASE; (3) to remove a malignant tumour (cancer) from the vagina, uterus, Fallopian tubes, or ovaries. In addition, a hysterectomy may sometimes be necessary as part of surgery required to correct a life-threatening disorder elsewhere in the abdominal cavity, in the bladder, rectum, or intestines.

A second category of indications for hysterectomy is less clear-cut, the need for surgery depending on the severity of the condition. Among these are: (1) severe and recurrent attacks of pelvic inflammatory disease; (2) extensive ENDOMETRIOSIS with disabling symptoms that does not respond to other therapy (especially when the disease is so widespread that pregnancy is very unlikely or the woman is past childbearing age); (3) uterine FIBROIDS that are very large and/or pressing on other organs, and/or causing recurrent, very profuse menstrual periods, and/or showing sudden marked growth, and that have not responded to hormone therapy; (4) when both ovaries must be removed (bilateral OOPHORECTOMY); (5) the presence of PRECANCEROUS LESIONS; (6) prolapse of the uterus, bladder, or rectum that is severe enough to interfere with bladder or bowel functions and is not correctable by lesser surgery.

For pelvic pain or backache, irregular periods, menstrual cramps, small fibroids, uterine polyps, or ovarian cysts, hysterectomy should *not* be undertaken until alternative, lower-risk treatment has been tried. In addition, unless a woman faces an acute emergency (as with a massive haemorrhage) where immediate treatment is imperative, she is well advised to get at least one more opinion from a second doctor concerning the best course of treatment for her. Finally, hysterectomy should *never* be done for sterilization alone (TUBAL LIGATION is easier, cheaper, and safer) or to eliminate the risk of uterine cancer when no disease is actually present.

Where hysterectomy is the appropriate treatment, the kind of surgery performed depends on a number of factors. In women past menopause, removal of the ovaries is often recommended, since they no longer produce hormones and can possibly become cancerous. In women who are still menstruating regularly and whose ovaries are not diseased, oophorectomy is more controversial. Advocates say that in women over forty in particular the ovaries will soon cease functioning and present a risk of cancer, and therefore should be removed; they are less dogmatic concerning younger women. Opponents point out that ovarian cancer is rare, and surgically induced menopause is a violent shock to the endocrine system, often resulting in severe menopausal symptoms; further, oestrogen replacement therapy, which can mitigate that shock, is in itself risky.

The choice between abdominal and vaginal hysterectomy is usually easier to make. *Vaginal hysterectomy* is usually preferred when the main indication for surgery is prolapse of uterus, bladder, or rectum. The principal advantages are a hidden incision (and therefore no visible scar) and faster healing. The disadvantages are that the operation is more difficult to perform, especially if adhesions (scar tissue) are present; it is harder for the surgeon to see where he or she is working; and there is danger of shortening the vagina when the incision is closed, making for painful intercourse. There is also a 50 per cent greater risk of postoperative infection, which can, however, be offset by administering antibiotics both before and after surgery. The procedure is straightforward. After anaesthesia (general or regional), the patient is placed in the same position as for pelvic examination. The surgeon makes an incision inside the vagina near the cervix, which is extended through the uterus into the abdominal cavity. The uterus is then gradually cut free from the pelvic structures to which it is attached by ligaments and blood vessels and is removed, along with the cervix, through the vagina. The surgeon then repairs each layer of the incision and closes it.

Abdominal hysterectomy is always chosen when the ovaries and Fallopian tubes also must be removed, when a fibroid is too large to remove through the vagina, and when there are many adhesions (scar tissue) from previous pelvic infection or previous surgery. The principal advantage is that the surgeon can see the entire abdominal cavity. The disadvantages for the patient are a longer recovery period, more postoperative pain (because the abdominal muscles must be cut and then must heal), and a higher probability that adhesions will develop. Two kinds of incision are used, either a vertical (midline) incision extending from the pubic bone toward the navel, or a curved transverse incision below the pubic hairline and extending up on both sides toward the hipbones. The transverse incision allows the scar to be partly or wholly hidden by pubic hair, but the vertical incision affords the surgeon better visibility and more room in which to operate.

Hysterectomy is major surgery, requiring hospitalization for five to eight days. After the patient is anaesthetized, the incision is made into the abdomen and the bladder is separated from the uterus so that it will not be injured. The ligaments connected to the uterus are divided, the blood vessels clamped and tied, and the vagina is cut from around the cervix and uterus. Both uterus and cervix are removed, with or without the tubes and ovaries. Sometimes an appendicectomy is performed at the same time. A hysterectomy for cancer may be still more extensive. In a *radical hysterectomy* (also called *Wertheim procedure*) the surgeon removes the pelvic lymph nodes and ligaments and the upper portion of the vagina, along with the cervix and uterus. Even in this extreme procedure, however, the ovaries, if they are definitely not involved, may be left intact.

Although the risk of death from hysterectomy is fairly low, that of complications is quite high. Up to 10 per cent of women have postoperative infections that require treatment, and, though antibiotic treatment alone is often sufficient, some do develop large abscesses that require further surgery. Haemorrhage occurs during surgery in up to 15 per cent of cases, sometimes requiring blood transfusion, and heavy bleeding may occur,

usually one or two weeks following surgery, when the internal sutures begin to dissolve. Problems with the urinary tract are common during the first few postoperative weeks, with about half the women developing bladder or kidney infections. Danger signs after the patient returns home, any one of which should be reported to the surgeon immediately, are: fever (over 104°F. oral); pain not relieved by medication given when leaving the hospital; bright red vaginal bleeding with large clots (small ones alone are common) or bleeding that soaks one or two pads per hour; constipation (more than three days without a bowel movement); persistent bladder discomfort, bloody urine, or inability to urinate; pain, swelling, tenderness or redness in a leg; chest pain, cough, difficulty in breathing, or coughing blood; odourous and/or copious vaginal discharge.

In addition to the above-named complications, fatigue and minor discomfort affect most women for some weeks. Some women feel depressed and weepy. They may also experience HOT FLUSHES, even if their ovaries were not removed; the reason is not known, but presumably their hormone balance is temporarily upset by surgery. Recovery time varies, depending on the individual's age and general physical condition. Most women return to regular activities in four to six weeks, but some recuperate much more slowly. In premenopausal women, if the ovaries have been removed they will experience some or all of the symptoms of MENOPAUSE caused by greatly lowered oestrogen levels.

Many women tend to gain weight postoperatively, chiefly because they are so much less active during the period of recuperation. Such weight gain can be avoided by reducing caloric intake. Conditioning exercise will help retone muscles flabby from inactivity and usually may be begun four to six weeks after surgery. Vaginal sexual intercourse may usually be resumed after six weeks. Some women experience a change in their sexual functioning. The removal of uterus and cervix leaves less pelvic tissue to become engorged during sexual arousal. There no longer can be any sensation of expansion in the uterus, nor the contractions of the uterus normally felt during orgasm. These changes may be very apparent to some women and scarcely noticeable to others. In women whose ovaries also are removed, the consequent loss of oestrogen may make the lining of the vagina thinner and less readily lubricated, making intercourse more difficult and sometimes uncomfortable. (See VAGINAL ATROPHY.) Oestrogen replacement therapy relieves such dryness but is not without risk and may not be used at all by some women.

The drawbacks of hysterectomy are, for many women, partly or entirely offset by the relief following surgery that has eliminated a previously painful (and sometimes life-threatening) disorder, along with the nuisance of menstruation and the risk of pregnancy. Thus, although some women feel a profound sense of loss, others (and sometimes even the same women) regard it as a relief from the burden of illness, menstruation, and unwanted pregnancy.

Hysteria, conversion Also *conversion disorder, hysterical neurosis, hysteria syndrome.* An emotional disorder that is expressed as (or 'converted into') a severe bodily dysfunction without any physical cause. It occurs far more often in women than in men. It may take the form of *paresis* (partial paralysis) or complete *paralysis* (inability to move) of a limb that is physically quite healthy, or loss of sight when nothing organic is wrong with the eyes. Other common manifestations are *aphagia* (inability to swallow food or water), *aphonia* (inability to tense the vocal cords to utter sounds, although the person can usually whisper), sensory disturbance (loss of vision or sensation), and pain. Such symptoms, crippling as they may be, are often accompanied by a seeming indifference to them, which psychiatrists call *la belle indifférence* (French for 'beautiful unconcern').

Conversion hysteria was first described by the Greek physician Hippocrates, who believed it to be caused by a uterus that somehow became detached and moved around inside the body, obstructing the particular area in which the symptoms appeared. Indeed, 'hysteria' comes from *hysterikos*, the Greek word for 'uterus'. The condition was described by Sigmund Freud, who added the term 'conversion' and believed that it expressed a repressed psychological conflict, usually one of a sexual nature. For example, repressed guilty feelings about masturbating might be expressed as paralysis of the hand used to masturbate. Most modern psychiatrists have broadened this concept to include psychological conflicts other than sexual ones. Treatment is directed at uncovering the underlying cause which, when recognized and acknowledged by the patient, usually eliminates the symptoms.

Hysterosalpingography The injection of dye and subsequent X-ray study of the uterus and Fallopian tubes, usually to determine whether a woman's inability to become pregnant is caused by an obstruction. This procedure usually performed in the outpatient X-ray department of a hospital involves the injection of special dye through a small tube inserted in the cervix. The radiologist watches on an X-ray screen as the dye fills the uterus and is forced up into the Fallopian tubes, revealing abnormalities in shape as well as any obstruction in these organs. A second X-ray may be required twenty-four hours later. By then the dye will have spread throughout the pelvic area, and a residue of dye near the end of either Fallopian tube may indicate scar tissue near the ovary, which may be obstructing the passage of an egg into the tube.

Hysterosalpingography involves some discomfort, usually resulting from the dilatation of the cervix to enable inserting the dye. Also, the cervix must usually be held steady by means of a clamp (tenaculum; see under D AND C), which may cause cramping, and a pinch when it is first applied. The procedure, which is best performed after a menstrual period but before ovulation, is accurate in detecting tubal obstruction in about 75 per cent of cases. Its chief drawback is that it delivers a high dose of radiation to the ovaries, and therefore many doctors consider the minor surgery involved in LAPAROSCOPY safer.

Hysteroscopy The insertion of a visualizing instrument, called a *hysteroscope*, through the cervix into the uterus. It is used to locate and remove, by means of a special forceps attachment, an INTRAUTERINE DEVICE (IUD) that has perforated the uterine wall. It can also be used to effect TUBAL LIGATION by means of a cauterizing instrument that is passed through the scope and coagulates the tubal openings.

Hysterotomy Surgery through the uterine wall to terminate a prgnancy of sixteen to twenty-four weeks. It resembles the operation of CAESAREAN SECTION, the foetus and placenta being removed through a small incision in the uterus. In some cases the foetus is alive when removed, but usually it dies very quickly because it is too immature to sustain life. The complications and mortality rate of hysterotomy are high enough to make it a dangerous procedure, far more so than AMNIOINFUSION for a second-trimester abortion, so that it should be used only for women whose medical problems rule out safer methods.

I

Iatrogenic disorder Any disorder directly resulting from medical treatment. Until modern times it was commonplace for physicians and surgeons to do more harm than good, and today medical care itself is still sometimes responsible for new illness. For example yeast infections of the vagina may follow the use of anti-biotics for unrelated infections.

Identical twins See under MULTIPLE PREGNANCY.

Idiopathic Having no known cause. Menstrual irregularities often are idiopathic.

Ileostomy A permanent surgical opening on the abdomen, where the ileum section of the small intestine, through which solid wastes (faeces) are eliminated, is brought to the surface. Usually the entire colon and rectum are removed. The end portion of the ileum is brought through the abdominal wall to form a *stoma* (opening), usually on the lower right side of the abdomen. An appliance (bag) must be worn over the stoma at all times to collect faeces and control odour. With a somewhat different procedure – the *Kock internal reservoir* operation – the diseased portion of intestine is removed and an internal sac is fashioned from some of the tissues; this sac, or reservoir, collects faecal matter,

which the patient must remove with a catheter four or five times a day. This method avoids the use of an appliance but can be used only on certain patients.

About 80 per cent of all ileostomies are performed for ulcerative colitis, a chronic inflammation of the colon characterized by bloody diarrhoea. Usually ileostomy is performed only when medical treatment over a period of time has failed to control the condition. Other indications are birth defects, familial polyposis (the formation of numerous polyps that may become cancerous), injury, cancer, and Crohn's disease or regional enteritis, a chronic inflammation of unknown cause that most often affects the lower ileum. The ileostomy substitutes for the elimination functions formerly performed by the colon.

Ileostomy involves major surgery and a period of recovery and readjustment afterward. It need not interfere with leading a normal life; only a job that requires heavy lifting may be contraindicated lest the stoma be injured. Sexual function in women is not at all impaired, and sexual potency in men only rarely (see also under OSTOMY). Bathing or showering can be done, with or without the appliance in place. Although a low-residue diet is usually recommended for the first few weeks after surgery (including only easily digested foods and no raw fruits or vegetables), a largely normal diet can usually be resumed fairly soon. Some, although not all, persons have excessive gas following ileostomy; it can usually be relieved by eliminating certain foods entirely, and by chewing all solid foods slowly and thoroughly

Immunotherapy Treatment of cancer that attempts to stimulate the body's immune system to produce cancer-fighting cells. For example, a strain of tuberculosis bacillus used to vaccinate human beings has shown some ability to kill cancer cells when administered in conjunction with levasimole, a drug used to treat certain parasitic infections. Another approach to immunotherapy uses actual tumour cells, or extracts from them, that are treated in various ways (by radiation or chemicals) and then rein-jected into patients. In one kind of such *radioimmunoglobulin therapy*, certain antibodies that react strongly with a protein found in many cancers are pro-duced in test animals, tagged with a radioisotope that makes them powerfully radioactive, and injected into cancer patients. The antibodies concentrate on the protein in the cancers, which are then bombarded with powerful radiation; the radioactive antibodies have little effect on other, healthy tissue and consequently cause less discomfort and fewer side effects than RADIATION THERAPY nor-mally does. Still another approach uses antibody cells from experimental animals, which are fused in the laboratory with cancer cells that enable them to grow indefinitely. These hybrid cells are then made to reproduce by cloning and are injected into cancer patients. In most instances immunotherapy is still highly experimental and therefore is used only in patients with advanced inoperable cancers.

Imperforate hymen See under HYMEN.

Implantation Also *nidation*. The attachment of the fertilized egg, or zygote, to the endometrium (wall of the uterus), which takes place seven to ten days after fertilization. During that period the fertilized egg travels through the Fallopian tube into the uterus. It then penetrates the soft uterine lining by means of enzymes that break down the endome-trial tissue. The outside layer of cells forms tentacles called *villi*, which dig into the endometrium and start to draw nourish-ing elements from it. By about the twelfth day after fertilization a rudimentary PLACENTA has begun to form at the site of implantation, and in the next week or two the zygote begins to develop a circu-latory system whereby nutrients and oxygen from the mother's body will be absorbed by the foetus through the thin-walled villi. Some women experience slight vaginal staining, called *implantation bleeding*, around the time of implantation, owing to the formation of new blood vessels there.

Impotence In men, a SEXUAL DYSFUNCTION that occurs during the excitement phase of sexual response, in which the man loses his ERECTION. A man may have difficulty in achieving or maintaining an erection with his partner, or he may lose the erection during penetration, or he may lost it after pene-tration but before ejaculation. Temporary impotence affects practically every man at one time or another; it can be caused by fatigue, anxiety, fear, grief, overin-dulgence in alcohol or drugs, or some other transient condition, and rarely persists long enough to require treatment. Impotence can have organic causes, representing a by-product of such diseases as sickle cell disease, leukaemia, diabetes, syphilis, endocrine disorders, vascular disorders, and neurologic disorders, or the side effect of certain medications. *Potency*—the ability to have and sustain an erection—is not impaired by masturbation or too frequent intercourse; conversely, there is no physical reason for male athletes to avoid sex before an important competitive event. Most prostate surgery does not affect potency, although afterward men may experience retrograde ejaculation (see EJACULATION, definition 4). Age also does not necessarily affect potency, although it may lengthen the time needed to achieve erection and nearly always lengthens the time of recovery after ORGASM. Sex therapists and other mental health professional prefer to avoid the term 'impotence' altogether because they believe it has excessively negative and perjorative connotations. Instead, they prefer the term SEXUAL DYSFUNCTION. See also SEX THERAPY.

Impregnation See FERTILIZATION; also ARTIFICIAL INSEMINATION.

Incest A sexual relationship between two persons who are so closely related that marriage between them would be prohibited by law and/or cultural taboo. The most common such combinations are parent and child, and brother and sister. A child born of two such closely related parents is far more likely to have serious birth defects.

Incompetent cervix Also *incompetent cervical os.* In pregnancy, the dilation of the cervix during the second trimester (fourth to sixth months), followed by rupture of the amniotic membranes and expulsion of the foetus, which is nearly always too immature to survive. Generally neither bleeding nor pain occurs, so there is little or no warning of the condition. The cause is not known, but since it rarely happens in a first pregnancy it is believed to result from injury to the cervix during a previous delivery, or during a D AND C or other surgical procedure. Moreover, it tends to recur with each subsequent pregnancy, making incompetent cervix one of the more common causes of HABITUAL MISCARRIAGE. Treatment consists of reinforcing the cervix with sutures that, in effect, tie it into closed normal position. This procedure is usually performed between the fourteenth and eighteenth weeks of pregnancy, before the cervical os has dilated to 4 centimetres (½ inches). The sutures must be removed before the onset of labour, usually during the thirty-eighth or thirty-ninth week, unless Caesarean delivery is planned (in that case they can be left in place). In the majority of cases this procedure will prevent miscarriage. If, however, it fails, the sutures must be removed as soon as there are signs of imminent miscarriage, lest the cervix be injured (see MISCARRIAGE, definition 2 and 3).

Incomplete miscarriage See MISCARRIAGE, definition 4.

Incubation period The time lapse between the moment an infectious agent invades the body and the first appearance of symptoms and signs of infection. In the common infectious diseases of childhood it varies from about three to five days for scarlet fever to as long as two to three weeks for rubella (German measles). The incubation period is not identical to the period of *communicability,* that is, the period during which another person exposed to the patient can be infected. Measles, for example, can be communicated to another person two to four days before a rash has appeared, but the incubation period ranges from seven to fourteen days.

Induction of labour Also *induced labour.* Stimulating uterine contractions in order to start or speed up labour and delivery. The two principal means of inducing labour, frequently used together, are rupturing the membranes (also called AMNIOTOMY) and administering the hormone oxytocin. (Another means of inducing labour that is performed much earlier in a pregnancy, in order to terminate it, is AMNIOINFUSION.) To induce labour successfully by merely rupturing the membranes, the cervix must be *ripe*; that is, the front must be soft, it must be more than 50 per cent effaced (altered in preparation for delivery), and it must be sufficiently dilated to admit an index finger easily (2 centimetres, or ¾ inch). If any of these conditions is absent, rupturing the membranes will probably not succeed in starting labour or, even if contractions do begin, the labour is likely to be prolonged (see PROLONGED LABOUR). Also, some doctors believe that premature rupture removes the baby's protection against strong uterine contractions, since there is less amniotic fluid to cushion it.

If the cervix is not ripe and labour needs to be induced because of PRE-ECLAMPSIA or some other serious condition, it is occasionally can be helped to dilate more by *stripping the membranes*. However, this can be done only if the cervix is already dilated enough to admit the doctors index finger. When it is, the doctor places a finger between the cervix and membranes and rotates the finger around the cervix to loosen the membranes. This may cause the cervix to dilate more quickly, but sometimes not for several days.

The other principal means of induction is by administering OXYTOCIN, usually in the form of an intravenous drip. Again, this procedure is only effective if effacement of the cervix has occurred and the cervix is dilated at least 3 (some say 4) centimetres. If labour has begun and the baby is in good position (not in any ABNORMAL PRESENTATION), the intravenous drip is carried on for as long as eight to ten hours if necessary, along with careful checking of the foetal heartbeat (see FOETAL MONITORING) and constant observation of uterine contractions. If there is foetal distress or the contractions become too strong, a Caesarean section may have to be performed.

Inevitable miscarriage See MISCARRIAGE, definition 3.

Infection The invasion of the body by micro-organisms, such as bacteria and viruses, that multiply and damage its cells and tissues. Many such organisms normally reside in the body, in the abdominal and uterine cavities, in the lungs, on the skin, and elsewhere. However, they are prevented from multiplying to an extent where they can cause damage by the activity of mucus and other natural body substances that kill some of them, as well as by bacteria-fighting white blood cells. Occasionally, however, such organisms do overcome the body's natural defence systems and an infection results.

The overall process of bacterial infection is similar no matter what kind of organism is involved or where it attacks. Bacteria are nourished by the very fluid or tissue they attack, and produce waste products that are released into these same tissues. White blood cells are sent into the area to defend it. The area becomes warm, red, and swollen, both from increased circulation and from the accumulation of pus (made up of dead bacteria, dead white cells, and fluids). The bacterial waste products meanwhile enter the blood stream and exert a poisonous effect on the body, which may be manifest in fever, chills, and generalized aches and malaise. Meanwhile some normal cells are being destroyed, either by bacteria directly, or indirectly by the excessive swelling and poisonous bacterial wastes. Even after the bacteria are eradicated by drugs such as antibiotics, body tissues may take some time to heal completely, and some many never return to normal, being replaced by so-called *scar tissue*.

Virus-caused infections, which range from the common cold to HERPES INFECTION, are not susceptible to antibiotics. Effective antiviral agents are still few in number, and those that do work often produce adverse reactions and undesirable side effects, and therefore require careful monitoring of patients who receive them. However, vaccines against a number of virus infections have been developed, and they have been used so successfully that in some areas these infections have virtually disappeared; among them are vaccines for smallpox, yellow fever, measles, mumps, rabies, poliomyelitis, and rubella (German measles).

The principal kinds of infection that attack women in particular are vaginal infections (see VAGINITIS), urinary infections (see CYSTITIS), breast infections (see MASTITIS), and infections of the pelvic organs (see ENDOMETRITIS; PELVIC IN-FLAMMATORY DISEASE). In addition, sexually active women are vulnerable to various sexually transmitted infectious diseases (see VENEREAL DISEASE). See also ABSCESS.

Infertility Inability to become pregnant after one year of regular intercourse, a condition that affects an estimated 15 per cent of British couples. In *primary infertility* there has been no preceding pregnancy; *secondary infertility* follows one or more pregnancies. In approximately 40 per cent of cases the cause lies in the man and usually is poor SPERM production; in about 40 per cent of cases the cause lies in the woman; and in the remaining 20 per cent the cause is either a combination of factors in both or is never determined. In women common causes of infertility are: hormonal dysfunction, so that ovulation does not take place or the eggs produced are not viable; blockage in the FALLOPIAN TUBES, so that the eggs cannot enter or pass through them, usually owing to scar tissue resulting from PELVIC INFLAMMATORY DISEASE; malformation of the uterus or Fallopian tubes; disorders affecting the cervix, so that sperm cannot move up through it, because of either local inflammation or hostile secretions; an immunologic reaction, resulting in the production of antibodies to the partner's sperm; and inability to remain pregnant (see HABITUAL MISCARRIAGE).

Determining the cause of infertility is the province of the fertility specialist, usually a gynaecologist. It begins with a careful history and physical examination of both partners, including blood and urine tests. Among the routine tests usually made are semen analysis (see under SPERM), BASAL BODY TEMPERATURE charts or an endometrial biopsy (see BIOPSY, definition 8) to find out if and when the woman is ovulating, a SIMS-HUHNER test to check the cervical mucus, one of the various tests to determine if the Fallopian tubes are obstructed (see RUBIN TEST; HYSTEROSALPINGOGRAPHY; LAPAROSCOPY), blood tests to measure hormone levels, and a test for sperm incompatility (see DUKE'S TEST), which is usually performed last because it is least likely to be correctable.

If the partner's semen analysis is normal but the cervical mucus test shows few or no sperm, different timing, techniques, and positions for intercourse may be suggested. If none of these is effective, ARTIFICIAL INSEMINATION with either the partner's sperm or, if semen samples show insufficient healthy sperm, a donor's sperm may be considered.

In the woman, cervical mucus consistency can be changed by oestrogen therapy and cervical infections cured by antiobiotics or other treatment. Also, artificial insemination involving insertion of the partner's sperm directly into the uterus may overcome problems in the cervix. Ovulation can be induced or improved by treatment with Clomid (see FERTILITY PILL). Uterine fibroids preventing the egg's implantation in the uterine wall may be corrected by surgery. Sometimes obstructed tubes can be corrected by surgery (see TUBEROPLASTY) but often they cannot be reconstructed successfully; then an embryo transplant procedure may result in a successful pregnancy (see TEST-TUBE BABY). Antibody formation against the partner's sperm sometimes is reduced by using a condom for intercourse for a period of six months, during which the antibody level may decline markedly; if this measure does not help, artificial insemination direct into the uterus normally will. See also OLIGOSPERMIA; STERILITY.

Inflammation   The body's protective response to injury or destruction of its tissues by micro-organisms such as bacteria, a foreign body (such as a splinter), poison, or some other trauma. In effect the body walls off the injured tissue (and, somtimes, the agent causing the injury) from the rest. The classic signs of inflammation are pain, heat, redness, swelling, and loss of function. Not all these signs are present with every inflammation. The presence of inflammation does not necessarily signal INFECTION, but neglected inflammation will often become complicated by infection.

Inherited disorder   See under BIRTH DEFECTS.

Infusion   See under HERBAL REMEDIES.

Insemination   The EJACULATION of semen into the vagina. See also SPERM; ARTIFICIAL INSEMINATION.

Insomnia   Also *sleeplessness*. Persistent lack of sleep or disturbed sleep patterns. A very common complaint, it is associated with a number of physical and emotional disorders. Insomnia is also common in late pregnancy, when it may be difficult to find a comfortable sleeping position, or one that is comfortable for more than a couple of hours at a time. The safest solution is to make up for sleep loss by napping briefly whenever possible during the day and avoiding all sedatives (even mild ones should not be taken without consulting one's doctor). Insomnia is also common during menopause, particularly if sleep is interrupted by night-time hot flushes and sweats. At least one study indicated that oestrogen therapy can alleviate such insomnia, but whether it does so because it relieves the hot flushes or because it actually alters sleep patterns was not determined; the former is more likely. Sleeplessness or disturbed sleep may also be caused by physical pain (discomfort is usually worse at night, partly because there are fewer activities to serve as a distraction), increasing age, emotional distress of various kinds (anxiety, stress, depression), and shifting to a different time pattern or zone (jet lag, usually temporary). Older people tend to need less sleep and often experience interrupted sleep; this is thought to be perfectly normal, since metabolism in general slows down with advancing age. Worrying is a time-honoured cause of wakefulness. Also, severe depression can cause a person either to sleep excessively or to awaken very early (several hours before the accustomed time) and be unable to fall asleep again.

Most medications for insomnia are hypnotic sedatives that depress brain function. The principal *sleeping pills* are benzodiazepines (TRANQUILLIZERS), nonbarbiturates (bromides, chloral hydrate, and others), and antihistamines (most nonprescription pills are of this class). All of them involve some risk of habituation and tolerance (needing ever larger doses to be effective), and some are addictive. They should be used, therefore, in only the smallest possible amounts for the shortest possible time, and never without medical supervision. Before considering medication, it is advisable to try such old-fashioned and much safer approaches as vigourous exercise (outdoors if possible) on a regular basis, taking a warm bath (but not too hot) and/or drinking a glass of warm milk or mild herb tea before going to bed, and avoiding cola, coffee, tea, and other caffeine-containing drinks in the evening.

When one does have trouble sleeping, getting out of bed to do something productive or pleasant – writing a letter, reading, doing a chore – may relieve some of the anxiety often experienced with wakefulness. Some HERBAL REMEDIES taken for their soothing, sedative effect are teas brewed from valerian root (*Valeriana officinalis*), camomile leaves and flowers (*Matricaria chamomilla*), or catnip (*Nepata cataria*).

Insufflation, tubal See RUBIN TEST.

Intercourse, sexual Broadly speaking, any kind of sexual contact. In practice, the term most often means COITUS, involving a man and a woman. See also anal sex, under ANUS; ORAL SEX; ORGASM; SEXUAL RESPONSE.

Interstitial-cell stimulating hormone Also *ICSH*. Another name for luteinizing hormone (LH), which in men triggers the growth of interstitial cells in the TESTES and stimulates their production of testosterone.

Intraductal papilloma See DUCTAL PAPILLOMA.

Intrauterine device Also *IUD*. A device made of plastic, metal, or some other material that is inserted into the uterus and allowed to remain there for months or years in order to prevent pregnancy. It is a reversible contraceptive – that is, once it is removed a woman can become pregnant if she wishes – but it differs from other reversible methods like the diaphragm in that it must be both inserted and removed by a doctor. It is not exactly known how the device prevents pregnancy. It does not prevent ovulation, nor does it always prevent conception. It does, however, cause an inflammation of the endometrium (uterine lining), which may work in one (or more) ways: prevent IMPLANTATION of the fertilized egg in the lining; cause white blood cells to attack either the sperm or the fertilized egg; speed up the movement of the egg through the Fallopian tube so that it is not mature enough for fertilization to take place; change the chemical environment of the uterus so that implantation cannot take place. One kind of IUD is covered with copper wire, a material that also helps prevent pregnancy (though it is not known how) and permits the use of a smaller IUD; another kind releases synthetic progesterone (PROGESTIN), which helps prevent sperm from entering the cervix by altering the cervical mucus.

Before the insertion of an IUD a woman should have a check-up that includes a careful history to make sure she has no reason not to use such a device. *No IUD should be used* by women who have any of the following conditions: pregnancy or suspected pregnancy; a previous ECTOPIC PREGNANCY; abnormal anatomy, such as a double uterus or a very small uterus; PELVIC INFLAMMATORY DISEASE or a history of several severe pelvic infections; GONORRHOEA or any other venereal disease, or the possibility of exposure to one; one or more fibroid tumours large enough to distort the shape of the uterus; vaginal bleeding from unknown causes; a history of heavy menstrual bleeding and/or severe menstrual cramps; active cervical infection (cervicitis) or an abnormal PAP SMEAR; endometrial disorders, especially ENDOMETRIOSIS or ENDOMETRIAL HYPERPLASIA; heart disease; diabetes; current use of cortisone-type drugs or anticoagulants. In addition, copper-containing IUDs should not be used by women allergic to copper. These contraindications rule out the IUD for about one out of five women.

In addition, many doctors are reluctant to insert an IUD in young women (under twenty-five) who have had no children and have numerous sexual partners, because of their increased risk of contracting venereal disease. At the least, such women should have a gonorrhoea test (since gonorrhoea is often symptomless in women) before an IUD is inserted.

Once the decision to use an IUD is made, the particular kind must be selected. Older devices, such as the Lippes Loop, fill the entire cavity of the uterus and, being larger, are preferable for women who have had at least one child. A woman who has had no children probably should have a smaller IUD, such as Novagard, Minigravigard or Copper-7 (which releases copper).

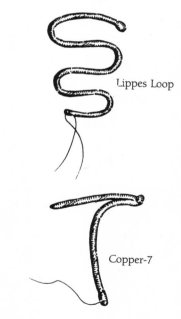

Lippes Loop

Copper-7

Two kinds of intrauterine device (IUD)

The timing of insertion is also important. Preferably it is done *during* a menstrual period, which indicates with some certainty that the woman is not pregnant (IUDs in pregnancy are dangerous; see below). Some doctors say it can be inserted immediately after an abortion, but others believe it then increases risk of uterine rupture, heavy bleeding, and infection. It is safe to insert during the first menstrual period following abortion. It can be inserted as early as eight weeks following vaginal delivery of a baby, even if the woman has not yet resumed menstruating, and three months after delivery by Caesarean section. Occasionally an IUD is inserted for morning-after birth control, that is, within five days of unprotected intercourse, to avoid possible pregnancy. However, this should be done only after a single instance of unprotected intercourse, because the insertion of an IUD after implantation of a fertilized egg can lead to serious damage. Some doctors consider it too risky.

An IUD can be inserted in a doctor's surgery, family planning clinic, or the outpatient department of a hospital. A pelvic examination is performed first to investigate the position of the uterus, and then a speculum is inserted. Local anaesthetic may be injected around the cervix; it takes effect in a few minutes. The cervix is then grasped with a clamp to hold it steady, and a long, thin uterine sound is inserted through the cervix to the top of the uterus, to measure its length. The sound is withdrawn, the IUD loaded into its inserter, and a stop is positioned on the inserter at the distance indicated by the sound. The loaded inserter is then passed into the uterus until the stop-mark reaches the cervix. The device is released by means of a plunger mechanism, and the inserter is withdrawn, leaving the IUD in place with its attached strings extending through the cervical opening into the vagina. The strings are cut so as to extend about two inches, and the woman should be told to feel them with her fingers once a week to make sure the IUD is still in place.

The IUD is effective against pregnancy immediately, but among the most common problems associated with it is spontaneous expulsion of the device from the uterus, which happens most often during the first three months after insertion. Therefore a back-up contraceptive is advisable during that period. Anywhere from 5 to 20 per cent of IUD users expel the device during the first year.

The insertion process ranges from being moderately uncomfortable to quite painful, with bleeding and cramping. After insertion, tampons and vaginal intercourse should be avoided for the remainder of that menstual period. The cramps gradually diminish. If they remain severe for more than twenty-four hours and/or there is fever, there may be an infection, and the doctor should be contacted immediately. Thereafter, most women find periods are heavier and longer than before, with more cramps as well. Also, many IUD users experience staining between periods, especially at midcycle; such bleeding should always be checked lest it be caused by some other disorder. BREAKTHROUGH BLEEDING after an IUD has been in place three months or longer is often an early sign of pelvic inflammatory disease.

Another complication is perforation, which most often happens during insertion. A puncture is made into the abdominal cavity (usually by the sound) and in time the IUD slips out of the uterus and into the abdomen, where it may cause no problem (unless it is copper-releasing) but can no longer, of course, prevent pregnancy. Absence of the strings protruding from the cervix therefore usually means either that the IUD has been expelled into the vagina, or it has moved elsewhere out of the uterus, and for this reason regular checking of the strings is important. Occasionally the strings become pulled up inside the uterus. Here, too, the doctor should check if the IUD is still in place and then attempt to pull the strings down again. If this manoeuvre cannot be carried out, the IUD may be removed and replaced with a new one, either at the same time or a month or so later.

If the IUD remains in position, it is about 96 per cent effective in preventing pregnancy. This means if one hundred women used it for a year, no more than four of them would become pregnant. For those who do become pregnant with an IUD in place, the consequences can be serious. The likelihood of miscarriage is very high – about 50 per cent – and if infection is present the situation can be very dangerous. Therefore, if a woman with an IUD skips a period or has other signs of early pregnancy, she should see her doctor very soon to rule out pregnancy; if she also has symptoms of infection, she should see someone immediately. If she is pregnant, the IUD should be removed within twenty-four hours to prevent infection, whether or not she intends to continue the pregnancy. If she then chooses to carry the baby, the risk for miscarriage is still higher than normal – about 30 per cent – but there is no other danger to the foetus. If she decides to terminate the pregnancy, the IUD can be removed at the time of abortion.

Another considerable risk is that of ECTOPIC PREGNANCY, which can be life-threatening. It is not known whether IUDs actually increase the risk of ectopic pregnancy or if they simply are less effective in preventing pregnancy outside the uterus than in it. In any case, the incidence in IUD users appears to be considerably higher than average.

Apart from pregnancy the principal complication of the IUD is a much higher incidence of pelvic infection. Again, it is not known whether bacteria can more easily enter the uterus by, in effect, climbing up the IUD strings, or whether the inflammatory effect of the IUD makes the uterus more susceptible to infection. Another hypothesis is that calcium deposits form around the device, as they do around many foreign substances, and create an environment favourable to bacterial growth. Such infections range from mild to severe, and can become life-threatening. Signs of infection should therefore be attended to promptly; they include abdominal pain or tenderness, pain during vaginal intercourse, fever or chills, and unusual vaginal bleeding or discharge (see also PELVIC INFLAMMATORY DISEASE). Infections of the cervix (cervicitis) also tend to occur more frequently in IUD users. Because of these complications and the side effects (chiefly more menstrual cramps and heavier flow), about half of the women who use IUDs have them removed within two years of their insertion. For those women who keep them, however, they represent a convenient and reversible form of birth control, without interfering with sexual activity before or at the time of intercourse, and without the need to remember to take a pill (see ORAL CONTRACEPTIVE).

Putting something inside the uterus to prevent pregnancy allegedly was first done by ancient camel drivers who inserted pebbles in their animals to prevent them from becoming pregnant on a long desert trek. Modern IUDs date from the early 1980s and a variety of materials have been used, ranging from silkworm gut to silver wire. Plastic IUDs were marketed in the late 1950, copper was added a decade later, and progestin in the 1970s. Since their development, a number of devices have been taken off the market. One was the Dalkon Shield (in 1974), which was linked to the death of a number of women and was thought to be responsible for uterine infection, septic abortion, and hysterectomy in more than 2,000 others. In 1968 the U.S. Food and Drug Administration already had recommended discontinuing IUDs that incorporate a closed design such as a circle or bow, and in 1973 a spring device (the Majzlin Spring) also had to be withdrawn because it tended to become imbedded in the uterine lining. IUDs available in 1987 included several open shapes and came in several sizes. However, the range of available IUDs is diminishing as manufacturers withdraw their products from the market because of the costs of defending themselves, even successfully, against litigation, mainly in the United States.

An inert plastic IUD can stay in place for years but should be checked at least once a year and removed within six months after menopause. A progestin-releasing IUD must be replaced yearly, and a copper IUD every two to five years. Despite their disadvantages, it was estimated that some 50 million women the world over currently use an IUD.

Intrauterine polyps See POLYP, definition 3.

Introitus An opening, specifically the opening of the VAGINA, which occupies the lower part of the VESTIBULE. It varies considerably in size and shape. In virgins it is hidden by the overlapping LABIA minora; when exposed, it may appear to be almost completely blocked by the HYMEN.

Intromission See under ERECTION.

Inverted nipple See under NIPPLE.

In vitro fertilization See TEST-TUBE BABY.

Involution, uterine The return of the uterus to its prepregnant condition following a pregnancy. It begins almost immediately after delivery of the baby, even before expulsion of the placenta (see under LABOUR), and is aided by continued uterine contractions for about forty-eight hours after delivery. From a two-pound mass of muscle immediately after birth, it changes back into a smooth, hard, gourd-shaped organ. By the end of a week it weighs one pound and has descended to about two inches above the pubic bone. Soon afterward it sinks within the pelvis and can no longer be felt by merely palpating the abdomen. The process of shrinkage progresses more rapidly when a woman breastfeeds. It continues until, after five or six weeks following delivery, the uterus is again the size and shape of a pear, weighing about two ounces. The growth of the uterus during pregnancy consists of an increase in size of each individual muscle fibre, which in turn must shrink again during involution. This process of growth and involution takes place with each pregnancy, making the uterus unique among body organs.

Iron See under ANAEMIA; DIET.

Irradiation See RADIATION THERAPY.

Irregular periods A widely varying MENSTRUAL CYCLE, with menstrual flow occuring at very irregular intervals, for example, 21 days, then 42 days, then 35 days, then 28 days, etc. This condition frequently occurs in girls during their first two or three years of menstruating, and in women approaching menopause. It is caused by hormone imbalance, particularly lack of progesterone in the absence of ovulation (see ANOVULATORY BLEEDING). Irregular periods can also be caused by stress, emotional problems, crash reducing diets, thyroid disturbances, iron or platelet deficiency (see ANAEMIA), any serious illness, and a variety of pelvic lesions ranging from endometrial hyperplasia to cancer. See also BREAKTHROUGH BLEEDING; OLIGO-MENORRHOEA; POLYMENORRHOEA.

Ischial spines See under PELVIMETRY.

Itching Also *pruritus*. An irritating sensation of the skin that is relieved by scratching. Although itching may be a symptom of skin disease as well as other disorders in both men and women, two kinds affect women only. One occurs during the latter months of pregnancy, when some women develop intense itching, sometimes accompanied by jaundice. Also called *cholestasis of pregnancy*, it is caused by the effects of increased hormone levels on liver function and disappears completely after delivery. However, it is apt to recur in subsequent pregnancies and also if an oestrogen-high oral contraceptive is later used. The other, itching of the vulva and vagina, is common in VULVITIS and VAGINITIS, which may be due to inflammation and infection from a variety of causes, as well as from dry skin and membranes (see VAGINAL ATROPHY). The itching from YEAST INFECTIONS often spreads to the area around the anus as well. Treating the underlying causes of infection usually cures the itching, but sometimes a topical cortisone ointment must be used for a time to clear up the skin involved.

IUD See INTRAUTERINE DEVICE.

J

Jelly, contraceptive See under
SPERMICIDE; also LUBRICANT.

K

Karyotyping A genetic study to diagnose problems leading to habitual miscarriage and possible birth defects. Chromosomes from a woman's tissue – usually white blood cells scraped from the lining of the mouth – are photographed, the photographs are enlarged, and the chromosomes cut out and arranged according to size and structure on a chart called a *karotype*. This process may reveal various chromosomal abnormalities such as the 'fragile X' trait responsible for a common form of mental retardation. See also CHROMOSOME.

Kegal exercises Also *pelvic floor exercises*. Exercises to strengthen the pubococcygeous muscle of the pelvic floor in order to reduce sagging, prevent urinary incontinence (see STRESS INCONTINENCE), strengthen orgasmic response, and prepare for and recover from childbirth. Named after their inventor, Arnold Kegel, an American doctor, they consist of alternately contracting (tightening) and relaxing the pubococcygeous muscle, which can be located by sitting on the toilet with legs spread wide and alternatively starting and stopping the flow of urine. The first exercise consists of alternate contraction and relaxation of this muscle, holding each for three seconds, working up to fifty times a day. When this has been mastered, a second exercise, called 'flicking', consists of alternate contraction-relaxation of the muscle as quickly as possible, up to fifty times per day. These can then be combined with a breathing exercise: take a deep breath and tighten the muscle, then relax the muscle while exhaling (ten times a day). Finally, there is an exercise consisting of alternately bearing down as though expelling something from the vagina and then tightening the muscle. This last exercise should not be performed during late pregnancy.

Kerr incision See under CAESAREAN SECTION.

Klinefelter's syndrome A congenital condition in which a male has three chromosomes, X, X, and Y, instead of one X and one Y chromosome, and therefore is usually sterile. He usually has a small penis and testes, and the secondary sex characteristics (deep voice, beard, pubic hair, chest hair, etc.) are weakly developed and do not respond to the administration of male hormones. There is a much higher than normal incidence of mental retardation as well. Some men with Klinefelter's syndrome develop breast growth at puberty, and, indeed, this syndrome is associated with a very high risk of breast cancer, an estimated sixty-six times greater than that of normal men. Klinefelter's syndrome occurs in about one of every seven hundred live male births, and, being a chromosomal defect, may be detected with AMNIOCENTESIS.

Kronig-Selheim incision See under CAESAREAN SECTION.

L

Labia *labium* (sing.). A Latin word meaning 'lips', referring to two sets of tissue folds that serve to protect the vaginal opening. The outer, larger pair of labia, or *labia majora* (*labium majorus*, sing.) are composed mostly of fatty tissue and correspond to the scrotum in men. Extending back from the MONS VENERIS to the perineum, they vary considerably in size and appearance, but on average they are 7 to 8 centimetres (3 inches) long, 2 to 3 centimetres (1 inch) wide, and 1 to 1½ centimetres (½ inch) thick. In children and virgins they usually lie close together, completely concealing what lies underneath, whereas in women who have borne one or more children they often gape widely. Their outer surface is dry, covered with skin, and after puberty, with hair. Their inner surface is moist, has little or no hair, and is richly supplied with sebaceous (oil) glands. After menopause the labia majora gradually shrink in size.

The inner pair of labia, or *labia minora* (*labium minus*, sing.), are two flat, firm, reddish folds that extend down from the clitoris. At their upper end each labium minus divides into two separate folds that form the prepuce (foreskin) surrounding the CLITORIS. They, too, vary greatly in size, and also in shape. Before childbearing they are usually hidden by the labia majora, but afterward they may project beyond them. Their outer cover-ing looks more like mucous membrane (like the inside of the mouth) than skin. They are hairless but have many seba-ceous glands and some sweat glands. The interior is supplied with numerous nerve endings and so is extremely sensitive.

Labour Also *accouchement, childbirth, confinement, parturition.* The process of giving birth to a baby, the actual birth being called *delivery.* In nearly all animals whose young are conceived and carried inside the mother's body, labour begins spontaneously after a more or less fixed period of time (GESTATION), when the baby is mature enough to survive in the outside world but still small enough to make its way out of the mother's body. What exactly triggers the onset of labour, in human beings or other animals, is not known.

Labour is quite literally physical work, that is, the generation of motion against resistance. The forces involved in labour are the muscles of the UTERUS, dia-phragm, and abdominal wall, opposed by resistance to the baby's passage by the structures of the BIRTH CANAL. Contrac-tions of the uterine muscles, aided by hormonal changes, cause the cervix to soften, thin out, and dilate to allow the baby through it. This process usually takes up most of the time of labour. Continuing contractions of the uterus and abdominal muscles then propel the baby through the bony birth canal. The muscles of the pelvic floor force the baby's head to rotate and extend as continued pressure from above expels the baby. This pressure often results in considerable molding of the baby's head in order to permit its passage.

Labour is divided into three stages. The *first stage*, which begins with the first perceived uterine contraction and ends with the full *dilatation* of the cervix to a diameter of 10 centimetres (4 inches; also called 5 fingers, since it is about the width of the average man's fingers held closed), involves both uterine contractions and the resulting hydrostatic pressure of the amniotic membranes against the cervix, or, if the membranes have already ruptured and separated, the pressure of the baby's presenting part against the cervix (see also AMNIOTIC SAC; DRY LABOUR). During this stage of labour the cervical canal is flattened and shortened to the point of disappearing altogether.

The *second stage* of labour, or stage of *expulsion*, begins with the complete dilatation of the cervix and ends with the expulsion of the baby (delivery). During this stage the baby descends – slowly but surely with a first baby, more rapidly in subsequent births – as it is pushed downwards by the uterine muscles with the help of the abdominal muscles and the diaphragm. The amniotic membranes usually rupture during this stage if they have not done so already. In a head-first, or vertex, delivery, the baby's head begins to distend the vagina and vulva, and eventually *crowns*, that is, appears in the vaginal entrance. Then the head, followed by the rest of the baby, is delivered. In a breech presentation the lower pole of the baby, that is, feet and legs, or buttocks, leads the way, followed by the trunk, shoulders, and head; this requires more active effort from the mother, since the head is the largest part of the baby, and is also more hazardous to the baby, because its oxygen supply may be compromised by pressure of the umbilical cord between its body and the birth canal. (See also PROLAPSED CORD.)

The *third stage* of labour involves the separation of the PLACENTA from the uterine wall and its expulsion. As the baby is born, the uterus shrinks to fits its diminishing contents. During the process the placenta is forced down until it separates from the uterine wall and is pushed out. The remaining amniotic membranes are stripped out along with the placenta, partly by the continuing uterine contractions and partly by traction exerted by the placenta. Some women cannot push the placenta out of the vagina, but they can be assisted simply by pressure of the birth attendant's hand over the fundus (top of the uterus), which stimulates the uterus to contract more.

The average duration of the first stage of labour with a first baby is about twelve hours, and with subsequent children about seven hours, but there is marked variation among indivduals, and the position of the baby also affects the time (see ABNORMAL PRESENTATION; PROLONGED LABOUR). Toward the end of the first stage of labour, when the cervix is dilated about 8 centimetres, the contractions become much stronger and longer, with less relaxation between them; this period is called the *transition* and is often accompanied by any of various symptoms, particularly nausea, vomiting, trembling, and irritability. However, the transition rarely lasts longer than half an hour with a first baby. The average duration of the second stage is one to two hours with a first baby, and twenty

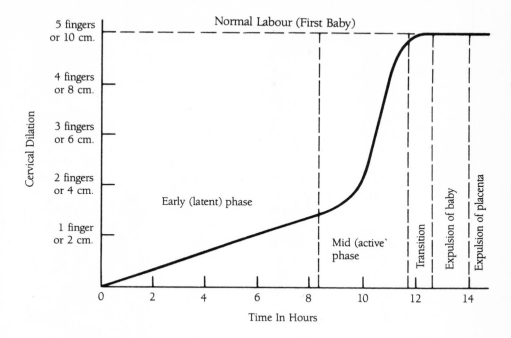

Normal Labour (First Baby)

Cervical Dilation

5 fingers or 10 cm.
4 fingers or 8 cm.
3 fingers or 6 cm.
2 fingers or 4 cm.
1 finger or 2 cm.

Early (latent) phase

Mid (active) phase

Transition

Expulsion of baby

Expulsion of placenta

0   2   4   6   8   10   12   14

Time In Hours

minutes or less with subsequent births. In the third stage, placental separation rarely takes more than two or three minutes, and placental expulsion about five minutes more. The reason for faster labour in multiparas (women who have given birth previously) is that the cervix, once dilated in labour, offers less resistance the next time; the same is true of the pelvic floor, which tends to be more relaxed. Labour also tends to proceed faster than normal when the membranes have ruptured before labour has begun, which occurs in about 12 per cent of all cases, lasting on average about ten hours with first pregnancies and six hours with subsequent ones.

See also ANAESTHESIA; CONTRACTION, UTERINE; DRY LABOUR; FALSE LABOUR; INDUCTION OF LABOUR; PREPARED CHILDBIRTH.

Labour, induction of See INDUCTION OF LABOUR.

Lactation The production of milk by the breasts, which is controlled by two hormones, prolactin and oxytocin. Prolactin is secreted by the pituitary gland. Except after delivery of a baby or under other special circumstances, it is inhibited (suppressed) by another substance, prolactin-inhibiting factor (PIF), secreted by the hypothalamus. After childbirth PIF is not produced and prolactin is released, stimulating the ACINI to secrete milk. As the baby suckles, more prolactin is released and more milk is produced, a process that continues until breast-feeding is discontinued. If a woman decides not to breast-feed, however, milk production will stop within a few days after delivery provided that her breasts are not stimulated by suckling. Binding the breasts, restricting fluid intake, or administering oestrogen, all measures formerly used to stop milk production, are not effective; only the lack of suckling stops lactation. Furthermore, the use of oestrogen for this purpose is associated with a higher incidence of blood clots. Stimulation from suckling also makes the posterior pituitary gland release oxytocin, the same hormone that stimulates uterine contractions during labour. It is oxytocin that is responsible for the LET-DOWN REFLEX which squeezes milk into and through the ducts in the breast.

The preparation of the breasts for lactation begins during pregnancy, when high levels of oestrogen and progesterone cause the growth of breast ducts and maturation of glandular structures. Because of the increased glandular mass, a pregnant woman's breasts enlarge significantly. During the second trimester of pregnancy the cells of the acini are stimulated to produce *colostrum*, a protein-rich yellowish fluid that also contains minerals, vitamin A, nitrogen, and antibodies. Colostrum continues to be produced until two or three days after delivery, when lactation begins; it is the baby's first nourishment. If lactation is suppressed by lack of suckling, colostrum production also ceases.

After delivery the production of pituitary prolactin increases rapidly, and milk is secreted on the third or fourth day after delivery. At this time the bulk of the breasts increases considerably, by as much as one-third, a phenomenon called *engorgement*. It may be accompanied by some discomfort (tenderness and pain) but generally disappears by itself within one or two days, particularly if breast-feeding is begun. Allowing the baby to nurse very briefly and/or manually expressing a little of the fluid can give some relief. If the mother decides not to breast-feed, firm breast support, ice bags, and mild analgesics will afford relief until engorgement subsides.

For centuries women have used HERBAL REMEDIES either to increase or to decrease their milk supply. An infusion of borage seeds and leaves (*Borago officinalis*) or fennel (*Foeniculum officinale*) eaten raw as a vegetable or fennel seeds steeped into a tea supposedly increase the flow of milk. To decrease the milk supply and assist weaning, teas made from cinnamon sticks or the powdered spice or from common sage (*Salvia officinalis*) have been used.

Normally prolactin is released only after childbirth. However, tumours of the pituitary gland, the oestrogen in oral contraceptives, and certain drugs can interfere with prolactin regulation, so that breast milk is produced without the stimulus of suckling. Also, severe emotional or physical stress can affect the hypothalamus and interfere with its production of PIF. Occasionally lactation has been deliberately induced in women who have not recently given birth – or, in rare cases, in women who have never been pregnant – in order to breast-feed an adopted child. Also milk production can sometimes be re-established after a long interruption owing to early weaning or a separation of mother and baby. Such lactation is usually induced by stimulation through suckling, massage, and the expression of milk by hand or mechanical or electric breast pumps. See also BREAST-FEEDING.

Lactobacilli See YOGHURT.

Lamaze method See PSYCHOPROPHYLACTIC METHOD.

Laminaria A species of seaweed that is very useful for dilating the cervix before D AND C or other procedure requiring the insertion of instruments through it. When wet, laminaria expands to a diameter three to five times greater than when dry. One or two thin rods of laminaria are inserted into the cervical canal, where, during the course of six hours or so, they absorb moisture from cervical mucus and gradually swell, thereby very gradually widening the cervical canal. A mild cramp or two may be felt when the laminaria are first inserted, but thereafter there usually is little or no discomfort when they swell, making this method, unlike other ways of dilating the cervix, practically painless. After insertion is is important to avoid douching, use of tampons, vaginal intercourse, or anything else involving putting something into the vagina.

Laparoscopy Also *Band-aid surgery, belly-button operation*. The insertion of a long, narrow optical instrument through a small (half-inch to one-inch) incision in the abdominal wall just below the navel (hence 'belly-button operation') in order to obtain a panoramic view of the pelvic organs and structures. It is used to detect adhesions (scar tissue), ovarian cysts, ectopic pregnancy, endometriosis, and other sources of acute abdominal and pelvic pain, as well as causes of infertility. The injection of two or more litres of carbon dioxide or nitrous gas into the abdomen lifts the abdominal wall up and away from the underlying bowel, exposing the uterus and Fallopian tubes. Specially designed instruments can then be passed through the laparoscope to remove a wandering IUD (see INTRA-UTERINE DEVICE), diagnose a tubal pregnancy or endometriosis, or perform a TUBAL LIGATION. When the laparoscopy is completed and the gas removed from the abdomen, the tiny incision can be closed with a single absorbable suture (stitch) and covered with a Band-aid (hence the name 'Band-aid surgery').

There are enormous advantages to laparoscopy as a diagnostic aid, since it can avoid a larger incision and major surgery (see LAPAROTOMY). For sterilization, it requires more skill of the doctor than an abdominal TUBAL LIGATION although it is easier for the patient. It is easier to perform immediately after childbirth, but most obstetricians wait eight weeks after delivery. Only regional anaesthesia is needed, but general anaesthesia is often used.

Regardless of the anaesthesia used, the woman may leave the hospital within eight hours, and the dressing (Band-aid) may be removed the next day. The patient may even have vaginal intercourse on the same day if she wishes. The principal discomfort felt is chest and shoulder pain caused by a residual pocket of gas in the abdomen, which stimulates a nerve that refers the pain to the chest and shoulder. Such pain usually lasts three to five days but can persist for a week. Air travel should be avoided for several weeks, however, because pressure changes may affect the residual carbon dioxide, causing pain.

Laparoscopy should not be undertaken in women with intestinal obstruction, extensive abdominal cancer or tuberculosis, or a serious heart condition. Previous surgery for a ruptured appendix or extensive intestinal disease, such as ulcerative colitis, are also contraindications, since scar tissue from these procedures can make laparoscopy useless. In women with an umbilical HERNIA laparoscopy can be performed but the incision should be made at least two inches lower than usual, farther away from the navel (umbilicus). Finally, for women in their late forties, close to menopause, laparoscopy for sterilization may not be worth the risk, since their chances of becoming pregnant are fairly small, and safer contraceptive measures are available. See also MINILAPAROTOMY.

Laparotomy Abdominal surgery that is usually performed for exploratory purposes, that is, to diagnose a suspected serious problem, such as ectopic pregnancy, an enlarged ovary that might be cancerous, or severe pelvic infection with suspicion of appendicitis or a pelvic abscess, or to assess the spread of some cancers. An incision about five inches long is made in the lower abdomen, enabling the surgeon to examine the uterus, Fallopian tubes, ovaries, and abdominal organs. Preparation for it and recovery are similar to abdominal HYSTERECTOMY and abdominal TUBAL LIGATION. See also LAPAROSCOPY; MINILAPAROTOMY.

Leboyer method Also *birth without violence, gentle birth.* An approach intended to ease the trauma of birth for the newborn baby by using a darkened room, eliminating harsh or sudden noises, and slowly and gently easing the baby from the mother's body. Frédéric Leboyer, the French obstetrician who promoted this approach in about 1970, also believed that the baby should not be swaddled in clothes but first be placed in a warm bath resembling its surroundings in the amniotic fluid, and slowly allowed to acclimatize itself to a stretched-out position before being dried and wrapped.

Leiomyoma Another name for FIBROID.

Lesbian A female homosexual, that is, a woman who prefers other women for sexual partners instead of men. The name comes from Lesbos, an island on which the ancient Greek poet Sappho lived and wrote of her love for other women. Until the latter half of the 20th century lesbians, like male homosexuals, were almost universally regarded as ill and/or insane.

Physically lesbians are in no way different from heterosexual women. They undergo puberty, menstruation, childbearing, and menopause in exactly the same way. The only difference is that sexually they respond to other women rather than to men. Some lesbians discover this preference in their early lives; others find out much later, sometimes after years of heterosexual marriage.

A number of health-care issues particularly affect lesbians, owing to their style of life. If they have exclusively lesbian relationships, they need neither birth control nor obstetric care; therefore they are less likely to seek annual gynaecological examinations and may become careless about procedures such as a regular PAP SMEAR. Furthermore, their experiences with conventional clinics and doctors, who are often intolerant of or insensitive to lesbians, may lead them to avoid such contacts whenever possible. Thus, when they contract a serious disease they run a higher risk of its being overlooked in its early, more readily curable, stages. Lesbians are less likely than heterosexual woman to become infected with syphilis or gonorrhoea, but they are just as likely to get some of the common vaginal infections, such as yeast infection, trichomonas, and herpes.

Another problem is childbearing. Women who discover they are lesbians after they have borne children and subsequently divorced from their husbands often have difficulty obtaining custody of their children, especially if they are living with another woman. Some lesbians who never married may still want children and wish to undergo artificial insemination. Lingering prejudice makes it difficult, sometimes impossible, to find facilities for this procedure. To overcome this some women have experimented with home methods of artificial insemination, using the sperm of a willing donor collected in a condom and inserting it into the vagina. Little is known about the outcome of these experiments.

Perhaps the most frustrating area for lesbians is that of mental health. Lesbians have the same emotional problems as heterosexual women; in fact, they may have more, simply because they are subject to considerable stress in a society that is, for the most part, different in its preferences and values. Yet many doctors are still in the foreground of those who consider lesbianism itself a disease and find it difficult to treat a lesbian with, for example, profound DEPRESSION without trying to make her change to a 'healthier' (that is, heterosexual) orientation.

Lesion Any change in tissue that differentiates it from the same kind of tissue in surrounding areas and that is caused by disease or injury. Examples include wounds such as a cut or burn, a pimple of acne, a chancre of syphilis, a wart, or an abscess. See also PRECANCEROUS LESIONS.

Let-down reflex The forcing of milk through the breasts, which may produce a momentary feeling of tightening or tingling. It is caused by the hormone oxytocin, whose production in turn is stimulated by suckling – or a baby's cry, or even the mere thought of suckling –

in a lactating woman. Oxytocin causes the smooth muscle fibres surrounding the ACINI (milk ducts) to contract, so that they are compressed and the milk secreted is forced into and through the big ducts of the breasts and in the nipples. The sensation stops as soon as milk is released. The let-down reflex is strongest during the first few weeks of breast-feeding, and usually occurs simul-taneously in both breasts. Some women, however, do not notice it at all. If the let-down reflex is triggered while a breast-feeding mother is away from her child, she may be able to prevent milk from leaking by exerting light pressure on the nipple area with the palm of her hand, fingers, or arms. See also LACTATION; BREAST-FEEDING.

Leukoplakia, vulvar The formation of white patches on the vulva, which may or may not be forerunners of cancer (see PRECANCEROUS LESIONS). Since they are difficult to distinguish from scar tissue formed after chronic infection in the area, and from the thinning and drying of tissue associated with ageing, the term is not very exact. The observation of leuko-plakia should be followed with tests to determine the cause and what treatment, if any, should be undertaken. See also PAGET'S DISEASE, definition 2.

Leucorrhoea   See   DISCHARGE, VAGINAL.

Libido Also *sex drive*. The desire to engage in sexual activity. It varies greatly in intensity and frequency both from one individual to another, and within a single person. The range of what is 'normal' libido is so broad that it defies definition. The biochemical changes of puberty, particularly the enormous increase in sex hormone production, usually result in a surge of libido during adolescence, especially in boys but also in girls; the difference apparently is due to increased levels óf ANDROGEN in boys. However, just as SEXUAL RESPONSE is governed by conscious thought and feeling, so is libido; consequently increases or decreases in sex drive can be caused largely or entirely by psychological or external factors, and not only by the body's chemistry. Seemingly insatiable libido (formerly called *nymphomania* in women) leading to more or less indiscriminate choice of sexual partners (so-called *promiscuity*) is nearly always the result of emotional problems and leads to physical problems only in that it exposes a woman to a much greater risk of VENEREAL DISEASE.

Fatigue and mental preoccupation are major factors in reducing sexual desire in both men and women. So are fear of pregnancy, intense involvement in work, serious personal problems, and marital conflict. When reduced libido becomes a chronic problem, it is considered a form of SEXUAL DYSFUNCTION and may be helped by sex therapy. Illness and certain medications, notably tranquillizers and some antihypertension drugs, also may diminish sex drive. Some oral contraceptives seem to increase the sex drive, and others to lessen it; use of an intrauterine device (IUD) has similarly mixed effects. In both cases increased libido may result from removing the fear of pregnancy, but with oral contraceptives changed hormone levels may be responsible as well. Similarly, pregnancy itself makes some women more interested in sexual activity and others markedly less so. After menopause, too, libido may be increased, decreased, or unchanged, and some women in their eighties or older – usually those who enjoyed sexual relations when younger – continue to enjoy them in old age.

The term 'libido' was used by Sigmund Freud and some followers of his theories in a broader sense to mean all physical energy controlled by an unconscious part of the mind that they called the 'id'.

Lightening Also *dropping*. In a pregnant woman, the descent of the fundus (top) of the uterus from the position it occupies at about thirty-six weeks of pregnancy to that of the month before (thirty-two weeks), caused by the gradual descent of the baby's head into the pelvic inlet. Most noticeable in a first pregnancy, lightening occurs a few weeks before labour begins. The abdomen changes in shape, the lower portion becoming more pendulous (droopy) and the overall shape less protuberant. The baby's head, which was freely movable until now, becomes fixed in the pelvic inlet. After lightening a woman often finds it easier to breathe, since the enlarged uterus no longer presses up against the rib cage, but she may find it harder to walk, may suffer from leg cramps, and may find she must void more frequently, all owing to pressure on the blood vessels of the legs and on the bladder.

Lipoma A benign (noncancerous) tumour of the breast, made up of fat tissue. If it can be established without a doubt that a growth is actually a lipoma, usually possible only by means of biopsy, it can simply be left alone. If the growth is unusually firm in consistency or has other characteristics making the diagnosis doubtful, it is usually surgically removed.

Lips, inner and outer See LABIA.

Lithotomy See DORSAL LITHOTOMY.

Liver spots Brown spots on the skin that resemble large freckles, occuring around and after menopause, particularly on the hands, forearms, face, and other parts of the body that are frequently exposed to the sun. They are caused by an increase in melanin, the pigment that influences skin colour and is itself influenced by hormones such as oestrogen, progesterone, and melanocyte-forming hormone. It is not known whether the formation of liver spots is related to cumulative sunlight exposure over the years, since melanin acts to keep the sun's rays from harming the skin, or the hormone imbalance associated with menopause, or both, or other factors not yet identified. However, even women who formerly were not especially sensitive to sunlight are advised to avoid direct exposure and overexposure from their middle years on.

LMP Abbreviation for *last menstrual period*, specifically the first day of the last menstrual period preceding a pregnancy. It is used in assessing the length of gestation. See also PREGNANCY TEST.

Local anaesthesia See REGIONAL ANAESTHESIA.

Lochia A vaginal discharge experienced after childbirth. For the first few days following delivery it consists of blood-stained fluid. After three or four days it becomes paler, and after the tenth day, owing to the presence of additional white blood cells, it becomes yellowish white or whitish. Normal lochia has a peculiar fleshy odour suggesting fresh blood; a foul smell signals postpartum infection.

Lubricant Any substance that reduces friction. During sexual arousal the walls of the vagina secrete a lubricant, mucus, to facilitate COITUS. Inadequate lubrication can make vaginal intercourse painful and can be a constant problem for some women. A longer period of foreplay for sexual arousal, or use of a little saliva to assist penetration, may be all that is needed. If these measures do not suffice, or if inadequate lubrication is due to hormonal changes, which for some women occur during every menstrual cycle and others only after menopause (so-called VAGINAL ATROPHY) and/or while breast-feeding, the use of a water-soluble lubricant such as K-Y jelly will usually solve the problem. Some women prefer to use natural vegetable oils, such as safflower or sunflower oil, and others use substances like yoghurt. Treatment with hormone creams or pills is also effective, since oestrogen promotes vaginal mucus production, but may not be worth its risks or side effects (see OESTROGEN REPLACEMENT THERAPY). Vaseline (petroleum jelly), although it does lubricate, is not water-soluble and does not wash off readily; furthermore, it damages the rubber of a condom, diaphragm, or cervical cap and should therefore not be used together with these birth-control devices.

Lumpectomy See MASTECTOMY, definition 7.

Lunaception A system of determining when OVULATION takes place that is based on the idea that exposure to sunlight and moonlight influences the timing of the MENSTRUAL CYCLE. Researchers have found that some women who sleep with a light on for several days at midcycle will begin to ovulate during those days.

The relation of light to body cycles had been observed by many ancient and primitive peoples – indeed, the words 'moon' and 'menstruation' have a common root – and modern research indicates that light may influence the reproductive system through the PINEAL GLAND. One woman, Louise Lacey, began to experiment on herself and discovered she could use light to regulate her cycle so as to make it a reliable means of birth control. However, much wider testing is needed to verify the effectiveness of this method. See also NATURAL FAMILY PLANNING.

Lupus   See   SYSTEMIC   LUPUS ERYTHEMATOSUS.

Lymph A pale, yellowish fluid that travels throughout the body by means of the lymphatic system and is derived from tissue fluids. Lymph consists of white blood cells in a plasma-like liquid. It is collected from tissues in all parts of the body and is returned to the blood via the *lymphatic system*, a circulatory network of lymph-carrying vessels, and the *lymphoid organs* – mainly the lymph nodes, spleen, and thymus – which produce and store infection-fighting white blood cells.

Lymphoedema Chronic swelling of the extremities owing to accumulation of fluid that results from obstruction or severance of LYMPH vessels and/or disorders or removal of the lymph nodes. It is characterized by puffiness and swelling of the affected arm or leg. Lymphoedema is a common after-effect of radical MASTECTOMY (definitions 2, 3, 4), which nearly always injures enough lymph vessels and nodes in the armpit near the site of the removed breast to create chronic swelling in the arm on that side. Moreover, that arm and hand become more vulnerable to infection, so that even a small burn or cut may lead to widespread infection and high fever. There is no effective cure for lymphoedema once it has occurred. Therefore, following a radical mastectomy, a woman is advised to wear gloves when gardening or using strong detergents, use a thimble when sewing, avoid touching harsh chemicals and abrasive compounds, take precautions against burns, including sunburn, have all injections, vaccinations, and blood pressure tests administered to the unaffected arm, avoid restrictive pressure on that arm and hand, and carry antibiotic ointment and bandages to treat unavoidable small injuries, hangnails, and scrapes. Postoperative lymphoedema can often be controlled by frequent and sustained arm elevation, regular use of a lightweight elastic, custom-fitted sleeve, and intermittent treatment with an inflatable sleeve called a pneumatic pump. Exercises, weight loss, and physiotherapy are also of some help.

Lymph nodes Small, bean-shaped masses of tissue situated along the vessels of the lymphatic system (see LYMPH). The nodes act as filters, removing bacteria or cancer cells from the lymphatic fluid.

Lymphogranuloma venereum Also *I.G.V.* A widespread VENEREAL DISEASE caused by an organism that has characteristics of both a virus and a bacterium, and is transmitted by vaginal, anal, and sometimes oral-genital sexual intercourse. It may also be spread by close physical contact other than intercourse. The organisms attack the lymph nodes. Symptoms appear five to twenty-one days (usually seven to twelve days) after infection, beginning with a tiny painless bump or pimple on the genitals, in men usually on the penis or urethra, in women anywhere on the vulva or in the vagina. The sore usually disappears by itself within a few days and, since it is painless, may not be noticed by the infected person. The organisms then spread from the initial site to nearby lymph vessels and glands, usually those in the groin. Ten to thirty days after the original infectious contact the lymph glands in one or both sides become swollen and tender. The swollen glands fuse together to form a single, painful, sausage-shaped mass called a *bubo*, which lies in the folds of the groin. The glands swell above and below the groin fold, giving the bubo a grooved appearance. The skin over the bubo becomes a bluish-red; some of the glands in the bubo are soft, others hard. In most cases these lymph glands are destroyed and several abscesses form that push to the surface and release pus. In about one-quarter of cases the bubo disappears spontaneously without treatment.

The formation of a bubo is more common in heterosexual men than in women or homosexual men. In women the original sore is often deep in the vagina, and the organism invades the deeper pelvic lymph glands. In homosexual men the sore may form in the anus and from there also invades the deeper pelvic lymph glands. In these instances visible bubos do not form, and the infected person remains unaware of the disease.

As the lymph glands are invaded, both men and women may have fever, chills, abdominal pain, loss of appetite, and joint pain. Backache often occurs when the deep pelvic lymph glands become infected. If treatment is delayed, complications may develop. Among them are anal and rectal problems when the anal area is invaded, especially rectal strictures (narrowing); blockage of fluid in the genital area and consequent swelling, called *elephantiasis* and more common in women than men; and cancerous and precancerous lesions, as a result of excess tissue growth in the rectal and genital areas.

Diagnosis of lymphoedema venereum is based on a skin test, involving injection of an antigen, or a blood test, called *LGV complement fixation test* (LGVC-FT); the latter is more accurate. Although the disease can be cured with antibiotics, it responds slowly and treatment must be continued for at least three weeks. The treatment of choice is a twenty-one-day course of tetracycline. For pregnant women or those allergic to tetracycline, one of the sulpha drugs must be substituted. Bubos that are on the verge of bursting should be surgically drained. In cases of genital elephantiasis plastic surgery may be performed to restore the vulva to normal size, and rectal strictures should be surgically repaired. Since LGV is difficult to eradicate, all patients should receive careful follow-up tests, every few months for the first year, and then once a year for several more years.

M

Maidenhead See HYMEN.

Make-up See COSMETICS.

Male contraceptive Interference with the production, storage, chemical constitution, or transport of sperm in order to prevent conception. The principal method of male contraception – and a completely reversible one – is the CONDOM, which simply collects sperm that are ejaculated in a rubber sheath. It is widely used in countries such as England, Sweden, and Japan, but much less in the United States and Canada. Various chemicals that inhibit production of sperm are also being studied. Among them are synthetic hormone compounds, including TESTOSTERONE, which inhibits the production of FSH, which in turn stimulates sperm production, but which has side effects similar to those of oral contraceptives in women; oestrogen and testosterone together; and an amoebicide, a drug used to control diseases such as amoebic dysentry, which also has serious side effects. Several researchers are experimenting with another class of hormones called PEPTIDES. In 1979 the Chinese announced they were testing a drug called *gossypol*, a derivative of cottonseed that appears to reduce both sperm count and motility in both rats and human beings and that is believed to be reversible, that is, sperm production resumes normal levels within a few months of discontinuing the drug. Gossypol reportedly has minimal side effects but high doses of it are toxic. Other methods of inhibiting sperm production still under consideration include THERMATIC STERILIZATION and ULTRASOUND (see definition 2). The principal means of permanent (non-reversible) male contraception – sterilization – is VASECTOMY.

Male menopause Also *male climacteric*. Strictly speaking, the end of male testicular function, meaning greatly reduced production of the principal male hormone, testosterone, and of sperm. As in women, declining production of hormones by the gonads (sex glands) makes the pituitary gland produce more gonadotrophic hormones to stimulate testosterone production. Hence the clinical signs of male menopause are low testosterone levels and high levels of gonadotrophin; in women the counterpart is high levels of pituitary FSH (see MENOPAUSE). However, unlike the end of ovulation in women, sperm production in men does not end abruptly except when surgery or radiation therapy has damaged the testes. Rather, men undergo a very gradual, long-term decline, which actually begins soon after the age of twenty but usually produces no noticeable symptoms of any kind until after the age of fifty or fifty-five. The first sign is usually diminished potency—decreased ability to have or maintain an erection. Occasionally a man may experience vasomotor symptoms similar to the HOT FLUSHES of menopausal women, but the majority of men note no change other than that it takes longer to achieve a full erection and ejaculation, and that the time between orgasms (the *refractory period*) lengthens. (See under ORGASM.) Because potency is so intimately related to psychological factors, including boredom, preoccupation with work, fear of ageing, mental or physical fatigue, and anxiety concerning sexual adequacy, it is not really known how much of this decline is due to lowered hormone production and how much to other factors. (See also IMPOTENCE.) Even clinical tests are not foolproof, because testosterone levels in a single individual vary considerably from month to month, and even from hour to hour, with no known cause or visible effect.

The most common physical problem men encounter after the age of fifty-five is prostate disorders. It is estimated that more than half of all British men over sixty have some enlargement of the prostate gland, and many encounter more serious disorders, ranging from inflammation and infection to cancer of the prostate, the fourth most common malignancy in British men. (The prostate is described under PENIS.) A significant number of men find their capacity to enjoy sexual intercourse unchanged in later life, despite decreased hormone levels and less frequent coitus.

Malignant Describing a growth or tumour that is cancerous. See CANCER.

Mammalgia Painful breasts. The pain may be caused by premenstrual oedema (fluid retention), poorly fitting bras, injury, or infection (MASTITIS). After childbirth a common cause of breast pain is the engorgement that occurs when milk is first produced (see LACTATION). Cysts in the breast often cause pain (see CYSTIC DISEASE) but breast cancer rarely does. However, there may be considerable post-operative pain following a MASTECTOMY.

Mammaplasty Also *breast augmentation, breast reconstruction, breast reduction*. Plastic surgery performed to increase or decrease the size of one or both breasts, or to restore breast form following surgery for cancer or other disease (see MASTECTOMY). Breast reduction surgery is not always a wholly cosmetic procedure. Extremely heavy breasts can cause chronic backache, breathing problems, and skin irritation from bra straps and perspiration. However, reducing breast size is a complicated surgical procedure and should not be undertaken lightly. Moreoever, if a woman considering breast reduction plans to breast-feed in the future, the surgeon must be particularly careful not to remove too much secretory tissue or cut through the major mammary ducts.

There are two principal techniques for breast reduction surgery. In one, the nipple and areola are removed, and excess tissue is taken from the lower portion of the breast, after which the surgeon replaces the nipple and areola as a skin graft. This procedure greatly reduces nipple sensitivity and also eliminates the possibilty of breast-feeding. In the other, the nipple and areola remain attached to the breast by a thin stalk of tissue, the surgeon removes excess breast tissue, and the nipple is then moved to a higher position on the breast. This technique preserves nipple sensitivity and in some cases enough tissue to allow breast-feeding. Reduction surgery takes three to four hours and is performed under general anaesthesia in a hospital. The woman remains hospitalized for three to four days and can generally resume most activities within two or three weeks. Any such surgery is best performed by a plastic surgeon, or a general surgeon with special experience.

Surgery to enlarge breast size or to replace tissue lost through disease or mastectomy generally involves implanting a pouch filled either with silicone gel or with a saline (salt-water) solution. Injecting liquid silicone directly into the breast, a procedure used in the 1950s and 1960s and subsequently outlawed in many places, is extremely dangerous, frequently resulting in infection, poisoning, and even the development of cancerous tissue. Silicone gel, which is an inert material that rarely produces inflammation or other reactions and is similar in consistency and resilience to the normal breast tissue, is contained in soft, seamless silicone or polyurethane pouches, so that it cannot migrate into other parts of the breast. A solid piece of silicone can be inserted without a pouch, but in most cases surgeons prefer to use internal prostheses, or sacs. The gel-filled pouch is inserted through a small incision at the base fold area of the breast, and positioned under the breast skin. Sometimes, however, it is placed under the major pectoral muscle. With inflatable implants, which are used less often than silicone-gel pouches, a saline solution is injected after implantation through a valve into the saucer-shaped implant and the wound is then closed. Additional saline cannot be injected, however, as increased pressure on the implant walls would cause leakage. Indeed, leakage and deflation are the chief disadvantages of this technique.

In some cases the nipple of a diseased breast can be saved by 'banking', that is, when the breast is removed the nipple is temporarily grafted to another part of the body and is later attached to the reconstructed breast. Or an artificial nipple can be constructed from either part of the remaining nipple or from the vulva or some other part of the body.

Opinion differs as to how long a woman should wait after mastectomy before undergoing reconstructive mammaplasty. When a cancer is localized and non-invasive (see CANCER), reconstruction is sometimes done at the same time as the mastectomy. When a tumour is larger, most surgeons prefer to wait three months to a year until the mastectomy wounds have healed completely. Some advocate waiting up to three years, because if a cancer will recur locally it most often (80 to 85 per cent of the time) does so within two years of the mastectomy. There is no maximum time limit for reconstruction following mastectomy, and some women have undergone mammaplasty ten or even twenty years after their mastectomies.

A woman can usually leave the hospital two to three days after mammaplasty but generally must keep her arm close to her side for a few days longer. Within a month she should have complete use of her arm, although she might not yet be able to undertake vigorous exercise, such as golf, tennis, or swimming. Some surgeons ask patients to wear a specially fitted bra day and night for the first few months so that the new breast takes on the desired shape.

The most common complication of implant breast surgery is necrosis (death) of the covering skin. If the flap of skin covering the implant is thin, there may be gradual thinning or discoloration of the skin over a large area of the implant. Occasionally sloughing of skin will require removing the implant. Other possible complications are blood clots, haemorrhage, infection, and oedema (fluid retention). Another problem is hardening of the breast into a baseball-like shape, caused by the formation of a capsule of scar tissue around the implant. These contractures, which can occur months or years after surgery (since scar tissue may take a long time to grow), can result in abnormalities of breast shape and position, including lumps. They can, however, be treated by methods ranging from massage to separate scar tissue from the implant to manual rupture by the surgeon to minor surgery. A more serious objection to mammaplasty following mastectomy for cancer is that a silicone implant may make it hard to detect a new tumour growing behind it.

Not every woman can have breast reconstruction surgery following mastectomy. Most surgeons do not recommend mammaplasty for women with large tumours, or with extensive involvement of underarm lymph nodes, or women of advanced age, extreme obesity, or suffering from other serious disease. The best candidates are those whose cancer was smaller than 2 centimetres (¾ inch) with fewer than three positive lymph nodes. Some surgeons, however, feel that even women with uncontrolled cancer (spreading to other parts of the body) should have mammaplasty if it will make their remaining lifetime happier.

Women who have had a radical mastectomy in which too much skin and muscle were removed to permit inserting silicone-gel pouches must undergo *flap methods* for breast reconstruction. Breast mounds are created from skin and tissue that are transferred to the chest from other parts of the body (abdomen, buttocks, etc.), and chest muscle may be replaced by muscle tissue from the back. Such reconstruction usually requires numerous hospitalizations, as opposed to the single one generally sufficient for implant surgery, with follow-up procedures to reconstruct the nipple and areola and, as is often necessary, to increase or reduce the size of the remaining breast in order to match the reconstructed one.

Mammary duct ectasia Dilation of the milk ducts within the breast, which then fill with debris. It usually occurs in numerous ducts and is often associated with the formation of cysts (see CYSTIC DISEASE). If the ducts fill enough to rupture, they may become inflamed and infiltrated by plasma cells, and consequently become swollen and painful. This condition, which is relatively uncommon, is called *plasma cell mastitis* and affects mainly older women. Symptoms include one or more hard, poorly defined, immovable masses in the breast (usually both breasts), and a recurrent greenish or brownish nipple discharge. Treatment is palliative—hot compresses and analgesics until the inflammation subsides—but sometimes infection develops, and surgical excision may be required.

Mammary duct fistula A false passage (*fistula*) or tunnel extending from one of the main milk ducts in the breast out to the surface of the nipple. It usually requires surgical repair.

Mammography An X-ray examination of the breast that is used to detect and diagnose disease, including cancer. It is considered the most reliable mechanical method available for detecting a breast cancer before it can be felt. However, it does overlook some cancers; one study estimates that it misses about 20 per cent. Nearly half the tumours detected by mammography are too small to be felt on physical examination. Since X-rays themselves are carcinogenic (cancer-causing), caution must be exercised to avoid too much exposure, and mammography should not be used indiscriminately.

Mammography is a valuable diagnostic tool for women who have a palpable lump in the breast or under the arm, in order to determine whether a biopsy should be performed or the lump is a cyst that should simply be aspirated (drained) and observed. It is similarly useful for women who have noticed changes or abnormalities in the breast skin (dimpling, discoloration, puckering), in the nipples (scaling, discharge, sudden inversion), or in the size or shape of either breast. It is also recommended as an annual procedure for women over thirty-five who have had breast cancer, and for women over forty who have a close relative (mother, sister) who had it.

Manic-depressive illness Also *bipolar depression*. A severe emotional disorder that is twice as prevalent in women as in men and is characterized by recurrent cycles of mania and depression. Like some other kinds of DEPRESSION, it is believed to have biological basis; it tends to run in families, and possibly it is transmitted by a dominant gene. The mood changes occur for no apparent reason and are often accompanied by a specific physical change, that is, there is an increase in body sodium. Moreover, the condition can often be controlled by treatment with lithium (see under ANTI-DEPRESSANTS), which, however, can have toxic effects as well.

Manic-depressive illness can begin at any time but tends to strike around the age of thirty. Untreated, the depressive phase is characterized by extreme despondency, especially early in the morning, and progressive withdrawal from work, social affairs, and other human contact. Many patients become suicidal. Typically, after six to nine months of acute depression, a manic phase begins. There is an apparent sense of well-being and heightened self-confidence, as well as increased energy. Most patients become hyperactive, uninhibited, and extremely talkative. They often exhibit inappropriate behaviour, such as spending sprees, bizarre clothing, or the like, and sometimes they become very irritable. After three to six months, this mood is again replaced by depression.

In most patients the frequency and duration of these attacks increase with age, although depression becomes more common and mania rarer in elderly patients. Treatment usually requires hospitalization for at least a time, and attempted control of symptoms with a variety of drugs—lithium controls only the manic phase—and sometimes also electroconvulsive, or shock, therapy.

Mask of pregnancy See CHLOASMA.

Mastectomy 1 Surgical removal of the breast. It is usually undertaken as a treatment for cancer, but occasionally a very large benign (noncancerous) tumour cannot be removed without removing the entire breast (as in CYSTOSARCOMA PHYLLODES) or the high risk of cancer warrants surgery (see under definition 8 below). There are several different kinds of mastectomy, depending on the amount of tissue that is removed. From about 1895 to 1970 most breast cancer patients who were operated on underwent the Halsted radical mastectomy (definition 2 below), which removes not only the breast but underlying muscle and adjacent lymph nodes, on the theory that cancer cells spread to other parts of the body through the LYMPH. In recent years, there has been a growing tendency to regard CANCER as a systemic disease that should be treated locally by removing only the tumour and then systemically by subjecting the patient's body to radiation and/or chemotherapy (anti-cancer drugs); hormones, and other treatment. This theory has led to the development of various less extensive operations as well as approaches involving nutritional, manipulative, and psychological treatment (see under CANCER, BREAST). Increasingly, it has been realized that the patient herself must decide not only whether to undergo surgery but what surgery should be done.

The after-effects of mastectomy can be as traumatic as the surgery itself, or even more so. Following surgery small drainage tubes are left in place for a few days. It usually takes ten to fourteen days for the scars to heal superficially. The adjacent arm is normally swollen for at least a few days, but simple exercises, such as squeezing a small rubber ball, help control the swelling. Feelings of mutilation, of being 'less feminine', and fear of pain and death may be difficult to deal with. Surgery must often be followed up with RADIATION THERAPY and/or CHEMO-THERAPY, which not only have unpleasant side effects but serve as a constant reminder of life-threatening disease. Many women lose considerable

mobility in the adjacent arm, and some suffer more or less permanent LYMPH-OEDEMA. Also, cut nerves and scar tissue in the breast area may produce a combination of numbness and oversensitivity there, making it painful or unpleasant to be touched.

In Britain many hospitals have a nurse who is available to give counselling and advice to those who undergo mastectomy. In addition The Mastectomy Association of Great Britain, 1 Colworth Rd, Croydon CR0 7AD, gives help to those about to have or who have recently had a mastectomy. Following mastectomy, a large proportion of women can, if they wish, have breast reconstruction surgery (see MAMMAPLASTY). Mastectomy may be followed by radiation therapy, chemotherapy, immunotherapy, and/or hormone therapy (the last if the tumour tissue removed indicates hormone dependency, a test that can and should be performed).

2 Halsted radical mastectomy Also *radical mastectomy.* Surgery involving removal of a cancerous breast and its skin, the underlying muscle of the chest wall (both major and minor), the lymph nodes in the adjacent armpit, and fat tissue. The physical results are a flattened and sunken chest wall and the potential for developing more or less permanent LYMPHOEDEMA and shoulder stiffness. This kind of surgery was first performed about 1882 by William Stewart Halsted who described it in a paper published in 1894, and soon became the most commonly used procedure for treating breast cancer. Halsted's technique reflected his concern over the high rate of local breast cancer recurrence observed in his day; he himself reduced local recurrence to 6 per cent and metastasis (cancer spread to other parts of the body) to 16 per cent in fifty patients. There is no evidence, however, that this technique improved survival rates. Halsted himself did not remove lymph nodes because he did not really understand their role. Today it is known that even if all the axillary (underarm) lymph nodes are removed, cancer cells may already have spread to other parts of the body. It is, rather, the number of positive (cancer-bearing) underarm nodes that appears to be directly related to recurrence and survival rates.

3 **Extended radical mastectomy** Also *extended thorough mastectomy, Urban operation*. Surgery identical to the Halsted radical mastectomy (see definition 2) but also removing the lymph nodes of the internal mammary chain, which usually requires removing a section of the rib cage.

4 **Modified radical mastectomy** Surgery to remove the breast, some fat, and most of the axillary (underarm) lymph nodes, but leaving the chest muscles intact. It is technically more difficult and time-consuming to perform than the Halsted procedure (definition 2) because the axillary lymph nodes are hard to get at when the chest muscles are not disturbed. It results in a cosmetically more pleasing appearance than the Halsted, and preserves normal arm and shoulder strength.

5 **Simple mastectomy** Also *total mastectomy*. Surgery in which only the breast is removed, leaving intact the axillary nodes and chest muscles. It avoids the sunken chest that results from more radical surgery (definition 2, 3) and greatly reduces the possibility of lymph-oedema. It sometimes is combined with *axillary dissection*, which is performed primarily for the purpose of STAGING, that is, to determine the extent of spread and if there is need for subsequent treatment with radiation and for drugs. It differs from the modified radical mastectomy (definition 4) in that it takes only the axillary lymph nodes closest to the breast. If cancer has spread to the nodes, either radiation is used or the affected nodes are removed. If there is no low axillary node involvement, only the breast is removed and the axilla (armpit) closely observed following surgery. If cancer later develops in the nodes, they are surgically removed at that time. Preliminary results indicate that axillary dissection, either at the time of mastectomy or afterward, and radiation is equally effective in controlling spread to the nodes.

6 **Partial mastectomy** Also *segmental mastectomy*. Removal of a breast tumour and two to three centimetres (one inch) of surrounding tissue, including some of the overlying skin and part of the lining of the underlying muscle. The rest of the breast, along with the connective tissue, remains intact. Although the breast is partially saved, it may still be markedly disfigured. If appropriate, it can later be enlarged through plastic surgery, or the other breast may be reduced to match the affected one more closely (see MAMMAPLASTY). Opponents of this procedure say it does not take into account the multicentric nature of breast cancer, that is, its tendency to appear in another part of the same breast. About 13 per cent of women undergoing more extensive surgery have been found to have one or more hidden cancers in the same breast, in addition to the one originally detected. To kill any cancer cells that may remain in the breast, partial mastectomy is followed up with radiation therapy. Also, many surgeons believe that this procedure should be supplemented with removal and examination of at least

some adjacent axillary lymph nodes, to gauge the progress of the disease more accurately.

7 **Lumpectomy** Also *local wide excision, quadrant excision, tumour excision, tumourectomy, tylectomy, wedge excision.* Removal of only the tumour mass and a small amount of surrounding breast tissue, leaving muscles, skin, and lymph nodes intact. Nearly all surgeons performing this operation follow it with radiation therapy lest some cancer cells remain hidden in the breast, and sometimes they use long-term chemotherapy as well. Recurrence-free survival rates seemed to be good for Stage I and some Stage II cancers (see STAGING), although many doctors advised combining lumpectomy with at least a biopsy on a low axillary lymph node and proceeding with this conservative surgery only if there is no nodal involvement.

8 **Subcutaneous mastectomy** Surgery in which about 95 per cent of the internal breast tissue is removed without disturbing the overlying nipple and surrounding skin, with its fat. It is performed chiefly as a preventive procedure when there is a high risk of malignancy. If, after careful examination of the excised tissue, an invasive cancer is found, both the remaining breast tissue and axillary lymph nodes are removed in a subsequent operation. Sometime after surgery, a silicone implant is inserted in the chest cavity to restore the breast contour.

Subcutaneous mastectomy has also been used as primary treatment for a CANCER IN SITU of the lobe or other non-invasive cancers not close to the nipple. The major objection to this procedure as treatment for invasive cancer is that breast tissue cannot be completely eliminated from the nipple area, so that there is risk of leaving some cancer cells. Subcutaneous mastectomy is occasionally recommended as a preventive measure for women who are at high risk of breast cancer, especially those with any of the following: severe CYSTIC DISEASE; a biopsy that shows moderate to severe noncancerous breast disease; a family history of breast cancer and progressively more nodular (lumpy) breasts; nodular breasts and cystic disease in one breast and cancer in the other breast.

Mastitis An inflammation of the breast, caused by infection, most often by *Staphylococcus aureus* but sometimes by another organism. It is possible to contract mastitis from a bite, as in love play, but usually the organism invades the nipple of a woman who is breast-feeding. The symptoms of mastitis are pain in the affected breast, particularly in one spot, tenderness, and swelling. There may be a chill and there nearly always is fever, sometimes quite high. Treated with warm compresses and oral antibiotics, mastitis often subsides within about forty-eight hours. When it does not, it usually becomes localized (*suppurative mastitis*), forming an ABSCESS that must be surgically opened and drained. Although at one time it was considered mandatory to stop breast-feeding lest the baby become infected, many women with mastitis have found that suckling relieves the pain somewhat by emptying the breast, thereby reducing the opportunity for bacteria to multiply; it does no harm to the child, since the bacteria are usually from its mouth. *Chronic cystic mastitis* is a name sometimes used for CYSTIC DISEASE of the breast, but it is not accurate because such cysts rarely involve either inflammation or infection. (For *plasma cell mastitis*, see under MAMMARY DUCT ECTASIA.)

Some women who prefer HERBAL REMEDIES use local applications of various herbs to ease the pain of caked nipples and mastitis. Among these are poultices made from elderberry blossom (*Sambucus nigra*) and olive oil; grated raw potato; fresh ginger root; and comfrey leaves (*Symphytum officinale*).

Masturbation   Also *automanipulation*. The practice of sexually stimulating oneself to ORGASM. According to most authorities today, masturbation is quite normal during adolescence, and many feel it is normal at any age. Apparently the orgasms that women experience with masturbation are often more intense, with stronger muscular contractions, than those experienced with a partner, although the doctors who observed this phenomenon also pointed out that measurable physical intensity is not necessarily identical to a feeling of satisfaction, which may be more profound with a partner. Mutual masturbation – of one sexual partner by another, at the same time or in turn – can be a satisfying means of sexual enjoyment. For heterosexual partners it provides an excellent alternative when illness, injury, or a fertile period rule out vaginal intercourse. It is also a means for partners to become acquainted with each other's sexual responses, and is frequently recommended by sex therapists to help women who have never achieved orgasm (see FRIGIDITY). Women masturbate in a variety of ways, but nearly all involve stimulating the CLITORIS, with their fingers, by crossing their legs and exerting pressure, with a stream of water, an electrical or battery-operated vibrator, a pillow, or any other object. Masturbation was

frowned on as an unhealthy outlet, especially for women, throughout the 19th and early 20th centuries, at least in Europe and America, and some doctors actually removed the clitoris (clitoridectomy) or its foreskin to curb the practice. Today, in contrast, some doctors actually recommend masturbation to postmenopausal women who have infrequent or no sexual relations with a partner, in the belief that frequent lubrication of the vagina through sexual arousal helps prevent excessive drying of the tissues (see VAGINAL ATROPHY).

Measles   Also *rubella*. A highly acute, contagious disease of childhood marked by fever, cough, inflammation of the eyelids (conjunctivitis), and a spreading rash. It is caused by a virus, lasts about a week, and can be prevented entirely by immunization with a live virus vaccine. It is not usually a serious disease in itself, but its complications, such as pneumonia and encephalitis, can be dangerous. It is important that it be differentiated from a similar disease, called German measles, or RUBELLA, which can cause birth defects in a baby if the mother becomes infected during pregnancy. Measles is rare in adults, but is likely to make a person acutely ill when it does occur.

Melanoma   Also *malignant melanoma*. A malignant (cancerous) tumour that arises out of pigment cells (melanocytes), mostly in the skin or mucous membranes but sometimes also in the eye and central nervous system. Some kinds of melanoma spread so rapidly that they are fatal only months after they are first detected. Most melanomas arise from melanocytes in normal skin but about one-third arise from pigmented moles. They are more common in pregnant women than in nonpregnant women; however, pregnancy does not increase the likelihood that a mole will become cancerous, and abortion will induce a remission. The fact that melanomas seem to have some link with pregnancy, and a study published in 1977 indicating that women who had used oral contraceptives were twice as likely to develop malignant melanomas as women who had not, suggests that some melanomas, at least, may be hormone-dependent. Pigment-cell reproduction is controlled by the pituitary gland, which also controls ovulation. It is not known if oral contraceptives directly stimulate pigment-cell production or if they affect pituitary hormones that control pigmentation (see also CHLOASMA). There may also be a connection between exposure of the skin to intense burst of ultraviolet light and the development of melanomas.

In women melanomas appear more frequently on the legs, in men on the torso; in women they may also occur on the vulva and inside the vagina. A melanoma often looks like a mole that is growing, that is, a quite dark flat or raised spot on the skin; sometimes it is deeply pigmented with multiple colorations of red, white, and black. Some melanomas grow more rapidly than others, involving large areas of the surrounding skin and underlying tissues, as well as spreading to distant parts of the body. Then even surgical removal of the tumours, adjacent skin, and nearby lymph nodes may not remove all the cancer cells. Therefore it is wise to check immediately on any suspicious growths, moles that change in size or colour, or other skin lesions, and undergo a biopsy if melanoma is suspected.

Melasma Another name for CHLOASMA.

Membrane rupture See AMNIOTOMY; DRY LABOUR.

Menarche The beginning of menstrual periods, which usually occurs any time between the ages of 9 and 16 and, in 5 per cent of girls, between 16 and 18. Menstruation beginning before the age of 9 may be either PRECOCIOUS PUBERTY or a symptom of endocrine disease. In middle-class girls the average of of menarche in 1980 was 12¾ showing a steady decline from the average age of 14 in 1870 toward an expected 11¾ in the year 2000. This decline is largely attributed to improved diet, whereby girls attain their CRITICAL WEIGHT earlier. Contrary to a widespread myth, extremes of climate tend to slow down the rate of maturation, so that girls in tropical climates do not mature faster than those in temperate ones. Race is also not a factor. However, poor health – physical or mental – can delay menarche.

Menarche usually occurs three to four years after the first signs of PUBERTY appear, when 90 per cent of the rapid weight gain and height growth have taken place. Most girls are close to their mature height by the time of their first menstrual period, thereafter growing only one or two inches more. The frequency and amount of menstrual flow during the first few years ranges from one period every few months and light staining to full-fledged periods similar to those of adulthood. Early periods are usually, but not always, ANOVULATORY. See also AMENORRHOEA; MENSTRUAL CYCLE.

Menopause Also *change of life, climacteric, the change.* Strictly speaking, the ending of menstruation. In common usage, however, the term describes the period immediately preceding the end of menstruation, which in most women lasts from a few months to a few years, although in some it takes only days and in others five or six years. It may also refer to castration or *surgical menopause*, that is, menopause induced by bilateral OOPHORECTOMY (removal of both ovaries). Although hysterectomy (removal of the uterus) ends menstruation, oestrogen production and ovulation continue until the time of natural menopause, provided that at least one ovary is intact. The average age for menopause in Britain in the 1980's is between forty-five and fifty-three, although the normal range was much wider. Menopause occuring before the age of forty is considered *premature menopause* and calls for careful investigation to make sure no underlying disease is responsbile for the symptoms.

Except when it results from surgery, menopause is usually not abrupt. More often the first signs are fluctuations in the menstrual cycle and menstrual flow. Periods may become lighter and/or less frequent, or a period may be skipped altogether, or periods may become heavy and/or more frequent, as often as every twenty-one days. Sometimes both kinds of change occur in turn in the same woman. Basically menopause is a reversal of puberty. Where in puberty the pituitary gland stimulates the ovaries to increase oestrogen production and release eggs, in middle age – usually sometime after the age of forty – oestrogen production begins to slacken, ovulation (egg release) becomes irregular and tapers off, and eventually menstrual flow ends. Men, who have more abrupt and disturbing symptoms than women at puberty – voice change, more acne and mood swings, strong feelings of aggession – experience a far more gradual decline in sperm and hormone production in their middle years (see MALE MENOPAUSE). When there has been no menstrual flow for twelve months, the reversal is usually, but not always, complete, and thereafter a woman is said to be *postmenopausal*.

It is hormonal imbalance that accounts for the irregular periods of menopause. Irregularities themselves are normal, but certain symptoms can signal the possibility of serious disease. Extremely heavy bleeding (faster and heavier flow than a heavy period, often with clots), bleeding at intervals shorter than twenty-one days, lengthy staining outside the menstrual period (for three to four weeks), and bleeding after there have been no periods for twelve months all warrant a prompt gynaecological examination to rule out fibroids, polyps, cancer, or some other lesion. Note, however, that both oral contraceptives and OESTROGEN REPLACEMENT THERAPY can give rise to similar symptoms.

Although ovulation after the age of forty gradually occurs less and less, birth control continues to be necessary until periods have ceased for at least one year. Even then, ovulation sometimes resumes, although the likelihood of becoming pregnant by then has become very small. Oral contraceptives and intrauterine devices (IUDs) are not advisable during the menopausal period; mechanical barriers such as a diaphragm or condom are much safer. The birth control methods of determining ovulation can be used to check whether a menopausal woman is still ovulating (see under NATURAL FAMILY PLANNING).

In addition to menstrual irregularities, HOT FLUSHES are the symptom most closely associated with menopause. They are experienced to some degree – ranging from very slight and infrequent to very severe and frequent – by about three-quarters of women, and can persist for years. They are believed to result from a disturbance of the HYPOTHALAMUS, which regulates body temperature, caused either by lower oestrogen levels or by high FSH levels. The exact mechanism is still not understood, but hot flushes can be relieved by oestrogen, indicating that their cause is hormone imbalance. Since oestrogen replacement therapy is not without risk, its use for this purpose is controversial.

Another change experienced to varying degrees by many women, although often only postmenopausally – typically, several years after periods have ended – is thinning, drying, and loss of elasticity in the tissues of the vulva and vagina, called VAGINAL ATROPHY. The labia gradually lose some of their fatty layers, making the clitoris appear more prominent, and the vaginal walls become thinner and produce less mucus. Secondary results of this process are painful intercourse (DYSPAREUNIA) and greater susceptibility to vaginal and urinary infections. Like hot flushes, vaginal atrophy responds to oestrogen therapy, including local applications of oestrogen creams and suppositories which are absorbed by the body. Here, too, the risks must be weighed against the benefits, although in some cases a single application each week may relieve symptoms and may be too small to cause side effects.

Still another symptom associated with menopause and the postmenopausal years is OSTEOPOROSIS, a chronic skeletal disorder of ageing that affects women sooner and more severely than men. There is still considerable disagreement as to whether or not oestrogen replacement therapy can slow down this process sufficiently to warrant its risks, some

studies indicating that it does not and others that it does.

Besides the menstrual irregularity and hot flushes directly attributable to changing hormone levels, menopause is associated with other symptoms, some of them by-products of hormone imbalance and others the result of general aging. Some women experience symptoms identical to those of premenstrual tension (DYSMENORRHOEA, definition 5), with oedema headache, abdominal bloating, constipation, and breast changes; they are probably due to the secretion of oestrogen in the absence of progesterone. Others are affected with dizziness and/or PALPITATIONS, thought to be caused by disturbance of the vasomotor system similar to those that cause hot flushes. In still others, frequent hot flushes and subsequent sweating at night give rise to nervousness and irritability as well as profound fatigue, brought on by constantly interrupted sleep. Continued discomfort of this kind, as well as hormonal imbalance itself, can bring on mood changes not unlike those of puberty, including anxiety and depression. Moreover, the mixed feelings of an adolescent girl approaching womanhood and its new responsibilities have a counterpart in the middle-aged woman who may be experiencing other life changes and must face the prospect of ageing, with its largely negative connotations in a society that equates attractiveness with youth.

Menopause does not affect a woman's sex drive, which depends on the production of androgens (male hormones) by the adrenal glands and ovaries and does not seem to diminish. Indeed, many women find their sex life improved when fear of pregnancy is removed. In general, if a woman had satisfactory sexual relations before menopause, it is likely she will continue to have them. If not, there is no reason (other than lack of fear of pregnancy) for them to improve.

Most women – an estimated 60 to 80 per cent – experience only minor discomfort during menopause. After a year or two of irregular periods and a number of hot flushes of mild to moderate severity they simply stop menstruating. About 10 to 20 per cent have virtually no symptoms. For the remaining 10 to 20 per cent, including the majority of those who undergo surgical menopause, symptoms – especially hot flushes – may be a major annoyance and occasionally incapacitating. A striking feature is the great amount of variation found among individuals, no doubt caused by enormous variation in hormone production. Some oestrogen continues to be secreted after menopause, by the adrenal glands and probably also by the ovaries (although it is in a different form and is converted into oestrogen elsewhere in the body). The amounts produced vary considerably from one woman to another. Postmenopausally, fat women seem to have higher levels of oestrogen (in the form of oestrone) than thin ones, indicating that fat cells may store it and release it as they are broken down. In any event, there is no doubt that the severity of menopausal symptoms is a physiological phenomenon and has little to do with a woman's emotional adjustment, satisfaction with her life, anxiety or tranquillity over ageing, or similar concerns.

Human beings are the only animal species in which the female outlives her reproductive capacity; other animals die soon after they stop reproducing. Moreover, until the 19th century few women lived past menopause. Medical knowledge of menopause, therefore, is still relatively new and limited. During the 19th century various attitudes toward – and treatments for – menopausal symptoms developed. Treatments included bleeding (used in London in the 1850s), hysterectomy (invented in 1872), radiation, monkey gland transplants, and injections with the cells of unborn lambs. One view that became common, among women as well as doctors and one that persists to the present day, is that menopausal symptoms are to be disregarded, that if one keeps busy and ignores unpleasant symptoms they will disappear. This view continues to be reinforced by some members of the health-care professions, whose image of the menopausal woman is that of a childish neurotic, a nuisance to her husband and doctor, casting a pall over family and friends. Menopausal symptoms do have a real basis in physiological malfunctioning and some women – fortunately only a minority – do need assistance in getting through the worst of them. Since oestrogen replacement therapy is risk-laden, and in any case not always effective – some believe it merely postpones the appearance of symptoms, which will occur as soon as therapy is stopped – it should only be used in severe cases. Tranquillizers and other mood-altering drugs may relieve anxiety but since they also have undesirable side effects, such medication should be avoided if at all possible. Certainly simpler and safer remedies should be tried first.

Among those widely recommended are changes in diet. Reducing salt intake may help relieve oedema (fluid retention) and other symptoms resembling premenstrual tension. Avoiding foods high in tyramine, a chemical that raises blood pressure and is present in red wine, chocolate, canned and dried fish, avocado, raisins, soy sauce, aged cheeses, and certain other foods, as well as increasing the intake of naturally DI-URETIC foods (cucumbers, celery, parsley) may also help. A well-balanced diet is always important, and the addition of certain vitamins appears to be particularly helpful during menopause. The B-complex vitamins combat stress (and B_6 particularly helps the premenstrual syndrome); brewer's yeast, whole grains, and seeds are good natural sources. Some women have found that vitamin E relieves hot flushes (it is found in wheat germ, whole grains, vegetable oils, peanuts, navy beans, and salmon; see also under HOT FLUSHES), but women who have diabetes, rheumatic heart disease, or high blood pressure are advised to *limit* their intake of vitamin E to 125 International Units per day or less. Vitamin C helps the absorption of vitamin E and may help prevent vaginal infection. The mineral calcium, the need for which increases with age, helps combat osteoporosis; it is best absorbed from natural sources such as milk, yogurt, and cheese, and requires adequate intake of vitamin D which assists calcium absorption. If menstrual flow is long and profuse, additional iron may be needed to prevent anaemia. Since individual nutritional requirements vary greatly, vitamin supplements (in pill form) should be used with caution.

Regular physical exercise, especially brisk walking (a fifteen-minute mile) and swimming, helps keep bones and muscles strong, counteracts osteoporosis and arthritis, maintains muscle tone and cardiovascular capacity, and also gives a sense of well-being and burns extra calories.

Extra lubrication, such as K-Y jelly or a plain vegetable oil applied to the vagina, can protect against irritation due to drying tissues.

Women have long used various homoeopathic and HERBAL REMEDIES to relieve menopausal symptoms. For the premenstrual tension symptoms, the same herbs used for congestive dysmenorrhoea (see DYSMENORRHOEA, definition 5) may give relief. Liquorice root (*Glycrrhiza lepidota*) contains a substance chemically similar to oestrogen, and sarsaparilla (*Smilax officinalis*) contains one similar to progesterone; a tea brewed from these is used to relieve hot flushes. GINSENG root (*Panax quinquefolium*), long used in China, is used by some women for hot flushes, as is dong kwai (or tang kuei; *Angelica sinensis*), a Chinese herb that can be chewed, boiled into a tea, or taken in powered form. Long profuse periods have been treated with a tea made from either shepherd's purse (*Capsella bursa pastoris*) or bearberry (*Arctostaphylos uva-ursi*).

After menopause, regular physical examinations should be continued, including an annual check-up for blood pressure, height and weight, breast examination (see also under MAMMO-GRAPHY), pelvic examination, and Pap smear. At that time routine blood and urine tests may also be done, and there should be an annual test for glaucoma, a potentially blinding eye disease that usually develops only after the age of forty and, if detected early, can be controlled. Women should continue to examine their breasts monthly – with no period to remind them, a calendar date should be substituted – and probably should, after the age of fifty, have an electrocardiogram every five years or so, and more often in the presence of heart disease, high blood pressure, or high-risk factors.

Menorrhagia See HYPERMENORRHOEA. Also see MENSTRUAL FLOW.

Menses See MENSTRUATION.

Menstrual cramps See DYSMENOR-
RHOEA, definition 4.

Menstrual cup A soft, plastic, bell-
shaped device for collecting menstrual
flow. It is inserted just inside the vagina,
where it is held in place by suction. Its
principal advantage is that it can be
removed, washed, and reused many
times, representing a considerable saving
in cost and convenience. Some women
prefer to use a DIAPHRAGM to collect
menstrual fluid. Like the menstrual cup,
it holds far more than a tampon or pad.
See also SANITARY NAPKIN; TAMPON.

Menstrual cycle The regular, periodic
process of preparing the lining of the
uterus for the implantation and support
of a fertilized egg, which, if no egg is
fertilized, ends in menstruation (the
shedding of extra uterine tissue in
menstrual flow). The cycle, roughly a
month in duration, is regulated by the
levels and interactions of certain hormones, which govern the release of an
egg from the ovary (see OVULATION), the
preparation of the endometrium (uterine
lining) for pregnancy, and the shedding
of endometrial tissue when no pregnancy
is begun (menstruation).

The length of the cycle varies from
woman to woman, and in some women
it varies considerably from month to
month as well. Most cycles are between
23 and 35 days long. The *average* cycle
is 28 days long, counting from day 1 of
a menstrual period up to (but not
including) day 1 of the next period. It is
divided into three phases: (1) *the
menstrual phase*, days 1 to 5; (2) the
proliferative phase (also called *preovulatory*
or *follicular phase*), days 5 to 13; (3) the

secretory phase (also called *postovulatory*
or *luteal phase*), days 14-28. Some
authorities do not distinguish between
the menstrual and proliferative phases,
simply calling days 1-13 the proliferative
phase.

Between the proliferative and secretory
phases, on or about day 13 or 14 (at
midcycle), ovulation – the release of an
egg from the ovary – takes place. In
women whose menstrual cycles are
longer or shorter than 28 days, it is nearly
always the menstrual and proliferative
phases that are longer or shorter; in 90
per cent of women the secretory phase
is 13 to 15 days in duration. One can,
therefore, determine when ovulation last
took place simply by counting back 14
days from the first day of menstrual flow.

The menstrual cycle begins on the first
day of menstrual flow. This shedding of
endometrial lining results from declining
levels of the hormones oestrogen and
progesterone toward the end of the previous cycle's secretory phase. These low
hormone levels also, it is believed, have
a positive feedback (or stimulating effect)
on the HYPOTHALAMUS that causes it to
produce follicle release hormone (FRH),
or follicle-stimulating hormone release
factor, and luteinizing release hormone
(LRH), or luteinizing hormone release
factor, which in turn act on the pituitary
gland to make it secrete follicle-stimulating hormone (FSH) and luteinizing
hormone (LH). FSH stimulates the
growth of several follicles (each surrounding one egg) in the ovary, one of which
will become the *Graafian follicle*, that is,
the one activated to produce a mature egg
cell. LH stimulates oestrogen secretion by
the follicles.

The follicles' secretion of oestrogen
begins the *proliferative phase*, which starts
with the end of menstrual flow and ends

The Menstrual Cycle

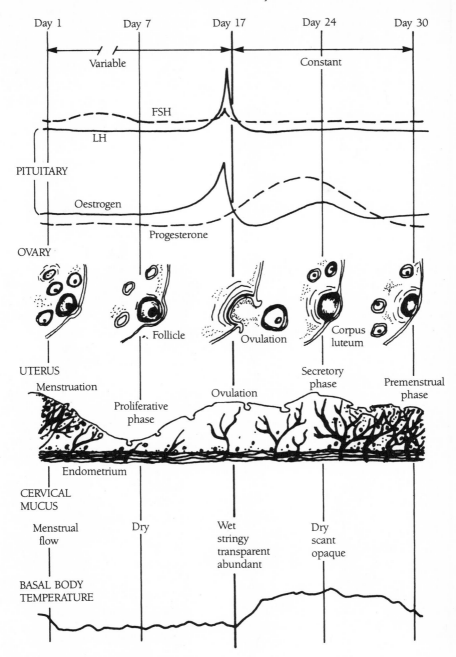

Adapted from *a book about birth control* by Donna Cherniak, Montreal Health Press

with ovulation. During this phase the levels of oestrogen increase, all but one of the follicles atrophy while the Graafian follicle continues to develop, and the endometrium thickens in preparation for the implantation of a fertilized egg. As oestrogen concentrations rise, FSH levels decline because, it is believed, the higher oestrogen level now has a negative effect on the hypothalamus. LH levels remain constant, however. At midcycle, the end of the proliferative phase, the high level of ovarian oestrogen causes the pituitary to release a large amount of LH, which in turn stimulates the Graafian follicle to reach maturity and release an egg (ovulation); the empty follicle is then transformed into the CORPUS LUTEUM, which secretes both progesterone and oestrogen.

With ovulation, the proliferative phase, which is dominated by the hormone oestrogen, ends. There follows the *secretory phase*, which is dominated by the hormone progesterone, secreted (along with oestrogen) by the follicle in its new form, the corpus luteum. During this phase the endometrium thickens still more and the uterine glands begin to produce their secretions of life-support-ing substances for the nurture of a fertilized egg. If fertilization does occur, the corpus luteum's secretions, are controlled by a different hormone, human chorionic gonadotrophin (HCG), manufactured by the placenta. If the egg is not fertilized, the secretions of the corpus luteum are controlled by LH. The higher levels of progesterone and oestro-gen produced by the corpus luteum now exert negative feedback (an inhibiting influence) on the production of LH and FSH, which begins to decrease. When the level of LH drops, the corpus luteum begins to atrophy and stops producing

oestrogen and progesterone. The thicken-ing of the endometrium can no longer be maintained and is therefore shed, along with some blood and mucus, in the form of the menstrual flow. The lowered hormone levels again trigger the hypothalamus to produce LRH and FRH, which in turn stimulate pituitary produc-tion of LH and FSH, and the entire cycle begins again. See also the separate entries on each of the hormones mentioned; also AMENORRHOEA; ANOVULATORY BLEED-ING; FOLLICLE; GRAAFIAN FOLLICLE.

Menstrual   flow Also   *menstrual discharge.* The vaginal bleeding that occurs on a more or less regular monthly basis from MENARCHE until after MENOPAUSE. The duration of bleeding, called the *menstrual period*, lasts, on the average, from two to seven days. The total amount of discharge varies considerably among different women but 60 to 70 cc. (millilitres; ¼ to ⅓ cup) appears to be average for a single period. The fluid is dark reddish in colour but tends to be brighter red if it is very profuse. It consists of blood, degenerated cells from the endometrium (uterine lining; see MENSTRUAL CYCLE for explanation), mucus from the cervical glands and vagina, and bacteria. It usually does not contain clots, nor is the blood component in it capable of clotting. The blood in menstrual flow is actually serum, which already clotted while in the uterus and then was dissolved and reliquefied by enzymes.

In many women menstrual flow is heaviest during the first day or two of their period and thereafter gradually dimishes. This pattern is by no means universal. Some women barely stain for the first two days and then flow more heavily, while others always experience a steady flow (either light or heavy). Some women always have very heavy periods (requiring the use of more than eight sanitary towels or tampons per day) and some always have quite light ones (one or two towels per day). Since the normal range is so wide, a marked *change* in a woman's own pattern is more significant than differences among individuals.

The principal means of dealing with menstrual flow, in Western countries, are the SANITARY NAPKIN and TAMPON (see also MENSTRUAL CUP). The occurrence of menstrual flow need not prevent vaginal intercourse. In fact, for couples wishing to avoid pregnancy, it may be a satisfactory time, since few women ovulate while flowing. Those who find intercourse messy at this time might try using a diaphragm during intercourse to contain the flow.

Scanty flow or *hypomenorrhoea*, is sometimes caused by oral contraceptives and is usually no cause for concern. In contrast, *hypermenorrhoea* or *menorrhagia*, meaning very heavy menstrual flow, can result from a number of disorders and should be investigated. One common cause is the presence of a FIBROID. Another, often unsuspected, is ectopic pregnancy. Other causes include a cervical or endometrial POLYP, PELVIC INFLAMMATORY DISEASE, an ovarian CYST or other tumour, and ADENOMYOSIS. Occasionally thyroid disturbances or a platelet deficiency are responsible. In some women an intrauterine device (IUD) causes such heavy flow that it must be removed and another form of birth control substituted.

Often, however, hypermenorrhoea is simply the result of a disruption in hormone balance, which is most likely to occur at menarche and menopause. Such DYSFUNCTIONAL BLEEDING may be corrected either by a D AND C or by the administration of hormones, either progesterone alone or oral contraceptives containing both progesterone and oestrogen. Hypermenorrhoea is both more alarming and potentially more dangerous than scanty flow. It can result in enough blood loss to cause anaemia and occasionally even to necessitate a blood transfusion. If heavy bleeding and anaemia persist and no other measure proves effective, as a last resort, hysterectomy may be performed. See also BREAKTHROUGH BLEEDING; OLIGOMEN-ORRHOEA, POLYMENORRHOEA.

A number of nutritional and HERBAL REMEDIES have been used to deal with hypermenorrhoea. Some women find that calcium and magnesium tablets help both severe cramps and heavy flow; they recommend taking a tablet every few hours during the first day or two of such a period. Vitamin A supplements (but less than 25,000 International Units a day) have also been used. Herbal remedies include teas made from yarrow (*Achillea millefolium*; **avoid if pregnant**), red raspberry leaf (*Rubus idaeus*), shepherd's purse (*Capsella bursa pastoris*), or cinnamon bark (stick cinnamon).

For painful menstruation and other problems associated with menstrual periods, see DYSMENORRHOEA.

Menstruation Also *menses.* Regular monthly shedding of endometrial tissue and blood through the vagina. The beginning of menstruation is called MENARCHE, the end, MENOPAUSE. See also MENSTRUAL CYCLE; MENSTRUAL FLOW.

Metabolic toxaemia of pregnancy
See ECLAMPSIA; PREECLAMPSIA.

Metabolism A general term for all the physical and chemical processes whereby the body acquires and uses the foods and energy it requires for life, growth, and maturation. It includes the transformation of nutrients into living tissue and the processes whereby complex substances are reduced to simpler ones.

Metastasis The spread of disease from one part of the body to another that is not directly connected to it. The term is generally reserved for the spread of CANCER, which is said to *metastasize*.

Metrorrhagia See BREAKTHROUGH BLEEDING.

Midcycle The middle of the MENSTRUAL CYCLE, when ovulation takes place. See also MITTELSCHMERZ.

Midwife A person other than a doctor who has some training (formal or informal) to serve as the principal assistant at childbirth. Although there are some male midwives, the majority are women. Midwives have been used since ancient times. In Europe and in America they were often accused of witchcraft, and, indeed, the first witch executed in the Massachusetts Bay Colony, in 1648, was a doctor and midwife, Margaret Jones. In Europe midwifery survived the witchcraft craze and midwives were integrated into the health services. In Britain and America, however, men were encouraged to enter the field of obstetrics and gradually took it over, eventually as doctors. With the establishment of hospitals and the increase in hospital deliveries, midwifery died out in America except in rural areas, since midwives were not allowed to assist births in hospitals.

In Europe, Africa, and Asia, on the other hand, midwifery never fell into disrepute as it did in America, and even in the most advanced European countries midwives continued to account for the majority of deliveries, both in hospitals and at home. In Britain it was not until the end of the last century that formal training and examination in midwifery was started. An Act of Parliament in 1902 made it necessary to have a certificate to practise midwifery. At that time a three-month training was required. Nowadays an eighteen-month training is required after first qualifying as a nurse. In Britain most hospital deliveries are carried out by a midwife with a doctor only intervening if there are complications. There are also community midwives who attend home births or come into hospital with the woman when she goes into labour to deliver the baby in hospital. This is known as the Domino scheme (domiciliary midwife in and out) and allows women who are at risk from complications to be delivered by their community midwife but in a place where there are specialist facilities if needed. (See also BIRTH ATTENDANT.)

Migraine Also *sick headache*. A recurrent kind of HEADACHE that affects women more frequently than men (some studies say five times as much, others only one and one-half times as much). The headache tends to occur in two stages. In the first, called *premonitory stage* or *aura*, a person has various sensory aberrations or simply a sense of vague uneasiness. During this stage certain cerebral arteries constrict, reducing the blood flow and oxygen supply to the brain. If the constriction is severe, the brain areas that receive messages from the eyes and other sense organs are temporarily disturbed, a condition that persists for a few minutes. Common among such disturbances are seeing flashing lights or zigzag lines, or experiencing blind spots or blindness. The constriction of arteries is usually limited to one side, and the visual or sensory disturbance is limited to the same side. Thus a person may briefly lose vision in one eye, or feel numbness or tingling of the fingers in one hand. Other sensations are general dizziness, 'ringing in the ears', or tingling on the back of the tongue.

The second stage begins when, in apparent rebound, the arteries dilate, causing the pain itself, a severe headache. It can affect almost any part of the head except the lower jaw, and usually begins on one side (the same side affected during the premonitory stage), in the lower forehead or temple. It tends to move from there to the back of the head, remaining more severe on the side originally affected. The head pain is frequently accompanied by nausea, sometimes with vomiting, and a variety of other symptoms, including increased urination, pallor, abdominal pain, photophobia (intolerance to light), sweating, and/or fever. By the time the nausea passes the headache has usually ended. Typically a migraine lasts eight to twelve hours, but it may persist for several days.

Migraine can be brought on by such external factors as bright lights, noise, motion, and abrupt changes in weather. It may also be precipitated by a change in oestrogen levels just before a menstrual period, psychological stress, and food allergy (especially to chocolate, tea, coffee – including decaffeinated – alcohol, yoghurt, aged cheese, legumes, and cured or smoked meats). Migraine tends to run in families. It usually begins between the ages of ten and thirty and frequently ends after the age of fifty. Some women develop migraine when they take oral contraceptives – a history of migraine is a relative contraindication to the use of oral contraceptives – and in such cases the medication should be stopped immediately and another form of birth control substituted.

For mild attacks of migraine, aspirin, codeine, or a sedative taken early, when the symptoms are first felt, may be effective. For a severe attack ergotamine tartrate has long been the principal drug used (dissolved on the tongue, inhaled through the mouth, injected, or given by rectal suppository), and caffeine appears to enhance its effect. It, too, works best when taken early. The drug methysergide has been used to prevent migraine attacks, but it has serious side effects and its use calls for careful monitoring. Neither ergotamine nor methysergide can be taken by pregnant women. An antihypertensive drug, propranolol, appears to prevent migraine in some patients or at least reduce the frequency of attacks, but it cannot be used by persons with asthma, severe heart disease, and some other disorders. The antidepressant drug amitriptyline is also effective for some patients.

Milk leg See PHLEGMASIA.

Minilaparotomy Also *minilap*. A kind of abdominal TUBAL LIGATION in which the incision is much smaller, only local anaesthesia is required, and there are fewer unpleasant after-effects than with LAPAROSCOPY.

Mini-pill An ORAL CONTRACEPTIVE that contains only a small dose of progestin (synthetic PROGESTERONE). It does not, like other oral contraceptives, prevent ovulation. Rather, it changes the cervical mucus so that is it no longer hospitable to sperm. It also slows the transport of an egg through the Fallopian tube. Since it contains no oestrogen, the mini-pill does not produce many of the side effects of other oral contraceptives. It does, however, give rise to breakthrough bleeding (between periods) and irregular menstrual cycles. Taken daily, it is thought to be about 97 per cent reliable in preventing pregnancy, somewhat less than pills containing oestrogen. To enhance its effectiveness, some women use a second method of birth control, such as a diaphragm or condom, at mid-cycle.

Some women stop having menstrual periods entirely while taking the mini-pill, meaning they are never sure whether they have missed a period because of pregnancy or the medication. Also, the incidence of ECTOPIC PREGNANCY (outside the uterus, a dangerous condition) is higher in women who become pregnant while taking the mini-pill, possibly because of the egg's slower transport.

A woman should have a complete check-up before beginning the mini-pill, which is available only by prescription. She then takes the first pill on the fifth day of a menstrual period (counting the first day of bleeding as Day 1) and one a day therafter, whether or not she has menstrual bleeding. If she forgets to take a pill she should take one as soon as she remembers but should also immediately begin using a back-up method of contraception (foam, diaphragm, condom, etc.) for the rest of that cycle. If more than forty-five days pass without a menstrual period, she should have a pregnancy test.

Miscarriage 1 Also *spontaneous abortion, natural abortion.* The loss of a pregnancy, or expulsion of a foetus before it is sufficiently developed to survive. Such a foetus is defined as one weighing less than 500 grams (1.1 pounds), although some authorities define an infant weighing between 500 and 999 grams (1.1 and 2.2 pounds) as 'immature' and others as an 'abortion' (see also PREMATURE). The term 'miscarriage' is strictly a popular or lay term; doctors always use 'abortion', distinguishing only between *spontaneous* or *natural abortion*, which occurs through natural causes, and *induced, elective,* or *therapeutic abortion,* which results from artificial intervention. This book follows current popular usage: 'abortion' is used only for artificially induced abortion; 'miscarriage' is used for natural or spontaneous loss of a pregnancy.

An estimated 15 to 20 per cent of all known pregnancies in Britain end in miscarriage; in underdeveloped countries the rate is much higher. Moreover, presumably a still higher percentage of unknown pregnancies – very soon after conception – end in spontaneous abortion. The majority of miscarriages occur during the first three months of pregnancy, and in at least half of these the cause lies in the foetus itself, which has some anatomic or genetic abnormality. The mother's activities – jumping, falling, vigorous physical exercise, frequent vaginal intercourse – do not cause miscarriage. Neither does emotional shock or stress. On the other hand, hormonal imbalance, infection, or immunologic factors are sometimes responsible (see under HABITUAL MISCARRIAGE), although not nearly as often as was formerly believed. However, habits such as cigarette smoking and regular use of certain drugs, such as LSD, do increase the risk of miscarriage. Other causes for miscarriage in the first trimester are inadequate production of progesterone or some other hormonal lack that either prevents successful IMPLANTATION of the fertilized egg or supplies insufficient nutritional or hormonal support for its growth, or some defect in the endometrium (uterine lining) itself that prevents successful implantation.

Causes of miscarriage during the second trimester (13 to 24 weeks) include anatomical uterine defects (a double or divided uterus, uterine scar tissue from repeated infection, fibroids, endometrial polyps, or a similar problems), an IN-COMPETENT CERVIX, infections such as syphilis or genital herpes, or an immunologic reaction causing the woman's body to reject the foetus as though it were a foreign body (see also under HABITUAL MISCARRIAGE). Many if not most of these conditions can be corrected by medication or surgery, and therefore need not cause miscarriage again.

A single miscarriage does not usually warrant the performance of elaborate tests to determine its cause. However, the risk of miscarriage does rise with a woman's age; one study shows it roughly doubles between the twenties and early thirties, and doubles again between the early and late thirties. For women who have postponed motherhood until their thirties and have had one miscarriage, it therefore may be advisable to determine the cause somewhat sooner, that is, after one miscarriage rather than the three consecutive ones that are considered to constitute habitual miscarriage. Such investigation should include an X-ray of the uterus, an endometrial biopsy timed to detect hormonal deficiency following ovulation, blood tests for blood group and type as well as antibody levels of both parents, semen analysis of the father, and chromosome analysis of both parents.

The loss of a baby that was planned and eagerly awaited can be emotionally very painful for both mother and father, as well as other relatives. Moreover, because miscarriage has a long history of myths and misconceptions, the couple's natural feelings of grief and loss are often complicated by a sense of guilt (what did I do wrong?), anger (it's all his/her fault), and fear (what if I/we can never have a normal baby?). Even people with a rational understanding of the statistics and causes of miscarriage may suffer from nagging doubts and fears. Consequently it is highly advisable after any miscarriage for a woman to ask relevant questions during the follow-up visit with her doctor – with the father also present, if possible – as well as to discuss the suspected or known causes of this particular miscarriage and the chance of a successful future pregnancy.

2 Threatened miscarriage Symptoms indicating that a pregnancy may end prematurely, most often consisting of slight bleeding and mild cramps. Bleeding alone need not be a sign of threatened miscarriage. If the bleeding continues for a time, however, it is advisable to check for a cause other than threatened miscarriage, such as a cervical POLYP. Bleeding and cramps together nearly always constitute a threatened miscarriage, although the cramps are not strong enough to dilate the cervix. When they are, miscarriage is usually inevitable (see definition 3 below).

An early threatened miscarriage, after one or two missed periods, probably cannot be treated effectively, but nearly all doctors recommend bed rest for at least twenty-four hours and no vaginal intercourse for a few days. Since it is believed that most such early miscarriages are due to abnormalities in the foetus and are, in effect, nature's way of eliminating a defective baby, presumably no treatment for the mother would make much difference. For threatened miscarriage later in pregnancy, however, bed rest and the use of drugs to relax the uterus and stop contractions may indeed help save a normal foetus.

3 **Inevitable miscarriage** The occurrence of severe vaginal bleeding and/or cramps in a pregnant woman, indicating that no medical treatment can avert a miscarriage. At this point the amniotic membranes have ruptured, the cervix is dilated, and membranes, foetus, and placenta are on their way to being expelled. The woman's doctor should be contacted immediately, and hospitalization may be necessary. If the foetus and other material are expelled at home, they should be placed in a sterile container and brought to the doctor for examination, since they may reveal the reason for the miscarriage. If pain and blood loss are severe and prolonged, further treatment in the hospital may be necessary.

4 **Incomplete miscarriage** A miscarriage in which not all of the products of conception – membranes, foetus, placenta – are spontaneously expelled. Usually it is part of the placenta that is retained. Incomplete miscarriage is usually marked by continued bleeding, which can be severe enough to constitute a haemorrhage. Sometimes a drug such as oxytocin is administered to stimulate uterine contractions that may expel the remainder, but more often a D AND C or VACUUM ASPIRATION is performed to make sure all the material is out of the uterus. Incomplete miscarriage tends to occur most often in the second trimester.

5 **Missed miscarriage** The retention of a dead foetus inside the uterus for at least two months. Unlike other kinds of miscarriage (see above), the symptoms are barely noticeable. There may or may not be vaginal bleeding. Usually the breasts return to pre-pregnant size and the uterus stops growing; eventually it becomes somewhat smaller, owing to absorption of amniotic fluid. Many women report few or no symptoms, but some complain of lassitude, fatigue, depression, and a bad taste in the mouth. Usually uterine contractions eventually begin of their own accord, and the foetus is spontaneously expelled, as in other kinds of miscarriage. When, however, the mother is aware of the fact that the foetus is dead, waiting for spontaneous miscarriage can be emotionally devastating for both her and the family. Consequently many doctors advise emptying the uterus promptly by inducing labour with oxytocin, by AMNIOINFUSION, or by D and C, the choice depending on the size of the uterus. See also STILLBIRTH.

6 **Septic miscarriage** Any miscarriage (see definition 1 to 5 above) that involves infection of the uterus and/or the products of conception. Symptoms include, in addition to the usual vaginal bleeding, marked tenderness of the uterus and lower abdomen, chills, fever, and an elevated white blood-cell count. Septic miscarriage is treated with massive doses of antibiotics for twelve to twenty-four hours; if labour does not begin by itself, a D and C is performed. Such infections are commonly found following an induced ABORTION performed by an unqualified or sloppy practitioner – they are common where a proper medical abortion is illegal or unavailable – or by women on themselves with instruments ranging from coat hangers to knitting needles. They may also be the result of PELVIC INFLAMMATORY DISEASE or of an INTRAUTERINE DEVICE (IUD) that has

failed to prevent pregnancy. Unless treated promply, such infection may cause enough damage to require removal of the uterus (HYSTERECTOMY). See also PUERPERAL FEVER.

Missed abortion (miscarriage) See MISCARRIAGE, definition 5.

Mittelschmerz A German word, literally meaning 'middle pain', used to refer to a cramping pain on one side of the lower abdomen that some women regularly feel at OVULATION. Occasionally the pain is quite severe and mimics the symptoms of acute appendicitis. It may or may not be accompanied by slight bleeding and sometimes even severe bleeding. The reason for these symptoms is not known, especially since many women never feel anything when they ovulate. One theory is that it may be due to the irritation of the abdominal lining caused by fluid or blood released from the ruptured egg follicle; another is that follicle growth stretches the surface of the ovary, causing pain (see also GRAAFIAN FOLLICLE). Whatever the cause, Mittelschmerz usually persists no more than a few hours, and rarely more than twenty-four hours.

Mongolism, mongoloid See DOWN'S SYNDROME.

Moniliasis See YEAST INFECTION.

Mons veneris Also *mons pubis, pubis, pubic mound.* A cushion of fat that lies over the central portion of the pubic bone, or *symphysis pubis.* After puberty it is covered with PUBIC HAIR, usually forming a triangular pattern called the *escutcheon.*

Montgomery's glands See under AREOLA.

Morning-after pill Any medication prescribed within seventy-two hours of unprotected (against pregnancy) intercourse, such as rape. The medication, which generally consists of a combined oestrogen and progesterone preparation given within 72 hours of intercourse and repeated after 12 hours. Another possibility for preventing pregnancy after unprotected intercourse are the insertion of an INTRAUTERINE DEVICE within five days to prevent implantation, which some doctors consider both unsound medical practice and often ineffective.

Morning sickness Popular name for the nausea of early pregnancy, technically called *nausea gravidarum.* It is believed to result from the greatly increased levels of human chorionic gonadotrophin (HCG) secreted during the first trimester. It is generally confined to the first three and one-half months of pregnancy, although a small percentage of women continue to experience it either steadily or occasionally until delivery. Also, although many women find it occurs only in the morning, when they first get out of bed, others experience it at different times of day, such as late afternoon, and some intermittently throughout the day. Some women feel nauseated, vomit, and then are relatively comfortable; others vomit but continue to feel nausea; still others simply feel constantly queasy and never vomit at all. The remedies generally recommended are to eat lightly a number of times through the day rather than taking a few big meals, slowly munching dry crackers or toast before arising (nausea is thought to be worse on an empty stomach), and avoiding greasy spiced foods and any particular foods that seem to bring on nausea (many women find meat and other proteins the worst offenders). A variety of both prescription and over-the-counter medications, especially anti-histamines and other remedies for motion sickness, have been used over the years, but many of them have come under suspicion as possible causes of birth defects. Therefore, unless the condition is so severe as to cause dangerous malnutrition, dehydration, or fluid-electrolyte imbalance in the mother, probably no medication of any kind should be used. Women with very severe cases – where the condition is called *hyperemesis gravidarum* – usually require hospitalization and find relief only when fluid-electrolyte balance is corrected by administering intravenous fluids.

Motility, sperm   The ability of sperm to move, which is necessary if they are to travel from the vagina through the cervical canal to the uterus and Fallopian tubes to fertilize an egg. For a man to be considered fertile, 60 per cent of the sperm in a sample of his semen must still be moving after four hours (see under SPERM for semen analysis). The application of heat to the testes is believed to decrease sperm motility (see THERMATIC STERILIZATION). Hormonal factors, infections, and disease of the prostate gland may have a similar effect.

Mucous membrane   Also *mucosa*. Glandular tissues that secrete *mucus*, a thick, sticky, lubricating liquid composed of glandular secretions, salts, dead cells, and white blood cells. Mucous membranes line practically all of the body cavities with external openings (orifices), including the mouth, nose, rectum, and vagina, as well as the internal surfaces of many other organs.

Mucus method   See CERVICAL MUCUS METHOD.

Mucus plug   A small wad of mucus that fills the cervical canal during pregnancy. It is often expelled spontaneously as a thick fluid discharge, along with a little blood, as the cervix is slowly dilating. This phenomenon is called the *bloody show*, or *show*, and may occur weeks before the onset of labour, just before labour, or during the course of labour.

Multigravida   A woman who has been pregnant more than once.

Multipara   A woman who has completed one or more pregnancies to the stage of viability (when the baby could live).

Multiple pregnancy   A pregnancy with more than one foetus at the same time, that is, twins, triplets, quadruplets, etc.

By far the most common kind of multiple pregnancy is twins. Of twins born in Britain, about one-third are identical (monozygotic) and the rest fraternal. Fraternal twins are more like siblings of the same ages than twins; they may be of the same or opposite sexes and do not resemble each other more than other, single children of the same parents do. Identical twins are necessarily of the same sex (all the genetic material of the egg divided into two to form them, including the sex chromosomes) and resemble each other closely. Occasionally identical twins do not separate completely but are born conjoined and share some of the same organs; this is the phenomenon known as *Siamese twins* and is caused by failure of the embryo to split entirely in two.

The occurrence of identical twins is, so far as is known, entirely a matter of chance. It is not affected by any identifiable factors, and indeed is rare in all other mammals except the nine-banded armadillo, which routinely produces four babies from one egg. In human beings identical twins occur at random in 1 of every 200 pregnancies.

Fraternal twinning, on the other hand, is influenced by the pituitary gland's secretion of FSH as well as a number of other factors. It occurs far more often in blacks than in whites, and far less often in Orientals. It is more probable when there is a family history of fraternal twins, presumably because the trait of producing more than one egg at ovuation, called *polyovulation*, or its cause – higher secretion of FSH – is hereditary.

Since the 1960s the incidence of fraternal twins has risen markedly with use of various kinds of FERTILITY PILL, which stimulate FSH production. The chance of bearing fraternal twins also increases with the mother's age and the number of previous pregnancies: at age twenty the chances are 4 for every 1,000; at age forty they are 16 for every 1,000. After forty, however, they drop again. Fat women are more likely to bear twins than thin women, perhaps owing to higher hormone levels.

With fraternal twins the eggs may be released from one ovary or from both. Each twin has its own amniotic sac and placenta. Identical twins may be formed at various times in the early development of the fertilized egg, but it is presumed that the division usually occurs before the eighth day after fertilization. Some identical twins share a placenta but have separate umbilical cords; these babies do not often survive, because their cords become entangled, cutting off their oxygen supply. More often each twin has its own placenta and cord. Even so, sometimes only one twin is born alive.

In such cases the dead twin may be expelled early, in miscarriage, and the live one carried to term. More often, however, the twins will be born at the same time (or at least within one hour), one alive and the other dead, the latter having been carried dead for some months. This tends to happen more with identical twins than fraternal ones and often results from *transfusion syndrome*, in which the twins have an arterial connection whereby one twin in effect bleeds the other to death.

Multiple pregnancy is riskier for both babies and mothers. The rate of miscarriage and stillbirth is much higher than in single births, as is the rate of newborn mortality. The latter is at least partly due to the fact that twins, like all multiple pregnancies, are rarely carried as long as single pregnancies – an average of thirty-seven weeks for twins versus thirty-nine weeks for single births – and PREMATURE babies have a poorer chance of survival. Nevertheless, combined perinatal and neonatal mortality is four times higher than with single births. Other complications occurring more often with twins are HYDRAMNIOS, PREECLAMPSIA, PLACENTA PRAEVIA, ABNORMAL PRESENTATION, PROLONGED LABOUR, and POSTPARTUM HAEMORRHAGE.

Often the existence of a multiple pregnancy is not discovered until one baby has been delivered and the size of the mother's uterus indicates it is not yet empty. Some women have even been given oxytocin or another drug to help the uterus continue contracting and return to normal size before it was realized that another baby was still there; this is extremely dangerous to both mother and child, and can usually be avoided by palpating the uterus immediately after delivery, so that another foetus would be felt. Occasionally, however, it must be done because the overdistended uterus fails to contract, haemorrhaging begins, and labour stops, putting both the second baby and the mother at severe risk.

Multiple pregnancy is suspected when the uterus is much larger than normal for the length of gestation, based on the last menstrual period. Often foetal heartbeats cannot be detected as early, probably because the foetuses are smaller than in a single pregnancy of the same duration. ULTRASOUND can establish the presence of twins quite early; X-rays usually do not reveal it until the end of the fifth month. by the seventh month abdominal palpation will often reveal the presence of two foetuses.

Especially during the last two months, women carrying twins require extra care to avoid the two major complications likely to occur then, preeclampsia and premature labour. More frequent antenatal visits generally are advisable. Careful review of the mother's diet is important, as well as extra rest. Some doctors advocate near or complete bed rest from about twenty-eight weeks on to reduce the risk of PREMATURE labour.

Multiple sclerosis Also *MS*. A recurring disease of the central nervous system that attacks the myelin, or covering sheath, of nerve fibres in the brain and spinal cord, which become scarred with hard, sclerotic patches that interrupt message transmission in the nerve pathways of vision, sensation, and voluntary movement. As a result, there may be a variety of symptoms, principally ataxia (failure of muscle control, leading to spasm and disturbed co-ordination), muscular weakness and tremor, extreme fatigue, numbness and paralysis in the extremities, difficulty with bladder control, double or blurred vision or other visual disturbances, and speech difficulties. The disease affects women half again as often as men, and usually strikes between the ages of twenty and forty. Its course, however, is so variable that it is virtually unpredictable. A first attack, which usually runs its course in a few weeks, may be followed by no symptoms whatever for a period of fifteen or twenty years; or the disease may recur in months or even weeks, usually at increasingly shorter intervals. Eventually, however, permanent and progressive disability may occur.

The cause of multiple sclerosis is not known. In addition, the disease is difficult to diagnose on the basis of a single attack (or even several attacks) because its symptoms are so varied and often resemble those of cerebral vascular accident (stroke), brain tumours, syphilis, and other conditions. No cure is yet known, and research on different treatments has been greatly hampered by the frequent occurrence of spontaneous remission, making it impossible to tell whether a treatment was effective or the disease subsided spontaneously. In 1981 researchers reported promising results with interferon, a powerful new antiviral drug, which did not cure the disease but seemed to slow or halt its progression, and also led to the speculation that the cause was connected with a virus or viral infection. However, later studies have not confirmed these results. Other treatment is strictly palliative, including avoidance of overfatigue, massage for weakened limbs, physiotherapy for impaired co-ordination, and prompt attention to urinary infections and similar secondary problems.

In women, multiple sclerosis does not affect either menstruation or fertility. Pregnancy is possible, but there is some evidence that it worsens the disease's symptoms, perhaps because of increased hormone levels. For this reason also, oral contraceptives should be avoided. The sex drive may be diminished during periods of extreme fatigue, and orgasmic ability is impaired when there is lack of sensation. However, some women who lose senation in the pelvic area find that other areas of the body become more sensitive to sexual stimulation. During intercourse and masturbation there may be increased urinary incontinence, which can sometimes be prevented by making sure the bladder is quite empty beforehand. During periods of remission, however, many patients are able to lead normal or near normal lives.

Muscular dystrophy A hereditary chronic disease in which the voluntary muscles become progressively weaker. The most common form, *Duchenne muscular dystrophy*, is a sex-linked recessive-gene disorder (see under BIRTH DEFECTS for explanation) passed on by mothers to their sons. It usually appears before the age of seven, beginning with difficulties in walking and standing, and eventually affecting the shoulders and arms. By puberty most victims are confined to a wheelchair. At present, there is neither a cure nor a specific treatment.

Myoma, myomectomy See under FIBROID.

N

Nabothian cyst See CYST, definition 4.

Natural childbirth See PREPARED CHILDBIRTH.

Natural family planning Also *biological birth control, calendar method, fertility awareness, periodic abstinence, rhythm method.* A method of both birth control and pregnancy planning that is based on timing sexual intercourse so as to avoid (or seek out) a woman's fertile period, that is, her time of OVULATION. For preventing pregnancy the couple abstains from vaginal intercourse during ovulation and, for more safety, several days before and afterward. Since an egg remains viable for only twenty-four hours after its release from the ovary, sperm, which can live forty-eight hours after ejaculation, must be present in the Fallopian tube during that interval if fertilization is to take place.

Natural family planning is still the only means of birth control sanctioned by the Roman Catholic Church. Its success depends entirely on how closely one can estimate the time of ovulation and on avoiding intercourse during this fertile period. The interval between a menstrual period and ovulation is highly variable, both from one woman to the next and in the same woman (see MENSTRUAL CYCLE) but ovulation always occurs approximately fourteen days before the start of the next menstrual period; thus one can tell when ovulation last took place, but only *after* the fact.

The four main methods of calculating the fertile period are: the calendar method, temperature method, CERVICAL MUCUS METHOD, and combined or sympto-thermic method.

The *calendar method*, also called *rhythm method*, uses the length of past menstrual cycles to calculate the probable time of ovulation. For this purpose a woman must keep track of her cycle for at least six months. A cycle is said to begin on the first day of menstrual flow (day 1) and end on the last day before the next menstrual flow. One subtracts 18 from the shortest cycle to obtain the fertile day, and 11 from the longest cycle to obtain the last fertile day. To prevent pregnancy, one must avoid vaginal intercourse from the first fertile day to the last fertile day. The rest of the month is considered the *safe period*. Another mode of calculation is counting to 15 from day 1 of a period; from that date subtract 6 and also add 6; these 13 days are the possible fertile ones, and the rest are 'safe.' The calendar method is considered the *least reliable* method of natural family planning, and is totally useless for women with very irregular cycles, or following abortion or delivery, or during breast-feeding.

The *temperature method*, also called BASAL BODY TEMPERATURE (BBT), is based on the fact that progesterone, released by the corpus luteum after ovulation, causes a measurable increase in basal body temperature, which remains raised until the next menstrual period. It, too, is an after-the-fact method of determining ovulation, that is, it provides evidence that ovulation took place, and when. It is somewhat more reliable than the calendar method and can be used by women with irregular menstrual cycles but is inaccurate following abortion or childbirth. Over a period of six to eight months, it may give a good indication of a woman's pattern of ovulation.

The CERVICAL MUCUS METHOD is based on the fact that the cervical mucus in most women changes in consistency during the course of each menstrual cycle. After menstruation and before ovulation, the mucus is thick, sticky, opaque, and scant. A few days before ovulation the amount of mucus increases and it becomes clear and more slippery, not unlike raw egg white. A woman checks her mucus manually and keeps a record of changes in consistency to establish some kind of pattern for ovulation (she can also use one of several chemical tests on the mucus). This method has not been tested adequately over a long period of time, but it appears to work reasonably well once a woman has become thoroughly familiar with her own body patterns.

The *combined* or *sympto-thermic method* uses both changes in basal body temperature and changes in cervical mucus to estimate the fertile period. It appears to be the most reliable method of these four, but none is as reliable as oral contraceptives, a diaphragm used with a spermicide, or intrauterine devices. (See illustration under CONTRACEPTIVE for a comparison.)

Natural family planning does have certain advantages. For birth control these methods are all totally reversible. They work either for planning a pregnancy or for preventing one. They have no harmful side effects. They are free or require only very inexpensive equipment, and they involve the male partner's co-operation. Their chief disadvantages are their limited reliability (depending on how regular a woman's cycles are) and the need for self-control exercised by both partners to prevent pregnancy (unless an alternative method of contraception is used during fertile periods). One other risk has been suggested. When natural family planning fails and unplanned pregnancy occurs, there appears to be a much higher than normal rate of miscarriage and birth defects. It is suspected this is due to fertilization involving an old egg or an old sperm. The best chance for normal pregnancy is fertilization at the time of ovulation. A miscalculation by a couple using natural family planning may lead to fertilization twenty-four hours after ovulation, with increased risk of defects.

Nausea An unpleasant feeling in the upper gastrointestinal tract and abdomen, often associated with vomiting. In addition to being a symptom of gastrointestinal disorders of many kinds, ranging from mild to serious, as well as a side effect of radiation therapy and chemotherapy against cancer, in women nausea is associated with a number of conditions in which hormone levels are temporarily higher than usual. Chief among these is the nausea of early pregnancy, commonly called MORNING SICKNESS. Nausea is sometimes a symptom of spasmodic dysmenorrhoea, along with the cramps accompanying the first days of menstrual flow; a side effect of some oral contraceptives, usually those very high in oestrogen; and, rarely, a symptom of incomplete miscarriage, when some foetal or placental material has remained in the uterus. Nausea is also one of the symptoms of the secondary stage of SYPHILIS.

Necrospermia Absence of live sperm in the seminal fluid, rendering a man sterile. See STERILITY.

Needle aspiration, needle biopsy See BIOPSY, definition 3.

Neonatal jaundice Also *neonatal icterus, newborn jaundice, physiological jaundice, hyperbilirubinaemia.* Mild jaundice in a newborn baby, manifested in yellowing of the skin and the eyes between the second and fifth days of life. It is caused by a delay in the ability of the baby's liver to deal with bilirubin, a product of the breakdown of haemoglobin (the oxygen-carrying molecule of blood) from foetal red blood cells. Mild jaundice from this source is quite common and rarely lasts more than a week. However, jaundice occurring before the second day of life or after the fifth day is abnormal (it may be a symptom of ERYTHROBLASTOSIS), as is severe jaundice. If the yellow colour is particularly deep, a blood bilirubin level test should be performed; levels over 20 mg. blood bilirubin per 100 cc. of blood can cause permanent brain damage in the child. Causes of abnormal jaundice include infection, blood incompatibility, or a structural abnormality in the liver, among others. Frequently the cause is never determined. Treatment consists of placing the baby blindfolded under fluorescent lights to lower the blood bilirubin concentration, and this phototherapy is continued until levels are within safe limits.

Neonatology The medical speciality of caring for sick babies before, during, and after birth. With a HIGH-RISK PREGNANCY it is advisable for the mother to be near a medical centre with a neonatologist, if at all possible.

Neoplasm Another   name   for TUMOUR.

Neural tube defects A class of common, very serious birth defects that involve failure of the baby's spinal cord to close properly. When the tube does not close at the top of the spine, the brain does not develop properly, a condition called *anencephaly*, which is generally fatal within hours after birth. When the failure to close occurs lower down, the condition is called SPINA BIFIDA.

Nidation Another   name   for IMPLANTATION.

Nipple The specialized part of the female BREAST through which milk is expressed during lactation. The breast's milk-producing glands, the ACINI, are connected to the nipple by a complex network of ducts that enlarge as they enter the nipple. The enlarged portions are called *lactiferous sinuses*, and their external openings are the numerous pin-sized holes in the nipple. Usually the nipple is cylindrical, protrudes somewhat above the surface of the surrounding AREOLA, and is a brownish colour somewhat darker than the areola. However, in some women the nipple may be quite flat, almost flush with the areola, or inverted (turned inward), and approximately the same colour as the areola. The shape of the normal nipple varies widely. Usually both nipples are about equal in size and shape but if one breast is significantly larger the nipple may be larger, too. Occasionally a woman has one or more extra (*accessory*) nipples. They are usually located below the breast and are flat, as in a child before puberty.

The nipple is covered with a layer of hairless skin and contains many muscle fibres, through which pass the terminal milk ducts from each lobe of the breast. It is the contraction of these muscle fibres that causes the nipple to become erect during sexual arousal (cold can similarly stimulate erection) and, in lactating women, to expel milk.

An *inverted nipple*, in which the central portion of the nipple appears to turn inward, is also normal, although it may require a little manipulation if a woman is attempting to breast-feed. Surgical repair of this condition is possible but is often only partly successful. Frequently, however, flat or even inverted nipples begin to project somewhat during lactation, and the shape does not interfere with milk production. Using a special plastic shield called a Woolwich Shield during pregnancy and the breast-feeding period helps some women. Also, a nipple-rolling exercise done twice a day may change the shape enough so that the baby can grasp the nipple more easily.

An inverted nipple should be distinguished from a *retracted nipple*, where the nipple is pulled inward by an underlying tumour or inflammation. Usually in the case of a tumour the nipple becomes larger and flatter as the tumour grows; also, only the nipple of one breast will show this change, giving some warning. Reddening, ulceration, or scaling of the nipple, which is normally bumpy and wrinkled in appearance, are also signs of disease.

In the non-lactating woman discharge from the nipples may be caused by tumours within the breast, either benign or malignant, by disorders of the pituitary or hypothalamus, by infection, as a side effect of some drugs (especially the phenothiazine tranquillizers), or from chronic stimulation of the nipples, as in love play. A thin white discharge is probably milk caused by some endocrine disorders that is producing lactation abnormally. A purulent (pus-laden) discharge is usually the result of an infection, such as MASTITIS. A thick sticky discharge, which may vary in colour is usually a sign of inflammation involving the terminal milk ducts, whereas a serous (thin, clear, yellowish) discharge, with or without some bleeding, is usually caused by either a benign or malignant lesion, most often a benign DUCTAL PAPILLOMA. The most serious kind of tumour involving the nipple is PAGET'S DISEASE (definition 1). See also BREAST-FEEDING; BREAST SELF-EXAMINATION; LACTATION.

Nit The egg of a crab louse. See PUBIC LICE.

Node Also *nodule*. A small mass of tissue resembling a swelling, knot, or similar protrusion. It may be normal, as in the case of lymph nodes, which actually are glands, or it may indicate the presence of disease, as when nodes occur on the joints in rheumatic disease.

Nongonococcal urethritis (NGU), nonspecific urethritis (NSU) See under URETHRITIS.

Non specific vaginitis Also, *NSV.* See under VAGINITIS.

Non-stress test Also, *NST*. See under FOETAL MONITORING.

Nullipara A woman who has never completed a pregnancy to the state of viability (when the child could live).

Nursing See BREAST-FEEDING.

Nutrition See DIET; OBESITY; WEIGHT.

Nymphomania See under LIBIDO.

O

Obesity The condition of weighing 20 per cent or more over what is considered one's ideal weight relative to height and body build. Obesity is nearly always caused by overeating, but the factors that lead a person to eat far more than his or her body needs, so that the excess is stored as fat, are not completely understood. Some individuals do not seem to gain much weight no matter what they eat, whereas others gain weight very readily. Both men and women have a tendency to gain more weight as they grow older, particularly women after the menopause, but whether such weight gain is partly due to hormonal changes or is simply a matter of eating the same amounts of food while becoming less physically active is not certain. What is known, however, is that obesity is dangerous, particularly to postmenopausal women. It makes them more susceptible to a variety of serious and potentially life-threatening disorders, including diabetes, osteoarthritis, heart disease, hypertension and cerebral vascular accident (stroke), gall bladder disease, and breast and endometrial cancer.

There is no easy way to convert an obese woman into a slender one. It is estimated that 3,500 calories of food produce a single pound of fat. The person who is 50 pounds heavier than she should be must therefore reduce her usual food intake over a period of time by a total of 175,000 calories. In theory, at least, one can lose a pound of fat per week by reducing one's food intake by only 500 calories a day. Unfortunately the weight loss on such a diet is rarely constant, owing to fluid retention and metabolic factors that are not completely understood. Nevertheless, to avoid malnutrition – and even obese persons can be malnourished if they eat mainly junk food and get inadequate vitamins and minerals – the best diet for weight reduction for an adult woman in otherwise good health provides 1,000 to 1,200 calories per day and consists of small servings of a large variety of foods that meet the necessary vitamin and mineral requirements, with 20 to 25 per cent of the calories from protein, 30 to 35 per cent from fats, and the remainder from carbohydrates. Any such diet should be accompanied by regular and gradually increased physical exercise, preferably by making a conscious effort to change one's daily habits to include more physical exertion. For undertaking a more vigorous programme, cardiovascular and respiratory status should first be assessed (see also EXERCISE). Fad diets that emphasize eating one or a few foods and eliminating most others, and diet medication should be avoided. In general, even if fad diets and medication help a person lose weight, that weight is generally gained back very quickly when diet or medication is discontinued. Many people find group plans or behaviour-modification groups, which aim at reeducating eating habits, helpful as a long-term solution. For a time grossly obese persons, who weigh twice as much or more than they should, were sometimes treated with a surgical procedure called an *intestinal by-pass operation*. It involved eliminating a section of the small intestine from the normal flow, reducing its effective length and thereby diminishing the total absorptive surface for nutrients. However, the side effects from it were so severe that it has been largely abandoned. A similar procedure, called a *gastric by-pass*, which removes part of the stomach is occasionally performed but only as a last resort.

See also DIET; WEIGHT, BODY; WEIGHT GAIN.

Obstetrician A doctor who specializes in *obstetrics*, that is, childbirth including antenatal care, delivery (both vaginal and surgical), and postpartum care. See also GYNAECOLOGIST; MIDWIFE; BIRTH ATTENDANT.

Oedema Also *fluid retention, water retention, bloating, dropsy* (obsolete). An abnormal accumulation of fluid in the body, specifically in the spaces ouside the vessels of the circulatory system. The principal symptoms are swelling, particularly noticeable in the extremities (fingers, ankles), and weight gain. Mild oedema is commonplace in women at certain times, especially premenstrually (see DYSMENORRHOEA, definition 5) and during late pregnancy. It is not known just why or how the body accumulates more water at those times, but it is most likely the higher levels of oestrogen and progesterone are a factor. Severe oedema, on the other hand, is a symptom of a number of potentially life-threatening disorders, among them ECLAMPSIA in women who are pregnant or have just given birth, and liver, heart, and kidney disease. Acute pulmonary oedema, a complication of congestive heart disease, is an emergency requiring prompt treatment.

Oedema is commonly treated with a DIURETIC, a class of drugs that aim to improve the function of vital organs whose impairment is causing the oedema and/or relieve the distress of symptoms. Such treatment is nearly always combined with the restriction of sodium (salt) intake in the diet, since high levels of sodium make the body retain water.

Oestrogen General name for the principal female sex hormone, produced in women chiefly by the ovaries and placenta. In men some oestrogen is produced by the testes. There are three principal forms of ovarian and placental oestrogen – oestrone, oestradiol, and oestrol – and at least seventeen minor kinds. At puberty production of a hormone, FSH, by the pituitary gland stimulates the development of egg follicles in the ovary, which produce oestrogen. These increased levels of oestrogen account for pubertal development: growth of the breasts, uterus, Fallopian tubes, and vagina; increase in layers of fat and their pattern of distribution, producing the characteristic female figure; slowdown and eventually ending of growth of the long bones (arms and legs, hands and feet); and growth of pubic and underarm hair. For the next thirty-five or forty years, levels of oestrogen rise each month during the MENSTRUAL CYCLE and drop if fertilization does not occur. During pregnancy oestrogen production is taken over by the placenta and remains high until delivery. Some oestrogen is also produced by a woman's adrenal glands and by adipose (fatty) tissue, which apparently converts androgens (male hormones) produced by the adrenal glands into oestrogen. After menopause, when the regular monthly upsurge of ovarian oestrogen stops, adrenal production and fatty-tissue release of oestrogen continue (which may account for the fact that large, plump women often have fewer menopausal symptoms associated with oestrogen decrease than small, thin women).

The discovery of oestrogen dates from about 1915, and the first synthetic oestrogen was produced some fifteen years later. Both natural oestrogen (often obtained from the urine of pregnant mares) and synthetic oestrogen (made in the laboratory) are used in oral contraceptives to prevent pregnancy, to replace oestrogen after surgically induced or natural menopause (see OESTROGEN REPLACEMENT THERAPY), to treat menstrual irregularities, to suppress lactation after childbirth, and to treat some forms of cancer. Side effects from taking oestrogen include nausea and vomiting (from too high dosage), breast tenderness and enlargement (also in men), headache, vertigo (dizziness), fluid retention, and irregular vaginal bleeding. Moreover, the administration of oestrogen is considered a contributing cause in a number of disorders, especially in blood clots, high blood pressure, and some kinds of cancer, and its use is therefore controversial. Oestrogen therapy of any kind is contraindicated if there is a personal or family history of cancer of the breast or pelvic organs, or a history of thrombosis or high blood pessure. In addition, the presence of obesity, gall bladder disease, and diabetes indicates it should be used only with great caution. Also, see the specific contraindications under OESTROGEN REPLACEMENT THERAPY and ORAL CONTRACEPTIVES.

Oestrogen-receptor assay A diagnostic test to determine whether a cancerous tumour's growth is dependent on oestrogen. Some cancers of the breast are stimulated to grow by oestrogen, and others are not. For those that are, chemotherapy (anticancer drugs) is often not very effective, but *endocrine manipulation* – changing the body's level of hormones – may help control the cancer. Such manipulation includes removing or inactivating organs and glands involved in oestrogen production (ovaries, adrenal glands, pituitary gland) or administering large doses of hormone. The ovaries can be excised surgically, or their function can be ended by radiation treatment, and the adrenals can be removed surgically (adrenalectomy). In 1981 researchers announced that their experience with the drug aminoglutethimide showed it cut oestrogen production as effectively as adrenalectomy. However, fewer than half of all breast cancers are hormone-dependent, so it is important to establish whether or not they are before initiating such therapy. The oestrogen-receptor assay can be used not only to plan additional treatment after surgery but to help plan future treatment if the cancer recurs. The test itself is performed on the tumour tissue, taken by biopsy. If the hospital where the biopsy is taken is not equipped to perform the test (and many laboratories are not), it can freeze the tissue and send it on to a laboratory that is. About two-thirds of patients whose tumours contain oestrogen receptors (are oestrogen-dependent) respond to endocrine therapy. Currently similar tests and treatments are being devised for progesterone-dependent tumours.

Oestrogen replacement therapy Also *ORT, hormone therapy.* The use of oestrogen in any of several forms – natural or synthetic, oral, by injection, or in creams or suppositories – in order to 'replace' oestrogen no longer produced by the ovaries. It is used principally to relieve some of the unpleasant symptoms of MENOPAUSE that occur either naturally or following surgical removal of both ovaries (which brings on menopause very suddenly). It is indeed effective against HOT FLUSHES and VAGINAL ATROPHY, and appears to slow down bone resorption (see OSTEOPOROSIS). It is not effective, however, in preventing cardiovascular disease (heart attack or stroke), wrinkles, arthritis, or depression. Moreover, since the mid-1960s there has been mounting evidence that oestrogen use may increase one's risk of developing serious cardiovascular disease, especially potentially fatal blood clots. Consequently, it should never to used by women who have severe kidney or liver disease, phlebitis, sickle cell disease, very high blood pressure, cerebral vascular diseases (including arteriosclerotic disease), or a history of breast or pelvic cancer, and it should be used only with extreme caution by women who have a family history of breast cancer or have had fibroids, endometriosis, endometrial hyperplasia, cystic disease of the breasts, epilepsy, migraine headaches, and tuberculosis.

If menopausal symptoms are so severe that a woman is willing to face the risks of oestrogen therapy, frequent check-ups, including endometrial biopsy and breast examination every six months, are considered mandatory. The mode of administration makes little difference; indeed, vaginal creams and suppositories are absorbed more readily and faster than pills (because the liver apparently filters out a considerable amount when oestrogen is taken orally). Most often oestrogen replacement is prescribed on a three-weeks-on, one-week-off schedule, which in some women gives rise to periodical vaginal bleeding resembling menstruation (so-called *withdrawal bleeding*), usually near the end of the week without oestrogen. Some doctors advise a schedule of three weeks of oestrogen followed by one week of oestrogen plus progestin (synthetic progesterone) to prevent build-up of the uterine lining (endometrium). Obviously the lowest effective dose is the least hazardous, and therapy should be continued for the shortest time possible. Even with care, some women are unable to tolerate oestrogen replacement therapy owing to such side effects as headache, severe nausea, abdominal bloating or cramps, breast tenderness and engorgement, fluid retention, irregular vaginal bleeding and staining, and oversecretion of vaginal mucus (heavy discharge).

Oligomenorrhoea Infrequent menstruation, with intervals of thirty-eight or more days between menstrual periods. It is particularly common at MENARCHE, when intervals of two or three months between periods often occur in girls during the first few years of menstrual periods. It is also common during the menopausal years, from the age of forty-five onwards. In both instances it usually constitutes ANOVULATORY BLEEDING, that is, menstruation in the absence of ovulation, which is caused by hormone imbalance. Some women, however, regularly have a longer than normal cycle, and if they menstruate fairly regularly every two months instead of monthly, that alone need not be a cause for alarm or require treatment. Occasionally emotional problems, crash diets, and obesity can upset the hormone balance enough to cause oligomenorrhoea. See also MENSTRUAL CYCLE.

Oligospermia Also *subfertility.* A relatively small number of SPERM in a semen sample, usually defined as 20 to 40 million sperm per millilitre of seminal fluid. Most doctors believe that at least two analyses of seminal fluid must be performed for any evaluation of sperm. Oligospermia may result from nutritional problems, acute or chronic illness, general metabolic disease, specific poisoning or occupational hazards such as exposure to radiation, central defects in the pituitary or hypothalamus, specific disease in the genital tract causing blockage to the vas deferens and scarring of the tubes, varicose veins in the testes (see VARIOCO-CELE), or congenital defects such as Klinefelter's syndrome. Even with all these possibilities, the cause can never be determined in some men. Among the principal remedies recommended initially are attention to a proper diet and adequate rest, severe restriction of smoking and alcoholic drinks, and avoidance of heat in the genital area (no tight underwear or prolonged baths; see THERMATIC STERILIZATION for explanation). Clomiphene nitrate (see FERTILITY PILL) in low doses over a long period (three months to a year) sometimes effects an increase in sperm count; so may a daily vitamin supplement high in vitamin C (300 milligrams), the B vitamins, and zinc, and the decongestant pseudoephedrine (30 milligrams twice a day).

In cases where the volume of the ejaculate is large (more than 5 million millilitres) but the sperm count low, a technique called split ejaculation may be effective. The man deposits only the first portion of his ejaculate in the woman's vagina; since this portion often contains the majority of the sperm, this technique in effect concentrates it. For some men with oligospermia, however, ARTIFICIAL INSEMINATION may be the only way to fatherhood. See also STERILITY.

Oophorectomy Also *ovariectomy.* Surgical removal of one or both ovaries. The former is called *unilateral oophorectomy*; the latter is *bilateral oophorectomy* and is usually performed in conjunction with removal of the Fallopian tubes and uterus as well. Removal of both ovaries constitutes both *sterilization* and *castration*, since these organs are the source of both ova (eggs) and most of the body's oestrogen. Following bilateral oophorectomy a premenopausal woman will experience all the symptoms of MENOPAUSE, often in quite severe form owing to the suddenness of change in hormone levels. A postmenopausal woman should have no such problem. Many doctors prescribe OESTROGEN REPLACEMENT THERAPY to ease these symptoms. Removal of one ovary reduces a woman's chances of becoming pregnant but does not make her infertile, since eggs continue to be released from the remaining ovary, which also still produces oestrogen.

See also CANCER, OVARIAN; CYST, definition 6; PELVIC INFLAMMATORY DISEASE; STEIN-LEVENTHAL SYNDROME.

Oral contraceptive Also *the Pill, birth control pill.* A hormone preparation taken by mouth that interferes with ovulation, fertilization, or the implantation of a fertilized egg and therefore prevents pregnancy. Available only since 1961, it was the first method of birth control that was nearly 100 per cent effective (provided a woman *never* forgot to take her pill), and it was estimated that by 1980 some 80 to 100 million women in the world were using birth control pills. However, disillusionment with the Pill began as soon as women experienced its side effects, and many women abandoned it because they found them so unpleasant. One oral contraceptive, the SEQUENTIAL PILL, was found dangerous enough to be taken off the market. Moreover, because oral contraceptives work by interfering with the normal functioning of the endocrine system, their effects are not confined to the reproductive system. They have become associated with increased risk of certain potentially life-threatening disorders, including blood vessel and clotting disorders, hypertension (high blood pressure), and liver disease. Some studies indicate there may be increased risk of cancer, especially of oestrogen-dependent breast cancers and some skin cancers (see MELANOMA), associated with oral contraceptive use but other studies have not verified this connection.

Most oral contraceptives contain both synthetic oestrogen and progesterone, the two hormones basic in the MENSTRUAL CYCLE; one kind, however, contains only progesterone (see MINI-PILL; PROGESTER-ONE). By keeping body levels of these hormones constant, combined oral contraceptives block the feedback mechanism whereby rising and falling levels of the hormones trigger ovulation. The Pill is taken for three weeks and then stopped for a week. During the no-Pill week hormone levels drop, causing bleeding similar to menstruation but usually lighter, shorter, and with few or no cramps. The Pill provides a very

regular cycle; a woman who takes it at the same time each day can accurately predict exactly when her 'period' will begin. To change that day, she can omit one or more days of the Pill at the end of the cycle or add one or more days. She should not delay starting a new package of pills for more than seven days following the previous one, or her cycle may become very irregular. Sometimes there is staining or breakthrough bleeding between 'periods'; if it occurs in the first half of the cycle it is usually caused by not enough oestrogen; in the second half it is usually caused by not enough progesterone. If spotting occurs during the first three cycles of the Pill it may have no significance, but if it continues beyond that time a different kind, with a different combination of progesterone and oestrogen, will often eliminate the bleeding.

Some women have no 'periods' when taking the Pill. A woman who misses more than one period should have a pregnancy test; if she is not pregnant and continues to miss periods after three months on the Pill she may need a kind with more progesterone. Similarly, some kinds of Pill have androgenic effects, causing the growth of facial hair, oily skin, and acne; women already susceptible to these characteristics should switch to another kind of Pill.

The principal advantages of oral contraceptives are their high rate of effectiveness, simple method of use, ease of discontinuing use, and beneficial effects on the menstrual cycle, mainly regularizing the cycle and reducing premenstrual tension, menstrual flow, and cramps. Balanced against these advantages are certain absolute contraindications, meaning that no woman with the conditions should even consider oral contraceptives, as well as commonly experienced unpleasant side effects. *No woman should take oral contraceptives if she has any of the following conditions:*

pregnancy or suspicion of pregnancy
breast-feeding
known or suspected breast cancer or any oestrogen-dependent tumour
abnormal genital bleeding of unknown cause
circulatory disorders such as phlebitis or embolisms, or a past history of these disorders
disease of the blood vessels supplying the brain or heart (cerebral-vascular or coronary-artery disorders)
severely impaired liver function
cystic fibrosis
sickle cell disease.

Some authorities feel this list should also include any disease associated with a high risk of circulatory disorders, particularly hypertension (high blood pressure), diabetes, high blood cholesterol levels, heart valve disease, and obesity. In addition, epilepsy and other seizure disorders, migraine, asthma, and kidney disease may all become worse as a result of fluid retention caused by the Pill, and anyone taking oral contraceptives who has these conditions requires careful monitoring.

The greatest risk of oral contraceptives is their association with the increased occurrence of blood vessel and clotting disorders, which include superficial or deep-vein thrombosis (formation of a THROMBUS, or blood clot), pulmonary EMBOLISM (a blood clot blocking the lungs), and the blocking of an artery (as in heart attacks and stroke). These risks, high in all women taking oral contraceptives, are still higher in women who also smoke (especially smokers over thirty

who use fifteen or more cigarettes a day) and in all women over the age of thirty-five. Moreover, some studies show that the effects of the Pill on blood vessels and circulation persist even after the Pill has been discontinued. Furthermore, at least one study suggests that women whose blood is Type A are five times as likely to develop blood clots with oral contraceptives than women with other blood types. Other risks associated with the Pill are increased incidence of a rare liver tumour and increased risk of developing high blood pressure, gall bladder disease, and clinical depression.

Minor but unpleasant side effects are common. Sometimes they pass after a few months of medication, and at other times they can be minimized or eliminated by changing to a different kind of Pill. They include oedema (water retention), with associated nausea, leg cramps, bloating, weight gain, headache, vision changes, irritability, and breast tenderness (early in the cycle they may be due to excess oestrogen and during the no-Pill week they may be due to excess progesterone); skin changes, especially darkening of the skin around the eyes and mouth (CHLOASMA, due to excess oestrogen); androgenic changes such as oily skin and hair, acne, increased body hair (due to excess androgens); loss of hair (due to excess progesterone); changes in normal vaginal discharge (too much or too little oestrogen); depression (excess progesterone); and repeated yeast infections (excess progesterone). Some women experience changes in appetite and sex drive as well as mood changes. Pill users take twice as long to eliminate caffeine from their bodies as non-users, and therefore may develop insomnia, anxiety, and tremors from what for others would be moderate amounts of coffee, tea, soft drinks, and other caffeine-containing substances.

The results of numerous laboratory tests can be altered by oral contraceptives, so it is important that a Pill user reports this fact when being tested for thyroid function, liver chemistry, iron level, blood cholesterol and fat levels, glucose tolerance, blood sugar, white cell count, and tubeculin skin test. The Pill also interacts with other drugs, sometimes causing adverse drug effects or becoming less effective for birth control.

If a woman decides she wants a child, she stops the Pill but should use another method of birth control for at least one cycle before trying to become pregnant. The Pill may be associated with a slight increase in birth defects, and the body should be allowed at least that long an interval to flush out the medication. Some women do not ovulate for several cycles after stopping the Pill, and either have no periods or very irregular ones. In most cases this corrects itself within six months; for the 2 or 3 per cent of cases where it does not, and in which there is also secretion from one or both breasts, other medication may be needed after disease has been ruled out (see POST-PILL AMENORRHOEA). Some doctors believe this condition can be avoided by stopping the Pill for a couple of cycles every two years, which allows for early detection of a suppressed natural cycle, but there is no evidence for this.

A woman should not begin to use oral contraceptives until she has menstruated for at least six months, lest the oestrogen in the Pill prematurely stop her bone growth (see under PUBERTY). Before taking the Pill, which is available by prescription only, she should have a complete check-up, including weight, blood pressure, and a history that will rule out health factors contraindicating its use. In addition to the usual tests (see under GYNAECOLOGICAL EXAMINATION), black women should be tested for SICKLE CELL DISEASE.

About two dozen brands of oral contraceptives are available in Britain. Each contains one of two synthetic oestrogens, mestranol (weaker) or ethinyl oestradiol, and one of five or six different synethetic progesterones, varying in strength. Because these hormones interact with each other, brands must be compared as entities and not just according to their separate components. Oestrogen is responsible for most of the dangerous complications and many of the minor discomforts, so the less oestrogen a Pill contains, the safer it is. Progesterone accounts for a few of the dangerous side effects and some discomfort and, because more varieties of this hormone are available, is more readily changed to relieve them. Also, different brands may involve different modes of manufacture, so changing brands sometimes relieves discomfort.

In starting the Pill, a woman waits for her period, counts the first day of flow as day 1, and takes the first Pill on day 5. She continues taking one Pill a day for twenty-one days, takes no Pill for seven days, and then starts a new package. She continues the pattern of twenty-one days on, seven days off, which enables her always to start on the same day of the week. Some manufacturers package twenty-one Pills of one colour, which contain hormones, and seven Pills of another colour, containing only sugar or iron, so as to lessen the chance that a woman will forget to resume taking pills after a week off them. Her period will usually begin several days after the last hormone Pill of a cycle is taken. She starts the new round of Pills seven days later, whether or not her period has actually started. The Pill should be taken at nearly the same time every day to keep hormone levels in the blood as constant as possible.

If a woman forgets a Pill she should take it as soon as she remembers, even if that means taking two Pills in one day. The chance of pregnancy is still very small. The risk of pregnancy increases, however, if she forgets more than one Pill in a single cycle. She should take the Pill as soon as she remembers, but should not take more than two in a day, and must use a second, back-up method of birth control through the remainder of that cycle. Some doctors say if one misses three Pills in a row, one should stop the Pill until the next period and then start a new round; if the period does not come, a pregnancy test should be carried out.

Women who become nauseated sometimes find that taking the Pill with a meal or just before bedtime helps. If repeated vomiting persists for more than a day, a back-up method of birth control should be used for the rest of the cycle lest the Pill was not absorbed in the stomach.

Certain signs of serious complication warrant seeking *immediate* medical attention, even if it entails going to the emergency department of the nearest hospital. They are:

  severe leg pain (in calf or thigh)
  severe abdominal pain
  severe headache
  severe chest pain
  shortness of breath
  changes in vision (blurring, flashing
    lights, blindness)
  jaundice (yellowing of skin).

All women on oral contraceptives should return to their doctor or clinic within three to six months of the first prescription for a thorough check-up and review. If all is well, check-ups thereafter may be yearly. A woman who becomes pregnant while taking the Pill should stop taking it immediately. Also, women scheduled for surgery of any kind should stop taking the Pill at least one month before entering the hospital in order to avoid increased risk of circulatory complications. For women who like the method of oral contraceptives but cannot tolerate oestrogen, an alternative is the MINI-PILL, which contains only progesterone but is slightly less effective in preventing pregnancy. In 1982 a French biochemist announced development of a four-day Pill, a synthetic steroid that could be taken for four days at the end of each monthly cycle, but considerable testing would be needed before it could be approved.

The Pill was developed in the United States by Dr. Gregory Pincus, who in 1951 received seed money for this purpose from BIRTH CONTROL pioneer Margaret Sanger. By 1955 he had isolated steroids that inhibit ovulation, and in 1956 clinical trials were begun. It became available in Britain in 1961. In addition to their use for birth control, oral contraceptives have been used to treat ENDOMETRIOSIS, STEIN-LEVENTHAL SYNDROME, ovarian CYST and extremely heavy menstrual bleeding. See also OESTROGEN MORNING-AFTER PILL.

Oral sex Also *oral-genital intercourse*. A form of sexual intercourse in which one or both partners use their mouths (lips, tongue) to stimulate their partner's genitals. Oral sex may be performed in addition to or instead of other kinds of sexual intercourse (anal, vaginal). There is no medical reason for a couple who wish to engage in oral sex not to do so except in the presence of venereal disease.

Both SYPHILIS and GONORRHOEA can be transmitted by oral-genital contact, and HERPES INFECTION is thought to be, too. The two principal forms of oral sex are CUNNILINGUS and FELLATIO. See also anal sex under ANUS; COITUS; SEXUAL RESPONSE.

Orgasm Also *climax, coming* (slang). A sudden release of congestion and muscle tension, accompanied by a feeling of intense pleasure, that is the peak of physical gratification in a sexual experience. In women the lower vagina and surrounding tissues as well as the uterus contract rhythmically. In men rhythmic contractions of the pelvic muscles cause EJACULATION, the forcible release of seminal fluid. In men orgasm is usually sudden and quite brief. In women there is more variation, both among individuals and in one woman at different times; orgasm may be sudden and brief, or it may be long and slow. Also, with continued sexual stimulation, women are able to experience multiple orgasms, that is, a series of orgasms separated by only a few minutes or less. However, women tend to take longer than men to reach orgasm, on average fifteen minutes as opposed to three minutes for men. (Individuals vary widely, however.)

A woman's ability to experience orgasm does not alter with age. In men, however, the time between potential orgasms, called the *refractory period*, definitely increases with age, beginning with thirty to sixty seconds in an adolescent boy and becoming, on average, twelve hours in a fifty-year-old man; there is considerable variation among individuals and in the same individual at different times. To some extent a woman's ability to reach orgasm increases with practice; some women, however, have great difficulty reaching it, or never do so at all, and are said to suffer from FRIGIDITY. Orgasm in women is most easily achieved through stimulating the CLITORIS, which can be done manually by a woman herself (see MASTURBATION) or by her partner, as well as during vaginal, oral, or anal intercourse. Many women find that the penile thrusting of vaginal intercourse does not sufficiently stimulate their clitoris to bring them to orgasm and find that additional stimulation, manual or other, is necessary. A woman can enjoy sex without orgasm, and women who have no sensation in the pelvic area due to disease or injury may find other parts of their body capable of considerable response to sexual stimulation.

Although a person experiencing orgasm is nearly always aware of it, his or her partner often is not, and may need to be told when it occurs or has occurred. Regular sexual stimulation without orgasm (that is, stopping short of orgasm) can lead to pelvic discomfort and even to chronic congestion of the pelvic tissues when the engorged blood vessels in that area do not empty promptly. Indeed, for many women orgasm is an effective way of relieving pelvic congestion associated with menstrual cramps (see DYSMENORRHOEA, definition 4). For more information about the physiology of orgasm, see SEXUAL RESPONSE.

Os See under CERVIX.

Osteoarthritis Also *degenerative joint disease*. A gradual breakdown of the cartilage that faces the body's joints. The most common form of ARTHRITIS, it strikes nearly everyone sooner or later to some degree but rarely begins before the age of forty-five. The onset is gradual and restricted to one or a few joints, which feel painful after being exercised and stiff after a period of inactivity. Eventually the affected joints become enlarged. Almost any joint may be affected, but the principal ones are in the spine, hips, and legs, and, in women particularly, the fingers. Involvement of the knee and hip, more common after the age of sixty, can become increasingly troublesome and occasionally disabling. Osteoarthritis of the spine may be quite severe without many symptoms.

The cause of osteoarthritis is not known, and treatment is entirely palliative. Overweight creates further strain on the weakened joints, so weight loss is often recommended. Frequent rest of the involved joints may help, and canes or crutches may help take the strain off affected weight-bearing joints. Heat helps relieve pain and muscle spasm, and isometric exercises help maintain muscle tone (appropriate exercises should be prescribed by a doctor or physiotherapist, because some kinds that help maintain motion also further damage the joints). Aspirin both relieves pain and reduces inflammation, and two stronger anti-inflammatory agents, ibuprofen and indomethacin may also be effective in those who can tolerate them (the principal adverse reactions are gastrointestinal upsets and rashes). For advanced joint degeneration, orthopaedic surgery, ranging from simple joint debridement to replacement of the joint with a prosthesis (artificial joint, especially successful in the case of hip joints), may be required. See also RHEUMATOID ARTHRITIS.

Osteoporosis A general decrease in bone mass that appears to be part of the ageing process but that occurs more severely and far earlier in women than in men. At any age bone tissue is constantly being worn out, resorbed (absorbed into the bloodstream and eventually excreted), and replaced by newly formed bone. Both men and women are believed to attain their peak bone mass at approximately thirty-five, although one study showed the beginning of bone loss as early as age twenty-five in 10 to 15 per cent of the individuals studied. Thereafter bone mass either remains constant or more bone tissue is lost than replaced. As bone mass decreases, the bones become more brittle and more fragile, breaking easily (osteoporosis means 'porous bones'). The rate of loss in women is for a time considerably greater than that in men, though by the age of eighty men have caught up. Part of the reason is that women's bones are less dense to begin with than men's. Also, women tend to be less active physically than men, and exercise appears to slow down bone loss. Furthermore, bone loss in women speeds up after menopause apparently because the decline in oestrogen makes the body less able to absorb calcium from the diet and incorporate it into bone.

About one-quarter of British women suffer from osteoporosis of varying severity – as opposed to only one-eighth of British men. Most of them are past middle age and postmenopausal. Spinal osteoporosis is four times more common in women than in men (see COMPRESSION FRACTURE), hip fractures two and one-half times more common – they are often the start of permanent invalidism in the elderly, and may even precipitate death – and forearm and wrist fractures ten times more common. Black women, very tall women, and obese women are less susceptible, probably because, like men, they have more bone mass to begin with. Other, less crippling symptoms of osteoporosis are backache and loss of height (due to collapse of vertebrae in the spine, with as much as one to one and one-half inches lost during each decade after MENOPAUSE), abdominal distention, and DOWAGER'S HUMP.

The true cause of primary osteoporosis is still unknown, nor has any cure been found. (Occasionally the condition is secondary to kidney disease or specific endocrine disorders and is then treated by eliminating the underlying problem.) After significant bone loss has occurred, no treatment can restore normal density. Physical discomfort can be relieved with painkillers such as aspirin, heat, massage, and orthopaedic supports when needed. It is known that physical stress stimulates an increase in bone mass while bed rest leads to a decrease. Also, insufficient calcium in the diet – which is thought to be true for practically all British adults – accelerates bone loss, while too much phosphorus (found in meats, poultry, fish, carbonated drinks, and many processed foods) seems to impair the body's ability to use what calcium it does get. Therefore regular exercise and a well-balanced diet high in calcium (with milk and other diary products the best source; calcium supplements are far less effective) will at least strengthen connective tissue – muscles, ligaments, tendons – and thus slow down the osteoporotic process. It is believed that OESTROGEN REPLACE-MENT THERAPY slows down bone resorption in women temporarily, but it does not stimulate bone formation and is also not risk-free. A recent study shows promising results from large doses of sodium fluoride combined with calcium supplements, which stimulates bone-forming cells to produce new bone more quickly.

Ostomy A surgical opening in the abdomen through which waste material is discharged when the normal function of bowel or bladder is lost. There are three principal kinds of ostomy: COLOSTOMY; ILEOSTOMY; and UROSTOMY. The ostomy is fashioned by bringing the opened portion of the remaining intestine or urinary vessel through the abdominal wall. The technical name for the opening is a *stoma*. Elimination through the stoma cannot be voluntarily controlled. In most cases it is collected in a plastic or rubber pouch, called an *appliance*, which is attached to the abdomen at all times and is periodically emptied through a bottom opening. Some colostomies, however, are controlled by irrigation (enema) and require only a small gauze pad or plastic stick-on pouch to cover the stoma between irrigations.

Ostomy surgery of and by itself need not interfere with sexual relations or childbearing. In men, however, it may impair sexual functioning, at least for a time. About 10 to 20 per cent of men with ileostomies suffer some impairment of sexual function and potency. Such impairment may be temporary, but in some cases recovery takes as long as two years. For men with urostomies and colostomies, impairment tends to be more severe. Those who have had urinary surgery early in childhood can usually sustain an erection but may be sterile; men who have such surgery as adults usually become impotent. Men with colostomies vary anywhere from full potency to complete impotence. Often potency is retained but the man becomes sterile; in some cases surgery is so extensive that potency is permanently lost.

Ileostomy is the most common kind of such surgery in women of childbearing age (urinary ostomy is performed mostly in the very young and in those over fifty for cancer; most colostomies are performed in women over forty). Ostomy surgery does not alter the physical structure of the vagina or uterus. Immediately following surgery there may be local sensitivity and pain, but once the abdominal incision has healed normal sexual relations can be resumed. When the rectum has been removed, the perineal area may be sore for some months—in some cases much longer—but this varies with individuals.

So far as pregnancy is concerned, it was formerly feared that an enlarging uterus might compress the stoma, or that a woman's muscles, nerves, and digestive system might be damaged. Today, most authorities agree that although bowel or bladder surgery may have been extensive and any pregnancy may be physically taxing, an ostomy need not limit the number of children a woman bears unless other complications are present. Nor need there be a particular waiting period before pregnancy; some births have occurred within a few days of ostomy surgery, although more conservative doctors advise a wait of two years after surgery before conception, and most advise a limit of two pregnancies.

The most common problem during pregnancy is swelling of the stoma, which tends to become tender and protrude during mid-pregnancy whether or not the abdomen is much distended. Usually the stoma returns to normal size soon after delivery. Because of this change, however, the person with an ostomy who wears a resuable appliance must make sure the opening fits the enlarged stoma properly to avoid exerting damaging pressure on it. Although people with oestomies may be advised that delivery may have to be by Caesarean section, in most cases a normal vaginal delivery is possible.

Apart from the physical problems of such major surgery, ostomy can be emotionally devastating. For this reason, support groups have been formed, in which former patients help counsel individuals before and after surgery. In Britain the following organizations offer advice and support for those with an ostomy.

Colostomy Welfare Group
38/39 Eccleston Sq.,
London
SW1V 1PB

Ileostomy Association of Great Britain and Ireland
Amblehurst House
Chobham
Woking
Surrey
GU24 8PZ

Urostomy Association
8 Coniston Close
Dane Bank
Denton
Manchester
M34 2EW

Outpatient A person who receives treatment at a hospital without being admitted as a resident, or *inpatient*. Some surgical and medical procedures can be performed on an outpatient basis, at a considerable saving of time and money.

Ova The plural of OVUM, or egg.

Ovarian cyst See CYST, definition 6.

Ovarian dysgenesis See TURNER'S SYNDROME.

Ovariectomy Another name for OOPHORECTOMY.

Ovary The female gonad, or sex gland, primarily responsible for secreting the female sex hormones, oestrogen and progesterone, and for producing female germ cells (ova, or eggs). There are two ovaries, located at the back of the broad ligament on either side of the uterus, just below the Fallopian tubes, whose outer ends curve over them. In mature women each ovary is about 3½ by 1½ by 2 centimetres (1½ by ½ by ¾ inches) and is shaped like a flattened egg, covered by a greyish white membrane. Each of the ovaries is attached to its side of the uterus by a special ligament about 4 centimetres (1 to 2 inches) long, but they are suspended by other ligaments as well, and they can shift position somewhat.

Oviducts See FALLOPIAN TUBES.

Ovulation The regular release of an egg, or ovum, from the ovaries, which takes place more or less monthly, except during pregnancy, from soon after menarche until after menopause, or roughly from the ages of fourteen to fifty-four. At puberty the production of sex hormones is greatly increased, and the pituitary gland begins to produce FSH, which stimulates the growth and development of a number of follicles in the ovary. Each follicle contains an egg cell. As the follicles develop, they produce oestrogen which in turn stimulates the pituitary to produce LH. Now LH, together with oestrogen, suppresses the growth of the numerous follicles stimulated during this cycle except for one, or occasionally two. This follicle, the GRAAFIAN FOLLICLE, grows to maturity and moves toward the ovarian wall. As

it moves, that portion of the walls thins and bulges outward. In response to LH, the follicle ruptures, bursting through the ovarian wall and allowing the egg to move out through the opening. Fingerlike ends of the nearby Fallopian tube – the FIMBRIA – move toward the opening in the ovarian wall to catch the egg as it emerges and draw it into and through the tube. It takes an egg about four days to travel the length of the tube, but unless it is fertilized by a sperm that has travelled up the tube to meet it within twenty-four hours of its release from the ovary the egg will no longer be viable. Sometimes two eggs are released during a single cycle; such *double ovulation*, if both eggs are fertilized, results in the birth of fraternal twins (see MULTIPLE PREGNANCY).

Ovulation method See CERVICAL MUCUS METHOD; also under NATURAL FAMILY PLANNING.

Ovum *Ova* (pl.). The Latin word for 'egg', the female reproductive cell in all animals that reproduce sexually, including human beings. Unlike sperm – the male reproductive cells that are produced by the testes after puberty – the ova are already present in the ovaries at birth but only begin to mature and be released after puberty. The average ovum survives outside the ovary for about twenty-four hours before it degenerates; ideally fertilization (the union of ovum and sperm to form a fertilized egg) takes place within twelve hours after the release of an ovum from the ovary, the release being called OVULATION.

Oxygen, in childbirth the administration of oxygen to the mother during labour. It is also used to saturate the blood with oxygen when there is foetal distress or the mother experiences hyperventilation, nausea, or other discomfort. Oxygen may be administered to a baby after birth, especially a PREMATURE baby and/or one suffering from respiratory distress. However, if too much oxygen is given to a newborn baby, there is danger that the retinas of its eyes will be damaged, possibly resulting in blindness (see RETROLENTAL FIBROPLASIA), so the levels administered must be carefully monitored.

Oxytocin A hormone stored and released by the pituitary gland in response to stimulation by the HYPOTHALAMUS. Its main functions are to stimulate uterine contractions during labour and to contract the cells of the breast's milk ducts, causing the expulsion of milk (see LET-DOWN REFLEX).

P

Paget's disease 1 A form of breast cancer in which the NIPPLE and AREOLA become encrusted and look inflamed. The underlying cause is a cancerous growth between the milk ducts deep in the breast, from which malignant cells have spread upward along the ducts that end at the nipple. Paget's disease tends to occur in middle-aged women.

2 A CANCER IN SITU of the VULVA that is characterized by a reddish lesion interspersed with white epithelial 'islands', which under the microscope are revealed to be large, pale 'Paget' cells. It is usually not associated with an underlying cancer.

3 A progressive bone disease of unknown cause that affects more men than women, and that eventually causes distortion, thickening, and overgrowth of various bones. The bones most often affected are those of the pelvis, hips, and skull. The disease does not usually begin until middle age and progresses quite slowly. No cure is known, and treatment is directed principally at relieving discomfort from the distortions.

Palpate To press the surface of the body lightly with the fingers to determine the size and position of an underlying structure, such as the uterus or ovaries (see GYNAECOLOGICAL EXAMINATION) or to locate abnormalities like lumps, as in BREAST SELF-EXAMINATION. Palpitation is a basic technique in physical examination.

Palpitations The unpleasant sensation of one's own heartbeat, perceived as abnormally fast or unusually violent or somehow irregular. It may indicate actual *tachycardia*, that is, a rapid heart rate, but often it does not, and there are no demonstrable signs of any kind. Palpitations frequently accompany an ANXIETY attack and are also associated with MENOPAUSE.

Pancreas An ENDOCRINE gland situated behind the stomach, between the spleen and duodenum, whose principal functions are to secrete digestive fluids into the intestine and to secrete the hormone insulin. See also DIABETES.

Pap smear Also *Smear test, Papanicalaou smear, Pap test*. A valuable test for cancer named after its inventor, Dr. Geroge Papanicalaou, that should be performed on a regular basis. An annual Pap smear is advised for all women from the age of twenty or when they have been sexually active for three years. After three consecutive negative tests – that is, normal findings – they need be tested only every two or three years, provided they have only one sexual partner, have no history of HERPES INFECTION, first had sexual intercourse after the age of eighteen, and are not in any other respect at high risk of cervical cancer.

The test itself consists of scraping away

a thin layer of cells from the surface of the cervix, using a wooden or plastic spatula. The cells are placed on a slide, sprayed with fixative, stained, and examined under the microscope by a pathologist or specially trained technician. The test is quite sensitive, detecting the presence of abnormal cells on the cervix and reliably revealing early, precancerous or potentially cancerous changes. It also helps evaluate oestrogen production and determines the presence of common vaginal infections. It does *not*, however, reliably detect cancer of the vagina, uterus, or ovaries. If a Pap test picks up suspicious pre-malignant changes, it is usually is followed up with a biopsy to remove cervical and endocervical tissue for further examination (see BIOPSY, definition 7).

Papilloma, ductal (intraductal) See DUCTAL PAPILLOMA.

Paracervical anaesthesia Also *paracervical block*. A kind of local ANAESTHESIA that is administered chiefly for a D AND C or for an abortion. It involves injecting a local anaesthetic through the vagina into the area around the cervix, that is, the ligaments and walls of the lower part of the uterus.

Formerly used in labour, paracervical anaesthesia is now considered unsafe in childbirth because it lowers the mother's blood pressure, which may impair the baby's oxygen supply.

Paraplegia Partial or total paralysis of the lower extremities, with severe impairment or complete loss of sensitivity to touch, pain, and temperature in that area. It usually results from an injury to the spinal cord.

Parathyroid Four small ENDOCRINE glands located behind the thyroid gland. They secrete a hormone that, in conjunction with vitamin D, regulates the body's metabolism of calcium and phosphorus.

Parturition Another name for childbirth; see LABOUR.

Pediculosis pubis See PUBIC LICE.

Pelvic cavity See under PELVIS.

Pelvic examination See under GYNAECOLOGICAL EXAMINATION.

Pelvic exenteration Radical surgery formerly performed for very advanced cancer of the cervix. It involved the removal not only of cervix, uterus, Fallopian tubes, and ovaries, but also rectum and bladder, which were replaced by special openings in the abdomen (see OSTOMY). Today chemotherapy and radiation therapy have largely replaced this procedure.

Pelvic inflammatory disease Also *pelvic infection, PID, salpingitis*. Inflammation and/or infection of the Fallopian tubes, which often involves the ovaries and uterus as well. Strictly speaking, inflammation of the tubes is *salpingitis*, of the uterus *endometritis*, and of the ovary *oophoritis*. Some authorities use the term 'pelvic inflammatory disease' as another name for salpingitis, because it primarily involves the tubes; others use it more broadly, for any pelvic inflammation or infection, sometimes even including CERVICITIS.

Pelvic inflammatory disease can range from a mild to a very serious, even life-threatening disorder. It may be *acute* (a sudden, severe infection), *subacute* (less severe), or *chronic* (with persistent inflammation and low-grade infection). In its acute form it is characterized by severe lower abdominal pain and tenderness, felt especially on movement of the cervix. Other symptoms include high fever, chills, a purulent (pus-filled) cervical discharge, vaginal bleeding, and a raised white blood cell count, signalling an active infection. A frequent finding is the rapid development of adhesions (scar tissue) between any of the adjoining pelvic structures (ovaries, tubes, uterus) or between them and the small intestine, colon, or rectum. The pain felt on palpating these adhesions is similar to that felt with appendicitis and pyelonephritis (kidney infection), which therefore must be ruled out.

Diagnosis includes a pelvic examintion (to locate pain and swelling) and laboratory analysis of the cervical discharge. If there is doubt, an exploratory LAPAROSCOPY may be needed, and, should an abscess be suspected, ULTRASOUND may be used to locate it. An abscess is a serious complication; if it ruptures, the infection can spread through the tubes into the entire pelvic and abdominal cavity, causing peritonitis (the peritoneum is the lining of the abdomen), a medical emergency; it can cause death in as little as an hour. Because such an abscess does not often respond to antibiotic treatment, it may require surgical incision and drainage. Another serious complication of acute pelvic inflammatory disease is massive enlargement of a Fallopian tube with fluid (hydrosalpinx) or pus (pyosalpinx), which may cause it to rupture. Still another is septicaemia (blood poisoning), which usually occurs only when the disease is a sequel to childbirth, abortion, or miscarriage: the infection then spreads into the bloodstream

through open blood vessels in the uterus. Fortunately, the severe discomfort of acute pelvic inflammation usually prompts a woman to seek medical attention before these serious complications can develop.

Pelvic inflammatory disease is a bacterial infection. Usually the organisms responsible enter the body through the vagina and work their way up into the pelvic cavity. The gonococcus, which causes GONORRHOEA, and *Chlamydia trachomatis*, which can cause URETHRITIS and VAGINITIS, are thought to be responsible for the majority of cases. The rest are caused by other bacteria, principally *Escherichia coli*, which normally resides in the rectum, or streptococci or staphylococci, which may enter through the cervix during childbirth, abortion, miscarriage, or by means of an intrauterine device (IUD), either during insertion or, some authorities believe, up the device's string. Occasionally, although quite rarely, the disease is caused by tubercle bacilli (which cause tuberculosis) that have spread into the pelvix, or by some tropical infectious organism.

Once the diagnosis has been made, treatment with broad-spectrum oral antibiotics is usually begun at once and continued for about two weeks. In a severe acute case the patient may be hospitalized and antibiotics given intravenously. At home, bed rest is generally recommended, at least until the temperature returns to normal, to help prevent jarring of uterus and tubes, which may increase inflammation and slow down healing. Certainly all vigorous activities, especially any that jostle the pelvis, such as sexual intercourse, should be avoided. Heat is often beneficial, in the form of a hot bath, lasting fifteen to twenty minutes, taken four times a day. If the condition improves within two weeks, treatment is usually continued for another week to ward of a recurrence. If there is no improvement or the condition worsens, a new antibiotic will probably be tried. If three different courses of treatment fail to effect improvements, the disease may be termed a case of *chronic* PID (provided the original diagnosis was correct).

Chronic pelvic inflammatory disease is a low-grade infection that may persist from several weeks to many months. Symptoms may include more or less constant abdominal pain or discomfort, weakness, fatigue, and very heavy menstrual periods, often with severe cramps. A mild case, however, may give rise to few or no noticeable symptoms. Nevertheless, persistent pelvic discomfort should be checked, because even a subclinical (almost symptom-free) infection can give rise to the most common aftermath of pelvic inflammatory disease: partial or total INFERTILITY. The disease, even in mild form, can permanently scar the delicate tissues of the Fallopian tubes, so that bands of scar tissue (adhesions) distort the shape of the tubes or seal their open ends (near the ovaries). As a result eggs are blocked from passing into and through the tubes, and fertilization cannot take place. Also, partial obstruction of a tube can lead to an ECTOPIC PREGNANCY, because the fertilized egg, unable to pass down into the uterus, instead becomes implanted in the tube or elsewhere. Finally, the presence of scar tissue increases the risk of recurrent infection and, depending on its location and abundance, can cause severe pain during sexual intercourse and during menstrual periods. Early treatment, however, minimizes these complications.

Chronic pelvic inflammatory disease that does not respond to bed rest and oral antibiotics is treated in a number of ways. Hospitalization and intravenous antibiotics may be tried first. Sometimes the patient may decide to live with the disease and its potential risks. Some women have found relief through a variety of HERBAL REMEDIES, usually in conjunction with antibiotics. Among these are heat treatment with a poultice made from fresh ginger root or yucca plaster, made from coarsely grated yucca (a tuber; if not available, substitute red-skinned Irish potato). Herbal teas used include one made from goldenseal root (*Hyrastis canadensis*) and myrrh (*Commiphora myrrha*), and another from red raspberry leaf (*Rubus idaeus*), ginseng (*Panax quinquefolium*), comfrey root or leaf (*Symphytum officinale*), and cinnamon bark (*Cinnamonum zeylancium*).

Pelvic pain Discomfort, ranging from mild and intermittent to severe and unremitting pain, in the general area of the genital tract (ovaries, uterus, vagina). The pain may be felt principally in the lower back or, more often, in the lower abdomen. The site usually depends on the cause, but sometimes the discomfort is very generalized (widespread).

Sudden severe pain in the lower abdominal area may be caused by acute PELVIC INFLAMMATORY DISEASE (especially if an abscess forms), ECTOPIC PREGNANCY, the twisting on its stem of either an ovarian cyst (see CYST, definition 6) or a uterine FIBROID, or ovulation (see MITTELSCHMERZ). Sensations of painful pressure in the vaginal, urinary, or rectal areas may be caused by pelvic relaxation, that is, prolapse of the uterus, urethra, bladder, or rectum (see PROLAPSED UTERUS; URETHROCELE; CYSTOCELE; RECTOCELE) or by a pelvic tumour. Deep abdominal or vaginal pain felt during vaginal intercourse (DYSPAREUNIA) may

Side view of female pelvic organs

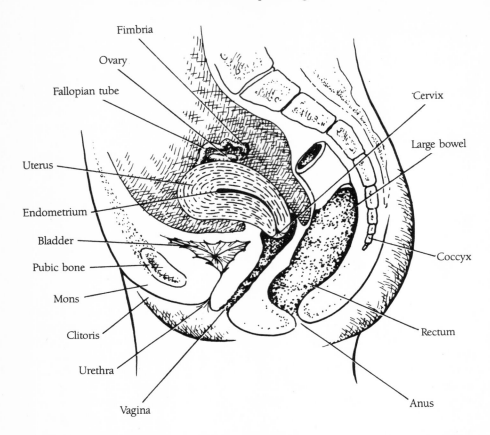

Fimbria

Ovary

Fallopian tube

Cervix

Large bowel

Uterus

Endometrium

Bladder

Pubic bone

Coccyx

Mons

Clitoris

Rectum

Urethra

Anus

Vagina

occur after surgery resulting in a short-ened vagina (such as a vaginal HYSTER-ECTOMY) or be a symptom of either pelvic inflammatory disease or ENDOME-TRIOSIS. Endometriosis causes pain and tenderness in various places, depending on where the endometrial tissue is growing, but characteristically it is most apparent in the days just before men-struation and in the early days of menstrual flow. Painful menstruation (see DYSMENORRHOEA, definition 4) may begin just before or during menstrual periods and may persist for a few hours or throughout the entire period; it may

focus in the abdominal area, the lower back, or both. Another source of pelvic pain is ENDOMETRITIS.

Not all pelvic pain is caused by dis-orders of the reproductive organs. Non-genital sources of pain usually involve the urinary tract (kidney, ureters, bladder), the gastrointestinal tract, or the skeletal system and supporting tissues. Pelvic pain thus may be caused by cystitis, a renal calculs (kidney stone), diverticulitis (inflammation of the large bowel), appendicitis, cholecystitis (gall bladder disease), colitis (inflammation of the large intestine), osteoarthritis or osteoporosis affecting the lower spine, a ruptured disc, poor posture, scoliosis, or a bone tumour.

Pelvimetry Measuring a woman's pelvis to determine whether or not there is room for vaginal delivery of a baby. Certain dimensions of the pelvis can be estimated manually, the doctor inserting his or her fingers into the vagina and/or rectum and also externally palpating the abdomen and lower back. Should more accurate measurements be needed, they can be obtained by X-ray.

Pelvis The bony girdle located at the bottom of the spinal column just above the bones of the thighs. It encloses the *pelvic cavity*, the lowermost portion of the abdominal cavity, which contains the internal reproductive organs (uterus, Fallopian tubes, ovaries) as well as the bladder and rectum.

Penis Also *phallus*; *dick*; *cock* (slang). The male organ of urination and copulation (sexual intercourse). It is made up of three sections of spongy erectile tissue. Two of them lie side by side, forming the upper part of the *shaft* of the penis; near the top they separate and anchor the penis to the underlying pubic bones. The central section runs between the other two and then forms the lower part of the shaft; it contains the urethra. At the tip it widens to form the *glans*, the dome-shaped, highly sensitive end of the penis; at the upper end, or root, it enlarges to form the *bulb* of the penis. The outside of the penis is covered with loose skin that is attached to the circumference of the glans, or *corona*. A fold of this skin, called the *prepuce* or *foreskin*, loosely covers the glans. It is this fold only that is removed in CIRCUMCISION. Uncircumcised men must regularly pull the

prepuce back to clear the glans of *smegma*, a waxy secretion produced by glands under the prepuce. At the tip of the glans is the urethral opening, through which both urine and sperm are transported to the outside.

The average penis is 3½ to 4 inches (8½ to 10 centimetres) long when not erect. During sexual arousal the spongy sections of the penis, which are rich in blood vessels, become engorged with blood, causing the penis, which normally hangs down, to become hard, erect (upright), and enlarged, on average 6 to 7½ inches (15 to 19 centimetres) long and about 1½ inches (4 centimetres) wide. This phenomenon, called *erection* enables the penis to be inserted into the female vagina. When the peak of sexual excitement and release, or ORGASM, is reached, the sperm and other secretions, together called *semen* or *seminal fluid*, are ejaculated through the urethral opening.

SPERM, which begin to be manufactured at puberty by the two testes in tiny adjacent tubes (the *seminiferous tubules*), pass up from each testis to a coiled tube behind it called the *epididymis*. From there they pass up through a second tube on each side, the *vas deferens*, each about 18 inches (45 centimetres) long. The vasa deferentia run from the groin up to the bladder, behind which each vas widens into an *ampulla* where the sperm are stored. Muscular contractions of the vasa deferentia push the sperm up to the ampulla. On the outer side of each ampulla lies a 2-inch-long gland called the *seminal vesicle*, which produces secretions important to the survival of the sperm. The duct of the seminal vesicle joins that of the ampulla to form the *ejaculatory duct*. It is here that gland secretions and sperm are mixed together into seminal fluid just before ejaculation

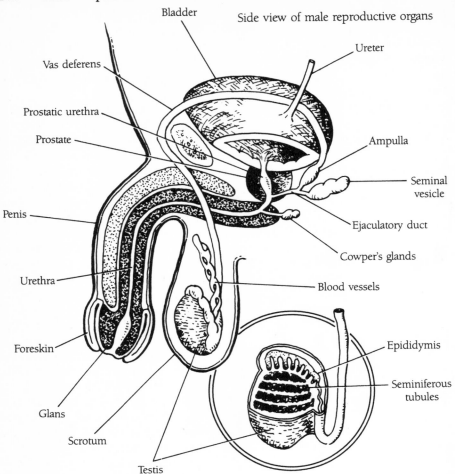

Side view of male reproductive organs

Bladder

Ureter

Vas deferens

Prostatic urethra

Prostate

Ampulla

Seminal vesicle

Penis

Ejaculatory duct

Cowper's glands

Urethra

Blood vessels

Foreskin

Epididymis

Seminiferous tubules

Glans

Scrotum

Testis

occurs. The ejaculatory ducts from each side join the urethra within the *prostate gland*. This gland, made up of gland and muscle tissue and located under the bladder, also produces an alkaline fluid that helps the sperm to propel themselves. The urethra runs from the bladder through the prostate, whose secretions enter it through many tiny ducts and mix with the sperm only seconds before ejaculation. One other structure, *Cowper's glands*, which join the urethra as it leaves the prostate, contributes lubricating fluid during sexual arousal.

Peptides Hormonal proteins that are currently being manufactured in synthetic form and studied for use as contraceptives in both men and women. The first peptide to undergo intensive study was an analogue of LRH (luteinizing release hormone), which sets off a kind of chain reaction resulting in androgen production by the male testes and oestrogen production by the ovaries. In addition to their possible value in BIRTH CONTROL, the peptides showed promise in correcting infertility, by inducing ovulation in women and increasing sperm production in men. The first results, reported in 1981, showed LRH to be effective in suppressing sperm production, nontoxic, and reversible, but side effects, which included loss of libido and potency, made it unacceptable in its present form.

Perforated uterus   See under D AND C.

Perineum   Technically, the muscles and fascia (fibrous tissue) of the entire region underlying the urethral and vaginal openings and the anus, as well as the pelvic floor. In common usage, however, the term is used for the area between the scrotum and anus in men, and in women for the section of fibrous tissue between the anus and vagina, which during childbirth may be stretched considerably and often tears. To prevent tearing, obstetricians may enlarge the vaginal opening surgically (see EPISIOTOMY). Some authorities believe that *perineal massage* – massage of the area between anus and vagina – during late pregnancy and during labour stimulates circulation there and decreases the risk of tearing and the need for episiotomy.

Pessary   A hard rubber or plastic device that is inserted into the vagina to support a PROLAPSED UTERUS and weakened vaginal walls. It usually must be removed by a doctor for cleaning every eight to twelve weeks. It has several other drawbacks as well: it may cause an irritating and smelly discharge, which then requires regular douching and the use of vaginal creams; it can abrade the delicate tissues inside the vagina; and it can interfere with vaginal intercourse, shortening the vagina and thus limiting penetration. For these reasons it is used mainly in women for whom surgery to repair a prolapsed uterus represents too great a risk. Occasionally a pessary is used to keep a repositioned RETRO-VERTED UTERUS in place. Pessaries have been in use since the 19th century.

Pethidine   A synthetic narcotic widely used for the relief of pain in childbirth as well as other severe pain. Formerly it was regularly used in labour together with SCOPOLAMINE (it replaced an even stronger narcotic, morphine) to induce a relatively pain-free twilight sleep. It is very effective as a pain reliever, but its principal disadvantage is that it has a depressant effect on the baby's respiratory centre if it is in the baby's bloodstream at delivery. Pethidine also makes a new-born baby sleepy for a day or more.

Pfannestiel incision   A horizontal incision into the lower abdomen, about 5 inches (12½ centimetres) long, over the pubis, near the top of the pubic hair, which is used for hysterectomy, Caesarean section, or abdominal tubal ligation. It leaves a less noticeable scar than the midline vertical incision formerly used exclusively.

Phallus   See PENIS.

Phenylketonuria   Also *PKU.* A hereditary disorder thought to result from lack of a gene needed to produce an enzyme that converts the amino acid phenylalanine to a similar acid, tyrosine. As a result of this chemical block, phenylalanine is converted to phenylpyruvic acid, which builds up in the body fluids and, frequently, causes severe mental retardation. PKU occurs in 1 of every 10,000 births and is detectable by means of a simple urine and blood test as soon as a baby begins digesting food. All babies born in

British hospitals today are tested automatically for PKU.

Phlebitis Also *venous thrombosis, thrombophlebitis.* An acute inflammation of the veins – most often the deep veins – characterized by the formation of small blood clots, or thrombi (see THROMBUS), in the veins. Depending on the severity of the inflammation, there may be no symptoms or there may be tenderness, pain, swelling, warmth, and redness of the overlying skin and/or prominence of the superficial veins in the area involved. Phlebitis most often affects leg veins and pelvic veins. Pain is usually felt when standing and walking but is relieved by sitting or lying down with the affected leg elevated. Even when there are no symptoms, if phlebitis is suspected it is important that it be correctly diagnosed particularly if deep veins are involved.

Phlegmasia Also *milk leg, white leg.* Inflammation of the femoral vein in one or both legs after childbirth (see also PHLEBITIS). The leg becomes swollen, tender, and usually bluish-white in colour owing to constricted blood vessels. Formerly very common, especially after a difficult labour, phlegmasia today is relatively rare. Treatment consists of bed rest with the leg elevated, elastic supports, pain relievers, and, if deep veins are affected, anticoagulants to prevent clot formation.

PID Abbreviation for PELVIC INFLAMMATORY DISEASE.

Pigmentation See CHLOASMA; LIVER SPOTS; SKIN CHANGES; also MELANOMA.

Piles See HAEMORRHOIDS.

Pill, the See ORAL CONTRACEPTIVES.

Pineal gland Also *pineal body.* A tiny, egg-shaped body located in the midline of the brain that secretes at least one hormone, *melatonin,* which is believed to inhibit (suppress) the function of the sex glands (testes, ovaries).

Pituitary gland One of the ENDOCRINE glands, located below the base of the brain, to which it is attached by a stalk. An oval structure about 1½ centimetres (½ inch) long and less than 1½ centimetres wide, it consists of two parts. The *adenohypophysis* or *anterior pituitary,* which constitutes three-quarters of the total gland, produces protein hormones that are trophic hormones – that is, they regulate the growth and hormone production of other endocrine glands – as well as hormones that directly influence body growth, metabolism, and lactation. The anterior pituitary was once believed to be the 'master gland' of the endocrine system, until it was discovered that most of its functions in turn are controlled by the HYPOTHALAMUS.

PKU Abbreviation for PHENYLKETONURIA.

Placebo Treatment that is not directly related to relieving the condition for which it is given. Placebos are often used in research to determine whether a medication being tested is actually effective. In a *double-blind* study, neither the doctors nor the patients (researchers nor subjects) know who is getting a medication and who is being given a placebo; often the placebo is a pill that looks real but contains sugar or some other harmless substance. Doctors also use placebos in general practice in order to obtain the *placebo effect*; that is, improvement that results from any therapeutic intervention (some patients get better simply because they believe a particular treatment or doctor will help them). A placebo usually takes the form of medication (powder, pill, capsule, liquid), but strictly speaking the term can be used for any treatment, including hypnosis, manipulation, surgery, or simply the presence and attitude of a doctor. From an ethical standpoint the use of placebos is controversial. Supporters point to their practical usefulness – they sometimes work very well – and the fact that interactions between the human mind and body are still poorly understood; opponents insist that their use involves deceiving a patient and consequently they are dishonest.

Placenta Also *afterbirth*. A highly specialized organ that connects a foetus to its mother and enables the exchange of soluble, blood-borne nutrients and secretions, including oxygen. The placenta usually lies at the top of the uterus and is connected to the foetus by the UMBILICAL CORD.

Without an intact, functioning placenta a foetus cannot survive. In ABRUPTIO PLACENTAE and PLACENTA PRAEVIA, where the placenta becomes detached from the endometrium, the foetus's oxygen and food supply are threatened. Once the placenta has separated completely, no oxygen can be transferred through it. Toxic wastes build up in the baby's tissues, and its brain, which can survive only eight minutes of oxygen deprivation, begins to suffer irreversible damage.

At term, after nine months' gestation, the human placenta is a disc shaped mass measuring about 15 to 20 centimetres (8 inches) in diameter and 2 to 3 centi-metres (1 inch) in thickness. It weighs about 500 grams (1.1 pound) and is located in the upper two-thirds of the uterus. The foetal side is covered by a transparent membrane (the amnion). Foetal blood flows to the placenta through the two umbilical arteries, which carry de-oxygenated (venous) blood. Maternal blood with a significantly higher oxygen content returns to the foetus from the placenta through the single umbilical vein.

During childbirth the placenta becomes detached in the course of labour and is expelled after the delivery of the baby, still attached to it by the umbilical cord. The openings of the uterine blood vessels where it is torn from the endo-metrium are closed by contractions of the uterine muscles; this is the reason why the uterus must continue to contract after delivery, and, if it does not, haemorrhage may occur. The delivery of the plancenta is called the third stage of LABOUR. Occasionally it is not completely detached during labour and must be removed either manually, by pushing down on the mother's abdomen near the top of the uterus to help expel it, or with instruments. The doctor, midwife, or other birth attendant should always examine the placenta after delivery to make sure it is intact; retention of part of the placenta can cause haemorrhage in the mother.

For *placental insufficiency*, see under POSTMATURE.

Placenta praevia Location of the PLACENTA over or near the internal cervical os (opening), that is, where the cervix widens into the body of the uterus, instead of near the top of the uterus. Placenta praevia is, along with ABRUPTIO PLACENTAE, one of the two main causes of haemorrhage in the latter part of pregnancy.

Placenta praevia is not very common – it occurs in about one of every two hundred pregnancies. Both age and parity (number of previous children) play a role: women over thirty-five and women with numerous children are three or four times more likely to develop placenta praevia than younger women and women who have had no children. Also, once it has occurred, it is quite likely to recur in subsequent pregnancies.

The chief sign of placenta praevia is painless bleeding (usually heavy but sometimes light) during the eighth month of pregnancy. The initial haemorrhage usually stops by itself and is rarely (if ever) fatal, but it may recur at any time. Sometimes, however, there is a continuous discharge of smaller amounts of blood. With low-lying placenta praevia, the bleeding does not usually occur until the onset of labour, and then may be light or very profuse.

With total placenta praevia delivery *must* be by Caesarean section, which is also indicated for any kind of placenta praevia with massive bleeding or foetal distress. Caesarean section results in less blood loss because delivery is so much faster, and therefore a Caesarean may be indicated even if the baby has died before delivery. However, for women who have had children previously, have a low-lying placenta, and are already well into labour, with the cervix dilated to at least 4 centimetres – conditions that apply to about half of the cases – a simple vaginal delivery may be possible, provided that bleeding is not too severe, delivery is imminent, and the baby is in no distress.

Plasma cell mastitis See under MAMMARY DUCT ECTASIA.

Polycystic ovaries See STEIN-LEVEN-THAL SYNDROME.

Polygalactia Excess secretion of breast milk. It usually occurs before breast-feeding is well established (immediately after birth), before the supply has been regulated by the infant's demand for milk, and during weaning, especially if there is some reason for weaning very quickly (rather than gradually reducing the number of feedings per day over a period of several weeks). See also BREAST-FEEDING; LACTATION.

Polyhydramnios Another name for HYDRAMNIOS.

Polymenorrhoea Frequent menstrual periods, with intervals of less than twenty days between menstrual flows. It usually signifies a hormone imbalance; that is, too much oestrogen in the absence of progesterone (or relative to progesterone), a condition found mostly in young girls who are not yet ovulating and in women approaching menopause (see ANOVULA-TORY BLEEDING). It may also be caused by a uterine FIBROID. For young girls threatened with anaemia from too frequent periods, progesterone alone or sometimes an oral contraceptive containing both oestrogen and progesterone may establish a more normal cycle. In older women fibroids and other growths, benign or malignant, should be ruled out before giving any medication. Some women routinely menstruate every nineteen or twenty days and, in the absence of anaemia or other problems, such a short MENSTRUAL CYCLE is no cause for alarm or for treatment.

Polyp 1 A soft, fleshy, easily crumbled, noncancerous tumour, usually attached to normal tissue by a stem or pedicle. Common sites for such growths are the nasal passages, vocal cords (larynx), gastointestinal tract, and pelvis.

2 **Cervical polyp** A polyp that develops high up in the cervical canal, near the entrance to the body of the uterus. It may occur singly or multiply, and is an overgrowth of normal tissue from the lining of the cervix or uterus. It may give rise to no symptoms at all, or it may cause bleeding between periods or staining in postmenopausal women. Very large polyps sometimes cause cramping as they push down through the cervical canal. Diagnosis is relatively easy, because such polyps usually protrude into the vagina and so can be seen on pelvic examination. Normally they can simply be removed in the doctor's surgery or in a clinic or hospital on an outpatient basis, but occasionally a D AND C may be needed to remove them completely.

3 **Endometrial polyp** Also *intra-uterine polyp, uterine polyp*. A polyp that develops inside the body of the uterus and can grow into and through the cervix. A long endometrial polyp may protrude all the way into the vagina. Like cervical polyps (see definition 2 above), it represents an overgrowth of normal endometrial tissue and may either be symptomless or cause bleeding between periods or after menopause, and cramping pain as it pushes down through the cervix. Also like cervical polyps, endometrial polyps may occur singly or in numbers. To remove them, a D and C must be performed, and sometimes a second D and C is required to locate an additional polyp that was missed the first time. Occasionally, if polyps continue to recur and/or if they persistently cause postmenopausal bleeding, a hysterectomy is performed to eliminate them entirely. See also ENDOMETRIAL HYPERPLASIA.

Pomeroy technique A method of closing the Fallopian tubes in TUBAL LIGATION. A small portion of each tube is raised, and a catgut suture is tied, forming a loop of tube. The loop is then cut off. By the time the catgut has been absorbed, in several weeks, the two stumps of the severed loop retract, leaving a gap between them. This method can be used with any kind of tubal ligation except LAPAROSCOPY.

Post-coital test See SIMS-HUHNER TEST.

Posterior presentation Also *posterior position*. In childbirth, the position of the baby, head first but with its face toward the mother's belly (instead of her back) as it comes down the birth canal. It is the most common form of abnormal position, the norm being *anterior*, or face down. In about 94 per cent of cases the baby eventually rotates by itself into the much easier anterior position, although often it may not do so until the head has reached the pelvic floor. Generally labour is somewhat prolonged with a posterior position, especially with a first baby, and frequently back discomfort (BACK LABOUR) is felt. If the baby does not rotate spontaneously and the doctor is unable to turn it manually or with forceps, a forceps delivery in posterior position may be necessary. Since the use of forceps nearly always requires enlarging the vaginal opening with a considerable EPISIOTOMY, it is preferable to turn the baby to an anterior position if at all possible.

Postmature The condition of an infant born more than two weeks beyond full term, that is, forty-two or more weeks following the last menstrual period. Approximately 4 per cent of all pregnancies are prolonged for more than two weeks. The effects vary. In some cases the foetus continues to grow at a significant rate and suffers no harm. In others, its growth stops as the pregnancy continues, and the foetus may show evidence of starvation, with loss of soft tissue and low birth weight at the time of delivery. In such cases, where the PLACENTA has become insufficient – that is, functions inadequately in transporting nutrients and oxygen to the baby – the baby's needs may not be met and the pregnancy must usually be terminated, either by INDUCTION OF LABOUR or by Caesarean section. *Placental insufficiency* is readily measured by the amount of oestrol (an oestrogen produced by the placenta) in the mother's urine or blood. A steady level of oestrol as determined by tests once or twice a week, shows that the placenta is continuing to function as before and there is no problem for the baby. If this test, combined with a weekly Non-Stress Test (see under FOETAL MONITORING) attests to the baby's well-being, no action need be taken. If the results of either test are poor, induction of labour or a Caesarean section should be done immediately.

Most postmature infants lack lanugo (soft down hair covering the shoulders of most newborns) and have long nails, abundant scalp hair, pale skin with some evidence of drying, and apparent increase of alertness. There may be little amniotic fluid, and it may be stained with foetal stools.

The reasons for postmaturity are not understood except in those cases where the infant is born severely damaged, when it is thought to be due to long-term malfunctioning of the placenta.

Postmenopausal bleeding Any staining or bleeding that occurs in a woman aged forty-five or older, twelve or more months after her last menstrual period. Such bleeding should be promptly investigated, even if it consists of only a little staining or spotting, because it can be a sign of cancer or some other serious disorder. An endometrial biopsy may need to be performed to rule out endometrial cancer; sometimes a D and C will be required. Some menopausal women do resume menstrual periods after an interruption of twelve months or so, usually on a quite irregular basis, until they finally stop menstruating. Consequently some authorities define menopause as the cessation of menstrual periods for two years. Nevertheless, to be on the safe side any bleeding after a full year's interruption calls for a prompt gynaecological check-up. See also MENOPAUSE.

Postnatal care See under POSTPARTUM.

Postpartum Referring to the period after childbirth, also called the PUERPERIUM or postnatal period. Routine hospital care during the first forty-eight hours after delivery involves taking the mother's pulse, temperature, blood pressure, and respiratory rate every six hours. In most hospitals a woman may get up and use the bathroom within one to twelve hours, depending on the mode of delivery (vaginal or Caesarean) and anaesthesia (none, local, regional, or general). A few women have trouble urinating after delivery, especially if the labour was difficult or forceps were used, and they may require catheterization intermittently until the bladder resumes normal function. Breast ENGORGEMENT normally occurs within two days after delivery; for women who decide not to breast-feed, the engorgement may take several days to subside. Uterine contractions (AFTERPAINS) continue for some days and are often triggered by breast-feeding.

If all goes well, most hospitals discharge women after three or four days (five to ten days following Caesarean section). Thereafter she may usually resume a fairly normal life, but should allow for more rest, take warm sitz baths if haemorrhoids from pushing or the stitches from episiotomy are uncomfortable, and drink extra fluids if she is breast-feeding. (Some doctors warn against baths, however, owing to danger of infection through the still dilated cervix.) Most doctors advise avoiding vaginal intercourse for six weeks, until after the standard postpartum check-up, but some women prefer to engage in it sooner and others to delay even longer.

The postpartum examination, usually performed six weeks after delivery, involves weight, blood pressure, and haemoglobin measurements, checking the breasts, and a pelvic examination. This is the time for discussing current and future methods of birth control, perhaps being fitted for a diaphragm since size may change after childbirth, and discussing future pregnancies if any are being considered.

Persistent pain of any kind during the postpartum period, both before and after hospital discharge, a smelly vaginal discharge, or a fever above 100.4 degrees Fahrenheit (38 degrees Centigrade) should be reported at once, since they may signal an infection. The principal medical complications following childbirth are bleeding and infection. See also POSTPARTUM HAEMORRHAGE; PUERPERAL FEVER; DEPRESSION (definition 2).

Postpartum depression See DEPRESSION (definition 2).

Postpartum haemorrhage Heavy bleeding during the postpartum period, that is, following childbirth. Such bleeding most often occurs when the uterus does not contract sufficiently after delivery of the PLACENTA. Other causes are failure to expel all of the placenta from the uterus; occasionally such retained pieces of placenta form growths similar to POLYPS in the uterine wall, causing menstrual irregularity, abdominal pain, and heavy bleeding.

Unlike other kinds of massive bleeding, postpartum haemorrhage usually involves no sudden gush of blood but rather constant moderate bleeding over a period of hours. A blood loss of 500 cc. (millilitres) or more during the first twenty-four hours after delivery is defined as a haemorrhage, since it is enough to be life-threatening at this stage. The principal danger to the mother occurs in situations where no blood transfusion is quickly available, as in a home birth.

Post-Pill amenorrhoea Also *post-oral contraceptive amenorrhoea*. Failure to resume menstrual periods within six months after stopping the use of ORAL CONTRACEPTIVES, in the absence of pregnancy or menopause. Some doctors believe that post-Pill amenorrhoea can be prevented by interrupting oral contraceptives for two to three months every two years to make sure that no such depression of hypothalamic activity has occurred.

Potency See under IMPOTENCE.

Poultice See under HERBAL REMEDIES.

Precancerous lesions Growths or other changes in tissue that may, under certain conditions, become malignant (cancerous). In the uterine area such lesions can be eliminated totally by hysterectomy (removal of uterus and cervix), but so radical a procedure may not be necessary. CANCER IN SITU of the cervix and uterus, often with no symptoms other than mild staining between menstrual periods or after intercourse, is confined to the surface cells. An even earlier precancerous condition is DYSPLASIA of the uterus and cervix, which may disappear spontaneously but sometimes develops into cancer (see also ADENOCARCINOMA, definition 2). Authorities do not always agree as to whether a lesion is precancerous or not. In the case of ENDOMETRIAL HYPERPLASIA – thickening of the normally thin uterine lining – some doctors believe that in postmenopausal women this condition readily develops into cancer and therefore recommend hysterectomy, whereas others prefer more conservative treatment, such as a D AND C. See also LEUKOPLAKIA, VULVAR; PAGET'S DISEASE, definition 2.

Precocious puberty The occurrence of sexual development and menstrual bleeding in girls before the age of eight or nine (and sexual maturity in boys before the age of ten). It is at least twice (some say three or four times) as common in girls as in boys, and 80 to 90 per cent of cases in girls are idiopathic, that is, no underlying cause can be found. Precocious puberty results from premature signals from the hypothalamus, pituitary, and adrenal glands, which trigger the growth of pubic and axillary hair, breast development and MENARCHE. Both careful explanation and emotional support should be given to the physically precocious girl and her family, since most such children have the psychological maturity appropriate for their actual age. Her breast development should be described as 'early' – not 'abnormal' – and the process of menstruation should be thoroughly explained, preferably before menstrual flow actually begins.

Preeclampsia Also *pregnancy-induced hypertension, PIH, metabolic toxaemia of late pregnancy, toxaemia.* The development, in the last trimester of pregnancy, of hypertension (high blood pressure), proteinuria (protein in the urine), and oedema (fluid retention) associated with a rapid weight gain. If not treated, this condition can progress to ECLAMPSIA and possibly death. Moreover, the progression from preeclampsia to eclampsia can be very rapid (a matter of hours), and therefore preeclampsia requires very prompt treatment.

The cause of preeclampsia, which develops in approximately one of every twenty pregnant women, is not known. It occurs most often in first pregnancies and in women who already have hypertension or vascular disease. Indeed, some authorities lump together preeclampsia, eclampsia, and hypertension that develops in late pregnancy, calling them 'hypertensive disorders of late pregnancy'. The hypertension of preeclampsia is caused by vasospasm, that is, constriction of the blood vessels that inhibits the flow of blood, especially to the liver, uterus, and kidneys.

The only specific treatment for severe preeclampsia is terminating the pregnancy; delivery alone can prevent convulsions and the death of the baby. Because the baby will usually be premature, there may be a temptation to delay till its chances of survival increase, but severe preeclampsia itself may kill the baby, and it is much safer for the mother not to wait.

Preeclampsia probably cannot be wholly prevented, despite the efforts of some doctors to do so by strictly limiting a pregnant woman's weight gain and sodium (salt) intake, and by almost routinely prescribing diuretics to prevent fluid retention. Indeed, these measures themselves can be dangerous, leading to protein deficiency, sodium-electrolyte imbalance, and other problems. Early detection, on the other hand, may prevent the development of life-threatening eclampsia. It is for this reason that good ANTENATAL CARE calls for increasingly frequent check-ups in the last trimester and routinely includes checking weight gain, blood pressure, and testing the urine for albumin (protein). Once symptoms appear, most doctors believe the woman should have complete bed rest on her left side, at home or in the hospital. Weight, blood pressure, and urine must be checked frequently. A protein-rich diet is used, and at least one authority believes that such a diet throughout pregnancy will prevent the development of pre-eclampsia. If the condition cannot be controlled with these measures, strong sedation and anticonvulsant drugs may be given to prevent eclampsia.

Pregnancy The condition of a woman who is carrying a fertilized egg (ZYGOTE) or embryo or foetus. She is also said to have *conceived*. An uninterrupted normal pregnancy, called a *full-term pregnancy*, continues for approximately nine months or thirty-nine to forty weeks, which for the sake of convenience can be divided into roughly equal three-months periods called *trimesters*.

Pregnancy is characterized by complex physiological changes, which begin almost immediately after conception. (The changes undergone by egg, embryo, and foetus are described under GESTATION). The earliest signs of pregnancy are usually a skipped menstrual period, somewhat swollen and tender breasts, nausea (so-called MORNING SICKNESS), sleepiness and fatigue, urinary frequency, increased vaginal discharge, and slight cramping in the area just above the pubis. The presence and intensity of these signs vary greatly from woman to woman, and also from pregnancy to pregnancy. Some women experience few or no symptoms during the first trimester other than absence of menstruation. Some even continue to have slight monthly bleeding resembling periods for two or three months after conceiving, although this is rare. Or, pregnancy may occur in a woman who has never menstruated but has ovulated.

These signs and symptoms all reflect hormonal changes in the body. Within five to seven days of conception chorionic gonadotrophins appear in the woman's blood and urine. Their presence or absence is the basis of every PREGNANCY TEST. Progesterone and oestrogen levels gradually rise. The blood supply to the pelvis becomes greatly increased, resulting in such early clinical changes as CHADWICK'S SIGN and HEGAR'S SIGN. However, none of this evidence is conclusive. Until recently pregnancy could be definitely established by clinical signs only during the second trimester, when the baby's heartbeat can be heard as distinct from that of the mother (today, use of a doppler or ultrasound can detect heartbeat at eleven weeks or earlier), the baby's movements can be felt by the examining doctor, and the foetus can be 'seen' by X-ray. Now ultrasound can detect pregnancy as early as three or four weeks after conception.

By the second trimester the abdomen is enlarged, and the shape, size, and consistency of the uterus have changed enormously. In many women there are pigment changes, especially darkening of the skin around the nipple and sometimes on the face (see CHLOASMA); also, a dark line from the navel to the pubic region may become evident. The skin over the enlarging abdomen is stretched, sometimes leaving pink stretch marks, or STRIAE. Some women, about midway through the second trimester, begin to leak a little fluid from their breasts (see LACTATION). There may be gastrointestinal discomfort from the enlarging abdomen, principally constipation and heartburn. As a result of pressure, VARICOSE VEINS may become troublesome in the legs, vulva, and/or rectum (HAEMORRHOIDS). The blood volume increases— by 30 to 50 per cent over the nine months of pregnancy—and the heart beats faster to pump the increased amount, causing some women to experience palpitations. There may be leg cramps and/or nosebleeds, the latter from congestion of the mucous membranes. Some women perspire and salivate more during pregnancy. Also, there is a growing tendency toward OEDEMA, especially swollen ankles, feet, hands, and wrists towards the end of the day. In general these discomforts are intermittent and not too severe; many (most) women regard the second trimester as the most comfortable period of pregnancy.

In the third trimester considerable enlargement of the uterus and abdomen begin to cause increasing discomfort. More striae appear. The baby is larger and its movements more evident, sometimes enough to cause night waking. Pressure from the growing uterus on other organs may cause shortness of breath, increased indigestion (especially heartburn, sometimes after every meal), constipation, urinary frequency, and more discomfort from varicose veins and oedema. Even without any of these symptoms, practically all pregnant women experience increased fatigue in the last trimester simply from carrying fifteen or more extra pounds.

Good ANTENATAL CARE is important from the moment pregnancy is verified, with special attention to DIET and EXERCISE. Except in unusual circumstances most women are able to continue all of their usual activities (including sexual relations) throughout the pregnancy, provided they get the extra rest they need. Even with good care and the absence of foreseeable special complications (see HIGH-RISK PREGNANCY), problems can arise. They include vaginal bleeding early or late in pregnancy, severe or persistent abdominal pain, urinary infection, premature rupture of the membranes, foetal death (see STILLBIRTH), PREMATURE LABOUR, ABNORMAL PRESENTATION, and PREECLAMPSIA. These situations rarely develop without some warning, so most doctors advise a woman to **seek emergency medical care at once if any of the following danger signals occurs:** severe persistent abdominal pain (no matter where in the abdomen, or in what stage of pregnancy); vaginal bleeding at any time during pregnancy (light staining in the first half of pregnancy can wait till morning; if it occurs during the second half, it is considered an emergency, even if the amount is slight, except for bloody show; see MUCUS PLUG); dimness or blurring of vision, especially in the second half of pregnancy; puffiness or swelling of the face, eyelids, or fingers, especially if sudden; fever and chills; severe persistent headache (especially during the last trimester); absence of foetal movement for twenty-four hours after the fifth month; membrane rupture (breaking of the waters; see AMNIOTIC SAC). See also LABOUR; PREGNANCY COUNSELLING; PREGNANT PATIENTS' RIGHTS.

Pregnancy, mask of See CHLOASMA.

Pregnancy counselling Assistance in deciding whether or not to continue an unplanned pregnancy, or to become pregnant, involving a careful review of the options available and their effect on the woman and her partner. In theory there are three basic options for a pregnant woman: continuing the pregnancy and keeping the child; continuing the pregnancy and giving the child up for adoption; and terminating the pregnancy by ABORTION. In practice, however, not every woman has all three options. Keeping a child fathered by a man other than the woman's husband (the result of rape, for example) might not be emotionally acceptable to both partners. Nor might continuing a pregnancy be an option when it is virtually certain that the child will be brain-damaged or carry some serious birth defect. Similarly, abortion might not be possible for a woman opposed to it on religious grounds, or for a woman who lives where it is not legal and cannot afford to travel elsewhere. A trained counsellor can help a woman (or couple) determine her (their) priorities and alternatives as well as refer her to appropriate agencies (an adoption agency, hospital, etc.) to help carry out her decision.

Because BIRTH CONTROL and legalized abortion have made parenthood an optional matter for many couples, an increasing number of women (and couples) seek advice *before* planning a pregnancy. They need to consider if having and raising a child fits in with their desired style of life (including professional and educational plans), whether their motives for childbearing are valid ones, how parenthood will affect their partner and their relationship, and similar questions. Increasingly, professional counsellors and therapists are helping find answers to these questions, so that the field of pregnancy counselling has been broadened to include pregnancy planning. See also GENETIC COUNSELLING.

Pregnancy-induced hypertension Also *PIH*. See PREECLAMPSIA.

Pregnancy test A test to determine whether or not a woman is pregnant. There are two basic kinds of pregnancy test: a blood test and a urine test. Both are based on the presence of human chorionic gonadotrophin (HCG), a hormone secreted by the fertilized egg during its journey from the Fallopian tube to the uterus, and later by the placenta. HCG is detectable in the mother's bloodstream as early as six to eight days after conception, and in the urine 21 to 28 days following conception. Its production reaches a peak 50 to 60 days later, and then steadily declines.

Urine tests are widely available and usually adequate for most women's needs. There are two principal kinds: tube tests (two-hour) and slide tests (two-minute). The former supposedly are accurate as early as 37 days after the last menstrual period (LMP; the first day of flow is Day 1) or about 14 days after the first missed period was due, whereas slide tests are rarely accurate before 41 days after the last menstrual period. Both are mor accurate if they are performed somewhat later – ideally, two weeks later, when HCG in the urine has reached its peak. All urine tests require use of the first urine voided in the morning after a night's sleep because it is more concentrated and so increases the chance of detecting HCG.

For all pregnancy tests, a *positive* result most often means a woman is pregnant unless the test is performed very early; only rarely do a tumour infection or medication cause false positive readings. As noted, however, a negative result is less certain, because HCG levels may be too low. The earlier the test is made, the less likely that a negative reading is accurate, and some doctors feel that every negative result calls for a repeat test one week later. For pregnancy tests one can perform at home, see EARLY PREGNANCY TEST.

Pregnant patients' rights   A general term that describes pregnant women's just claims on health-care services. Since about 1930 there has been increasing medical care (detractors call it medical 'intervention') in childbirth, at least in some developed countries. From the 1950s on, however, when the so-called natural childbirth movement gained momentum in these countries, there was growing scepticism about traditional hospital practices during labour and delivery, which involve various drugs and procedures (some of them not always necessary) that may be potentially damaging to the baby, the mother, or both. It was feared that increasingly widespread use of anaesthesia and forceps damaged babies, sometimes inflicting permanent brain damage. Some of the drugs used also could harm the mother. Consequently a number of groups, and organizations devoted to maternal and child health, have devised lists that spell out a woman's right to participate in decisions involving her own welfare and that of her unborn child.

These rights include the right to know about the direct or indirect effects, risks, or hazards to herself or her child that may result from the use of a drug or procedure prescribed for or administered to her during pregnancy, labour, birth, or lactation; and the right to be fully informed of any proposed treatment and its alternatives, including childbirth education classes that could help prepare her for labour and delivery and thereby reduce or eliminate the need for drugs and other intervention. Many of these practices have become the norm in some, but by no means all, hospitals. Some advocates go further, insisting that a woman has the right to have medical assistance no matter where she intends to give birth (at home); to refuse any drugs; to ask the birth attendant to avoid an episiotomy if possible; to labour at her own rate of speed, without intervention, and to give birth in whatever position she chooses; to keep the baby (if healthy) with her from birth on, nursing it immediately and whenever she wishes to; and to have her partner and/or friends with her throughout labour, delivery, and the hospital stay.

Premature   Describing any infant born before thirty-eight weeks of GESTATION, so that its chances of survival may be impaired. Infants born after thirty-five weeks of gestation usually do quite well. Some authorities believe that a birth weight of less than 2,500 grams (about 5.5 pounds) serves as a good definition of prematurity. Infants weighing more than this generally have as good a chance of surviving as any that are larger; infants weighing less do not.

Not all babies weighing less than 2,500 grams are premature in terms of development. Some suffer from intrauterine growth retardation, others from congenital malformation, and still others from intrauterine infection. Malnutrition before birth may be caused by inadequate blood flow or by placental insufficiency; that is, the nutrients from the mother do not reach the baby. Congenital defects such as DOWN'S SYNDROME are also associated with low birth weight, as are maternal infections such as RUBELLA. Conditions in the mother that seem to slow down the baby's weight gain include poor nutrition, hypertension (high blood pressure) and cardiovascular disease, preeclampsia, placenta praevia, and habitual cigarette smoking. Women whose mothers were given DIETHYLSTILBOESTROL during their pregnancies may be more likely to give birth to premature infants than unexposed women. MULTIPLE PREGNANCY usually involves premature labour and small babies.

The principal danger to the premature infant is respiratory distress. Other problems frequently occurring are inability to suck strongly and inability to maintain body temperature (hence the frequent use of warmers). In addition, premature infants are more apt to suffer from respiratory and gastrointestinal infections and, if they require high levels of oxygen, risk developing RETROLENTAL FIBROPLASIA. See also MISCARRIAGE.

Premature ejaculation See EJACULATION, definition 2.

Premenstrual tension Another name for congestive dysmenorrhoea; see DYSMENORRHOEA, definition 5.

Prepared childbirth Also *natural childbirth, childbirth education*. A system of preparing a woman (sometimes also her partner) for labour and delivery, through education concerning the process of birth, exercises to be used antenatally and during labour, and other means. A number of different methods are in current use, but their overall objective is essentially the same: to eliminate a woman's fear of childbirth by replacing it with knowledge of what to expect, and to prepare her mentally and physically for the sensations she will encounter during labour and delivery in order to avoid, as much as possible, the use of pain relievers, anaesthesia, forceps delivery, and other medical intervention that could possibly harm her or the baby.

The earliest method of prepared childbirth to become popular was devised by an English doctor, Grantly Dick-Read; later a method devised by a French doctor, Fernand Lamaze, the PSYCHOPROPHYLACTIC METHOD, virtually replaced the Dick-Read method. Still another method, devised by an American obstetrician, is called *husband-coached childbirth* or, after its inventor, the *Bradley Method*. Each of these methods not only has its advocates but has attracted teachers who have invented variations of their own. There is also a version of yoga devised by a Danish-trained teacher called *prenatal yoga* or the *Euronie method of yoga*, which involves exercises alone (no education concerning birth).

Prepuce Also *foreskin*. A sheath of skin, partly retractable, that covers the penis in men and the clitoris in women. The operation called CIRCUMCISION, performed for hygienic or religious purposes, surgically removes part of the prepuce.

Primigravida A woman pregnant for the first time. See also PRIMAPARA.

Primipara A woman who has delivered one child. See also MULTIPARA.

Progesterone A hormone produced after ovulation by the corpus luteum which builds up the uterine lining, or endometrium, for the reception and nurture of a fertilized egg and helps maintain a pregnancy. It is also released in tiny amounts by the adrenal glands in both men and women, in men by the testes, and in pregnant women in very large amounts by the placenta, which takes over progesterone production after the corpus luteum disintegrates. It was first discovered and isolated in 1934, but it was some years before its role in the MENSTRUAL CYCLE was understood. Progesterone production is triggered midway through the cycle by the pituitary hormone LH. In the absence of fertilization, the built-up endometrial tissue is shed during menstruation, and the lowered levels of progesterone and oestrogen stimulate the cycle to begin again. Progesterone causes the body temperature to rise about 1 degree Fahrenheit, making it possible to tell when ovulation occurs (see BASAL BODY TEMPERATURE). In pregnancy progesterone inhibits movements of uterine muscle, stops ovulation, and stimulates breast development.

Progestin Also *progestogen*. Synthetic (man-made) PROGESTERONE, used in oral contraceptives and other medications.

Prognosis A forecast as to the probable outcome of a disease. A favourable prognosis means recovery is likely; a poor prognosis means it is not.

Prolactin Also *luteotrophin*, *luteotrophic hormone*, *LTH*. A HORMONE secreted by the pituitary gland that stimulates the breasts to secrete milk and also inhibits the production of the pituitary hormones LH and FSH, which stimulate ovulation.

Prolapsed cord In childbirth, the condition existing when the umbilical cord lies ahead of or beside the presenting part of the baby (head, shoulders, buttocks) in the vagina. This phenomenon is extremely dangerous for the baby, whose oxygen supply and circulation can be impaired with any compression of the cord. It rarely occurs with vertex (head-first) presentation when the head is engaged by the time the membranes rupture because the head normally presses against the cervix, allowing no room for the cord. If for some reason the head is not engaged, or the baby is very small or the pelvis is too small, or if some other part, particularly a shoulder or foot, presents (leads the way), the cord can prolapse when the membranes rupture. Treatment depends on how much the cervix is dilated and on the position of the baby. If the cervix is fully dilated, the baby's life can usually be saved if it can be delivered immediately. If the cervix is only partly dilated and the baby is mature, an immediate CAESAREAN SECTION may save it. (Even if the cervix is fully dilated a Caesarean section may be performed because there might be too long a period of compression before delivery, so that the baby would be deprived of oxygen.) Even with prompt measures, however, the probability of the baby's death is fairly high (about 17 per cent).

Prolapsed uterus Also *fallen uterus*, *uterine decensus*. Partial descent of the uterus into the vagina, owing to pelvic relaxation, that is, weakening of the pelvic-floor muscles that normally hold the uterus in place. The condition usually results from childbirth (a long labour, large babies, many pregnancies) and tends to get worse after menopause. In severe cases the uterus drops completely out of the vagina, causing considerable irritation to the delicate cervix, which then rubs against clothing, and producing discharge and bleeding. Sometimes the uterus must be held in place with a sanitary pad or a special device called a PESSARY.

A prolapsed uterus may give rise to no symptoms at all, but usually there is a sensation of heaviness or pressure in the vagina. There may also be urinary incontinence (especially when coughing, laughing, or sneezing; see STRESS INCONTINENCE) and backache. The condition, which is often found in conjunction with a prolapsed bladder or rectum (see CYSTOCELE; RECTOCELE), can be readily diagnosed during a pelvic examination. In mild cases no treatment may be needed, or the prolapse may be partly corrected by trying to strengthen the pelvic-floor muscles with KEGAL EXERCISES; for overweight women, losing weight may also help.

In severe cases, the insertion of a pessary can alleviate the symptoms, and its use is advisable in women for whom surgery represents too great a risk or who want to bear more children. Otherwise, a vaginal HYSTERECTOMY (removal of the uterus through the vagina) along with any needed repair to the bladder or rectum may be the only means of correcting the condition permanently.

Proliferative phase The first portion of the normal MENSTRUAL CYCLE—usually days 1 to 14—when oestrogen secreted by the ovarian follicles causes the endometrium (lining of the uterus) to grow in preparation for the implantation of a fertilized egg. See also SECRETORY PHASE.

Prolonged labour Any portion of childbirth that lasts longer than the generally accepted established norm. The technical term for any difficult labour, whatever the cause, is *dystocia*. The causes fall into three general categories: ABNORMAL PRESENTATION, with the baby in a position from which it cannot be pushed out; *pelvic contraction* or *cephalopelvic disproportion*, where a part of the mother's pelvis is not large enough to permit the baby's passage; and, most often, *uterine dysfunction* or *uterine inertia*, meaning insufficiently strong or insufficiently regular contractions of the uterine muscles to dilate the cervix and expel the baby.

The duration of labour varies greatly. A first baby nearly always takes longer than subsequent ones, but even then there are exceptions. The first stage of LABOUR, which is by far the longest and involves dilating the cervix to a diameter of about 10 centimetres (4 inches), lasts, in an average first labour, about twelve hours (seven hours in subsequent deliveries). This first stage is often subdivided into a *latent phase* (*early labour*), characterized by weak, irregularly spaced contractions as the cervix is slowly dilated to about 3 or 4 centimetres, and an *active phase* (*hard labour*), where contractions are stronger, more regular, and dilatation proceeds more rapidly, until it reaches 10 centimetres. The latent phase may last six or seven hours, but the active phase rarely lasts more than four or five. It is followed by the second stage, the expulsion of the baby, which lasts two hours or less, and the third stage, delivery of the placenta, which lasts fifteen to thirty minutes (all these times refer to a *first* baby). See also the chart for 'normal labour' on page 179.

Given these average times, *prolonged latent labour* is defined as twenty hours for a first baby, fourteen hours for subsequent babies; *prolonged active labour* is marked by cervical dilation of less than 1.2 centimetres per hour with a first baby and less than 1.5 centimetres per hour for subsequent babies. Also, labour is considered prolonged if progress at any point comes to a halt. Prolonged labour tends to occur in older women (thirty-five or older for a first baby), with large babies in a first pregnancy, and with POSTERIOR PRESENTATION, the most common abnormal position, and with BREECH PRESENTATION.

Prophylactic 1 The medical term for 'preventive'. For example, penicillin or another antibiotic is often used following abortion to prevent the risk of possible infection; in this example penicillin is a prophylactic therapy, since no infection is present when it is given.

2 Another name for CONDOM.

Prostaglandins A group of fatty acids found in human and animal tissue that act on almost every organ system of the body. They play an especially important role in the reproductive, gastrointestinal, and cardiovascular systems that is not yet completely understood. Some of them are capable of stimulating uterine contractions and therefore have been used for abortion, principally by injection into the uterus (see AMNIOINFUSION). They have also been used in the form of vaginal suppositories, but though they work faster in this way they may cause violent nausea, intense uterine contractions,

diarrhoea, and sometimes fever. Prostaglandins are also suspected of being responsible for severe menstrual cramps (see DYSMENORRHOEA, definition 4), causing contractions of uterine muscle and blood vessels that are perceived as pain. Several drugs used for arthritis that also have antiprostaglandin properties appear to be effective in reducing severe menstrual discomfort.

Pruritis See ITCHING.

Pseudocyesis See FALSE PREGNANCY.

Psychogenic Describing a symptom or set of symptoms caused by emotional or psychologic factors, and having no objective manifestations. For example, a person may complain of a headache or stomach ache, or pain on urinating, and careful medical examination will uncover no physical reason for the pain. These symptoms may be a response to short-lived emotional distress or the expression of a severe emotional disorder, such as depression or anxiety. For an extreme example, see HYSTERIA, CONVERSION. See also PSYCHOSOMATIC.

Psychoprophylactic method Also *Lamaze method*. A method of PREPARED CHILDBIRTH that concentrates on teaching women about the physiology of reproduction and childbirth and instructs them in exercises to be used before and during labour and delivery, including special kinds of breathing (slow chest breathing, panting, blowing) to be used at various stages of labour.

The psychoprophylactic method is taught in a series of six weekly classes attended by the woman and, if possible, her husband or partner, beginning in the seventh month of pregnancy. The partner assists during labour by timing the length and frequency of contractions, massaging her back, wiping her face, reminding her of the responses she learned, and generally providing support and encouragement. The earliest and principal proponent of the psychoprophylactic method in America was Elisabeth Bing, who began teaching it about 1960 and over the years devised variations and refinements on it. In England the method of Erna Wright was based on it, as well as that of Sheila Kitzinger (who called her method *psychosexual preparation*); both introduced somewhat different breathing techniques, and Kitzinger a different method for bearing down during the second stage of labour.

Critics of the psychoprophylactic method say that it concentrates on blocking out pain instead of going along with body rhythms and 'riding with' the pain. Also, they say the light panting method of breathing may deprive the baby of needed oxygen.

Psychosomatic A broad term used to describe a physical symptom or disorder in which psychological or emotional factors play an important but not clearly understood role. The symptom or illness is physically present and demonstrable, but it is either precipitated by or aggravated by psychic factors. Among the disorders in which emotional factors are believed to play an important role are hypertension (high blood pressure), coronary artery disease, diabetes, rheumatoid arthritis, peptic ulcers, and asthma. However, the relative importance of psychological factors in such disorders varies greatly among different individuals;

besides, they are difficult to separate from other factors, such as hereditary predisposition, allergy, individual personality, individual responses to drugs, and social pressures. See also PSYCHOGENIC.

Psychotherapy Also *counselling, therapy*. A general term for the treatment of mental and emotional disorders that is based primarily on verbal communication between patient and therapist. Psychotherapy is conducted by psychiatrists and other doctors specially trained in this area, as well as by psychologists, social workers, psychoanalysts, lay analysts, nurses, pastoral counsellors, and others with professional training of various kinds in the technique. Psychotherapy may be conducted on a one-to-one basis (individual approach) or in a group with other clients (*group therapy*) and one or more therapists. Families and couples also may be treated together. In addition, some groups – *self-help* or *support groups* – function on their own, their members acting as therapists for one another.

Psychotherapy is most often performed in a surgery setting and on an outpatient basis, but seriously disturbed persons may require hospitalization, or they may use a day hospital (returning home every night) or residential programme in a hospital. Psychotherapy can be carried on alone or in conjunction with psychotropic drugs (principally TRANQUILLIZERS and ANTIDEPRESSANTS for outpatients), and/or electroconvulsive (shock) therapy, the latter usually performed only in a hospital setting.

There are many different psychotherapeutic approaches, ranging from classical psychoanalysis, developed by Sigmund Freud, and numerous therapies based on it (existential analysis, Jungian analysis, will therapy, etc.) to behaviourist therapy (and others based on it, including rational-emotive therapy, cognitive therapy, sex therapy, psychobiology, etc.) to purely group approaches, such as family therapy and psychodrama. See also FEMINIST THERAPY; SEX THERAPY.

Puberty The period during which sexual maturity is attained. In girls it begins several years earlier than in boys (at about the age of nine or ten) and lasts for about five years. (In boys the average age for onset of puberty is between twelve and fourteen, but a much wider range – ten to eighteen – is considered normal.) During this time girls experience a period of rapid growth in height and weight gain – the so-called *growth spurt*. Most women reach their mature height soon after the onset of menstruation, or MENARCHE, which occurs three or four years after puberty began (at an average age of 12.8 in Britain). At this time increased levels of oestrogen cause closure of the growth centres at the ends of bones, thus ending their growth. (Male sex hormones have a similar effect in boys, but much later.) Oestrogen also causes the deposit of increased amounts of fat in the subcutaneous tissue of the breasts, upper arms, buttocks, hips, and thighs, producing the characteristic shape of the female body. Influenced by oestrogen, the uterus enlarges and vagina lengthens; the inner lips of the vulva, the labia minora, begin to grow until they may protrude somewhat between the thick outer lips, or labia majora. The relative proportion of lean body mass (muscle and bone) to total body weight lessens, so that muscles look less prominent, masked by the higher proportion of fat. In boys, on the other hand, increased androgen levels produce both

greater muscularity and more prominent muscle definition, seen especially in the shoulders and chest. For these reasons women can rarely, if ever, develop the same upper body strength as men, though they are able to develop as much leg strength. Their larger proportion of fat, on the other hand, makes women better able to retain body heat in cold temperatures and also makes them more buoyant. (See also ATHLETIC ABILITY.)

Puberty is the time of developing *secondary sex characteristics*. In both boys and girls there is growth of pubic and axillary (underarm) hair, and the enlargement of axillary sweat glands, producing increased perspiration and also perspiration odour. In girls BREAST SIZE increases gradually, one breast often growing markedly faster than the other for a time; in boys the penis and testes grow, chest hair and facial hair appear, and the voice deepens. These changes takes place gradually, and at varying rates of speed in different individuals. Many adolescents worry about changing too soon (precocious puberty) or, more often, too late (delayed puberty). For most, little more is needed than frequent reassurance that their progress is 'normal'. *Delayed puberty* caused by later hormone production, although worrisome to children and parents, is in itself no cause for alarm, but when little or no pubertal change of any kind is apparent in girls by the age of sixteen (or in boys by the age of eighteen), medical investigation is warranted to rule out a tumour or serious disease. Total *pubertal failure*, which is more common in boys than in girls, is nearly always due either to a deficiency in the sex glands (testes or ovaries) or in pituitary stimulation of those glands, and usually responds to treatment with androgens or oestrogens. See also AMENORRHOEA, definition 2; PRECOCIOUS PUBERTY.

Pubic hair Hair that grows over the skin of the genital area during PUBERTY. In women it grows over the MONS VENERIS or pubis in a roughly triangular pattern (with the base of the triangle at the top), called the *escutcheon*. In men the pattern is less well defined and the hair tends to extend farther up toward the navel and down on the inner thighs, roughly diamond-shaped, as it is in some women, too. The pubic hair may be sparse or profuse, and straight or curly. Its function, like that of axillary (underarm) hair, is to absorb moisture and trap the scent secreted by the APOCRINE GLANDS. In girls it usually begins to grow about one year before menarche (the first menstrual period). If no pubic hair is evident by the age of sixteen (in boys, eighteen), it may be wise to investigate the cause of delay. Pubic hair sometimes becomes infested with tiny parasites (see PUBIC LICE).

Pubic lice Also *crabs, pediculosis pubis*. A parasitic infection that can be transmitted by sexual contact but also by infested bedding or clothing. The pubic louse (*Phthirus pubis*) is a tiny, yellowish-grey creature, about 1 millimetre long, with three pairs of claws and four pairs of legs, giving it a crablike appearance. It moves by swinging from hair to hair and then inserts its mouth into the skin, where it feeds on tiny blood vessels. If separated from human skin, it can survive only twenty-four hours at the most. During their thirty-day lifespan the adult lice mate frequently, the female daily laying about three oval white eggs called *nits*, which she cements to one side of a hair. They hatch in seven to nine days.

Symptoms of infection vary from none (rarely) to intense itching (usually). Scratching brings no relief and helps spread the lice via the fingers to other hairy parts of the body (thighs, underarms, scalp). Diagnosis is made by finding the lice or their nits attached to pubic hairs. Treatment is with carbaryl or a similar alternative available over-the-counter as a cream, lotion, or shampoo. After treatment, clothing and bedding should be changed and washed (though after twenty-four hours any remaining lice will have died), and non-washable items such as upholstery and mattresses should be sprayed with an appropriate pesticide to prevent reinfestation.

Pubis Another name for MONS VENERIS.

Pubococcygeous One of the important muscles of the pelvic floor that support the bladder, rectum, and uterus. It is the muscle used when one wishes to stop the flow of urine. It and the other pelvic-floor muscles often become over-relaxed after childbearing, leading to problems such as STRESS INCONTINENCE, RECTOCELE, CYSTOCELE, and PROLAPSED UTERUS. One way to strengthen the pubococcygeous is with KEGAL EXERCISES.

Pudenda Another name for VULVA.

Pudendal anaesthesia Also *pudendal block*. A kind of REGIONAL ANAESTHESIA administered during childbirth, when delivery is imminent (late in the second stage of LABOUR). The pudendal nerves around the vagina and vulva are injected through both sides of the vagina with a local anaesthetic that blocks their transmission of pain messages to the brain. These nerves are hard to locate and are placed differently in some women. Hence it takes considerable skill to block them, and as a rule the anaesthesia is only about 80 per cent effective. About the only risk of such anaesthesia, other than the slight one of an allergic reaction of the mother's, is injection of the anaesthetic into the pudendal artery, which can cause shock, and (rarely) death. Pudendal anaesthesia does not block the sensations of labour, only of delivery, and therefore is useful for low FORCEPS deliveries and the performance of a large EPISIOTOMY. It does not interfere with uterine contractions and the effects of the anaesthetic are not transmitted to the baby.

Puerperal fever Also *childbed fever, postpartum infection, puerperal sepsis.* Infection of the genital tract, usually of the endometrium (uterine lining), following childbirth. Its name comes from the fact that it is nearly always marked by a rise in body temperature (fever), and, indeed, the presence of fever after delivery is almost invariably a sign of infection. In this context, fever is interpreted as a temperature of 38 degrees Centigrade (100.4 degrees Fahrenheit) or higher on any two of the first ten days following delivery.

Puerperal fever was the leading cause of maternal death until fairly recently. It was first described in ancient times by Hippocrates and Galen, but its cause – wound infection – was determined only in 1847 by an Austrian physician, Ignaz Semmelweis, who believed that infection was introduced by the examining fingers of doctors, midwives, and students. He ordered all persons who examined women in labour to disinfect their hands with chlorine solution, and the mortality rate in his Vienna Lying-In Hospital dropped from 10 to 1 per cent almost

immediately. Nevertheless, his ideas were not widely accepted for many years. Epidemics of puerperal fever continued to occur in hospitals for another century although in the course of time aseptic techniques, antibiotic therapy, a reduction in traumatic deliveries and very long labours, and better general maternal health markedly reduced the death rate.

Puerperal infection can be caused by various organisms, but by far the most common source is the streptococcus. Infection usually occurs during the course of labour. Fortunately most such infections respond well to prompt antibiotic treatment, the choice of drug being based on the organism isolated by laboratory test. More recently, a sudden severe, potentially fatal infection in women who have given birth has been associated with *Staphylococcus aureus* (see toxic shock syndrome, under TAMPON).

Puerperium The period immediately following childbirth. A *puerpera* is a woman who has just given birth. See also POSTPARTUM.

Pulse See under ARTERY.

Purulent Also *suppurating*. Filled with or exuding PUS.

Pus A thick, yellowish liquid that forms in infected tissue. It consists chiefly of dead cells and white blood cells, and contains the bacteria causing the infection. See also INFECTION.

Pustule See under ACNE.

Pyelonephritis Also *kidney infection*. An acute infection of one or both kidneys, usually caused by bacteria that enter the body through the urethra and work their way up through the bladder and ureters to the kidneys. It is especially common in young girls and in pregnant women, and in both men and women who have diabetes or who have undergone catheterization or some procedure in which an instrument is introduced into the urinary tract. The most common cause is *Escherichia coli*, an organism that normally resides in the gastrointestinal tract. Typically, pyelonephritis comes on quite rapidly and is marked by fever, chills, and back pain on one or both sides near the waistline. There may also be nausea and vomiting. Bladder irritation from the infected urine may cause frequency and urgency of urination, which may also be painful, and haematuria (blood in the urine). Treatment should be promptly sought, because pyelonephritis can cause permanent kidney damage. The causative agent can be identified by testing the urine, but antibiotic treatment is usually begun before urine culture results are available. As with other urinary tract infections, drinking a great deal of water – at least six to eight glasses a day, and preferably more – helps by diluting the urine and so making it less hospitable to bacterial growth. Urinating frequently and completely emptying the bladder help keep bacteria from multiplying, and eliminating coffee, tea, and alcoholic beverages, which all contain kidney irritants, may also help relieve the symptoms.

Q

Quadriplegia Partial or total paralysis of all four limbs (both arms and both legs), usually resulting from injury to the spinal cord in the cervical (neck) segments. Such injury may occur in a traffic, industrial, or sports accident or in wartime; less often it results from tumours, infections, abscesses, and congenital defects. Once the spinal cord is injured, its nerve cells and fibres are unable to regenerate and the damage is irreversible, a permanent lesion now obstructing the paths of sensation and motor control. The extent of disability is determined by the extent and level of the lesion in the spinal cord. Quadriplegics suffer serious impairment or complete loss of sensitivity to touch, pain, and temperature in all the areas affected. Other problems are disturbances in blood circulation, loss of skin and muscle tone, and loss of voluntary bowel and bladder control. As a result, quadriplegics are apt to suffer from certain secondary complications, especially urinary infections and kidney and bladder stones, pressure sores (decubitus ulcer), muscle contractures of paralyzed joints (hips, knees, elbows), and fractures of weight-bearing bones. Another common complication is *autonomic hyperreflexia*: because the spinal cord, although cut off from the brain by injury, is still living tissue, when it is stimulated it generates a massive response that cannot be checked by the brain. Symptoms of hyperreflexia, which may occur alone or in combination, include throbbing headache, flushing of the face, neck, and upper body, sweating, seizures, nasal obstruction, chills, and hypertension. The most common precipitating cause of such violent reactions is retention of urine. Quadriplegics who have lost conscious urinary control normally live with an indwelling catheter (tube), which must periodically be checked for blockage.

In quadriplegic women, menstruation, fertility, and pregnancy are not affected. Oral contraceptives and intrauterine devices (IUDs) for birth control are generally contraindicated because circulatory problems are very likely to develop in paralyzed limbs and could go undetected due to lack of sensation, as could a pelvic infection. Sexual intercourse may be difficult in certain positions owing to hip and leg spasms, and there is increased risk of autonomic hyperreflexia during sexual arousal (and also during labour and delivery). There is also increased risk of urinary and bowel incontinence during masturbation and intercourse. Masturbating is difficult or impossible without assistance, and, depending on the exact location of the spinal cord lesion, there may be no sensation of orgasm, or no reflex sexual response with genital stimulation. However, other parts of the body (usually above the site of the lesion) may become highly sensitive to sexual stimulation, and some women report feelings identical to orgasm when these are stimulated. See also PARAPLEGIA.

Quickening The perception of the movements of the foetus by a pregnant woman. It usually occurs sometime between the sixteenth and twentieth weeks of pregnancy, and may be perceived initially as a very faint flutter or, especially later in pregnancy, as quite vigorous 'kicks'. The foetal movements can also be felt by placing one's hand over the lower abdomen. The movements of the foetus depend on the presence of the amniotic fluid, in which it floats. During the fourth and fifth months the foetus is small in relation to the amount of fluid. A sudden tap or simply pressure on the abdomen causes the foetus to sink in the fluid; it then rebounds to its original position, as though tapping back at the examining hand. This passive movement of the foetus is called *ballottement*. Both it and the more active movements can sometimes be felt upon vaginal examination to test for ENGAGEMENT; after engagement the foetus is fixed in the pelvis and cannot be ballotted. From the thirtieth week of pregnancy on, complete absence of foetal movements for a period of twenty-four hours or longer is a sign of possible foetal distress and should be investigated.

R

Radiation therapy Also *irradiation, radiotherapy.* Treatment of cancer by direct X-rays, cobalt, or other sources of ionizing radiation at specific parts of the body. If administered just as a cancer cell is ready to reproduce (divide in two), radiation will stop cell division and the cell will eventually die. Because cancer cells multiply faster than normal cells, they are more susceptible to radiation.

Radiation therapy is effective as a primary treatment – that is, used alone, without surgery – for many cancers, such as head and neck cancer and cancer of the uterus or cervix. Some specialists believe it can be used in this way for breast cancer as well, along with only minimal surgery (see MASTECTOMY, definitions 6, 7), but others disagree. However, it is the principal primary treatment for inflammatory breast cancer (see CANCER, INFLAMMATORY BREAST), for local control of inoperable breast cancers (in women who cannot or will not undergo surgery, or whose cancer is very advanced), as an adjunct to mastectomy, to shrink a large tumour to operable size, and to alleviate pain – especially bone pain – caused by distant METASTASIS. Implanting a radiation source temporarily at the side of a tumour can supplement external radiation in destroying cancer cells (also see below).

Like CHEMOTHERAPY (anticancer drugs), radiation also affects some healthy cells, particularly those subject to rapid growth, such as hair roots and gastrointestinal mucosa. Consequently it causes similar unpleasant side effects, the most common being hair loss, nausea, vomiting, and sores in the mouth. Radiation is usually less disfiguring than surgery. In the case of breast cancer, treatment may cause a temporary sunburn-like blistering but the final appearance of the skin will show minimal scarring in about 75 per cent of patients. Others have quite extensive scarring, however. Radiation occasionally leads to other complications. In breast cancer these include radiation-induced rib fractures, short-term lung inflammation, and, more rarely, scarring of the pericardium (the sac surrounding the heart). The major drawback to radiation therapy is that it itself is known to cause cancer; such cancers, however, may take many years to develop.

Radical hysterectomy Also *Wertheim procedure.* Surgical removal of the uterus, cervix, pelvic lymph nodes and ligaments, and upper portion of the vagina, and sometimes also the ovaries and Fallopian tubes. See under HYSTERECTOMY.

Radical mastectomy See MASTECTOMY, definitions 2, 3, 4.

Radioimmunoassay See under RADIORECEPTOR ASSAY.

Radioreceptor assay A PREGNANCY TEST developed in the mid-1970s that is so sensitive it can give a positive result in more than 99 per cent of pregnant women before a period has been missed. Like other pregnancy tests, however, it can also yield false negative results.

Radiotherapy See RADIATION THERAPY.

Rape Sexual intercourse without the woman's consent. Oral and anal sexual assault and penetration with objects are not recognized as rape in British law, and the maximum penalty is, in most cases, much lower than rape. All sexual intercourse with girls, below the 'age of consent' – 16 – whether or not she consents, is statutory rape. When rape and sexual assault happen in infancy and childhood, men take advantage of young girls' powerless position, their lack of information and fear of telling others. Age is only one of many factors that can increase vulnerability to rape.

The number of rapes reported to the police has increased greatly in recent years. On the one hand, rising poverty, financial dependence on men, and deteriorating housing, transport and other services, increase social tension and heighten the vulnerability to rape of many women and girls. On the other hand, women are now more likely to report rape because of the encouragement of the women's anti-rape movement. Nevertheless, Home Office statistics on the number of rapes still represent only the tip of the iceberg. *Ask any woman*, an independent survey of London women conducted by Women Against Rape, published in 1985, found that only 1 in 12 rape survivors reports it to the police.

While some countries have made rape in marriage illegal, in Britain it is not a criminal offence for a man to rape his wife, except where cohabitation has ceased and the couple are legally separated. Yet, rape in marriage is, in fact, the most common form of rape, with 1 in 7 women raped by her own husband.

Besides physical force and the threat of force, about a third of rapists abuse a position of power or authority, e.g. as employer, supervisor, landlord, carer, college lecturer, doctor, priest, babysitter, senior relative, even parent.

Women have been pressing for better protection from rape and a safer environment – in the home, street, campus and waged workplace. They are also pressing for more sympathetic treatment for *all* rape survivors, since many are deterred from reporting for fear of disbelief or a hostile response from the police, courts, doctors and other authorities, on the grounds of race, sexual preference, age, style of dress, etc. Women have campaigned to win and extend compensation from the State for survivors of rape. Women Against Rape has focused on women's right to financial independence as crucial in enabling women to leave situations where they, and their children, are in danger of rape, so that women are not made vulnerable to rape because of poverty and financial dependence on husbands, fathers, boyfriends, etc. In the absence of State provision, women's groups have established Rape Crisis Centres or Rape Crisis Lines in many cities, offering medical and legal advice and counselling, and have set up Women's Aid refuges for women escaping violent husbands. These numbers will be in your local telephone directory.

Rape survivors are urged to take the following steps:

1. If possible, call a local rape crisis line promptly for counselling on medical care, police and court procedures, and emotional problems resulting from the attack.

2. Get a prompt medical examination from a doctor trained in dealing with rape evidence. They should first treat any injuries sustained, all of which should be recorded in detail, even minor ones and then given a standard pelvic examination (see GYNAECOLOGICAL EXAMINATION) during which they should perform a PAP SMEAR and ask the pathologist to examine it for sperm cells, as well as test the cervix and vaginal walls for acid phosphatase, produced by the male prostate gland (and therefore present in ejaculated seminal fluid). For this test a small amount of saline solution is introduced into the vagina and then withdrawn with a syringe, and the fluid withdrawn is tested for both acid phosphatase and sperm. The clinician should record both the number of sperm seen and whether or not they were moving (evidence of sperm may disappear in eight hours, so promptness is important).

3. Tests for both GONORRHOEA and SYPHILIS should be performed. Since neither of these veneral diseases produces symptoms in the early stages, a second test for gonorrhoea should be done two weeks later, and a blood test for syphilis three months later. If the rape was oral or anal, specimens from the woman's mouth or rectum should be taken for gonorrhoea culture.

4. The woman's body and clothing should be checked for substances that could be used as evidence, such as blood or grass stains on clothes, scrapings from under the fingernails (especially if she resisted), pubic or scalp hair different from hers, etc.

5. If the risk of pregnancy appears to be considerable – if the rape occurred at mid-cycle and the woman was not protected by a contraceptive – use of the MORNING-AFTER PILL within 72 hours of rape might be considered. Another morning-after alternative, inserting an INTRAUTERINE DEVICE, is not advisable, because if the rapist was harbouring an infection, such insertion could carry infection into the uterus.

6. If the woman intends reporting rape to the police, she should report as soon as possible, going with a friend or other supportive person. The police may or may not decide to prosecute. She should give a full account of what happened and of the attacker's appearance, if possible. The earlier a woman reports, the more seriously her report is likely to be treated. If a woman does not report to the police immediately, she can do so later; although the police may be discouraging, there is no reason why a successful prosecution cannot follow a delayed report.

7. As well as taking these immediate measures, a woman may want to seek some kind of post-rape counselling. Such counselling is available through local rape crisis centres, through women's self-help clinics and other community organizations, and in some hospital psychiatric departments. Most women find that they have at least temporary emotional problems in the aftermath of a rape, and some develop long-term ones, especially in the area of sexual relations. Denial and depression often mask fear and anger, and it is easier

if these feelings are honestly expressed and worked out. Sometimes a professional therapist is needed. Even supportive friends, family and lovers may not be able to help enough. Children and teenagers particularly may need special care and counselling to face what happened and to resolve their own feelings.

Like many areas affecting women's health, rape prevention is far better than treatment. Among the suggestions made by anti-rape groups are:

1. Prepare yourself beforehand. Imagine what you might do (for example, fight, run, scream, talk to the attacker, disgust him by pretending to vomit).
2. If you live in a place with other vulnerable women (block of flats, nurse's homes, student residences, etc.) set up a rape squad to patrol the grounds as a deterrent, and/or a special call-for-help signal, such as a whistle.
3. At home, use mortis locks on outside doors, keep windows locked, especially at night, put iron grids on ground floor windows, keep curtains drawn at night, don't hide your key near the door or in any other obvious place.
4. If you live alone, list only your first initials in the phone book and by the doorbell.
5. Don't let strangers into your home; if you suspect someone has broken in while you were out, don't enter your home alone.
6. Acquire some self-defence skills; even if you can't use judo against an armed man, your knowledge will give you more confidence and also make you appear less vulnerable.

Rectocele A bulging of the wall of the rectum into the vagina, owing to pelvic relaxation, that is, weakening of the muscles that ordinarily hold the rectum in place. It may occur alone or in conjunction with a PROLAPSED UTERUS and/or CYSTOCELE (fallen bladder), and like them usually results from childbirth (long labour, large babies, many pregnancies). A rectocele usually causes discomfort during bowel movement, when pressure is felt. Some women must actually put a finger inside their vagina when they defaecate in order to hold back the rectal wall. The condition can be corrected by minor surgery, the surgeon making an incision along the back wall of the vagina, pushing the rectum back and up, and sewing it into place.

Recurrence The return of symptoms or signs of a disease. In the case of CANCER, the return of symptoms in the same general area as the primary tumour.

Regional anaesthesia Also *conduction anaesthesia, local anaesthesia*. Administering an anaesthetic that causes a loss of feeling in a particular part of the body by blocking the conduction of pain sensations from that part to the brain. The principal kinds of regional anaesthesia used to relieve the pain of childbirth and surgery in the pelvic area are CAUDAL, EPIDURAL, PARACERVICAL, PUDENDAL, and SPINAL.

Remission The decrease or disappearance of the symptoms and signs of a disease, either spontaneously or in response to medication or other treatment. Also, the period during which this change occurs. The term 'remission' is ordinarily reserved for serious illnesses that have a tendency to recur, or flare up, such as cancer or multiple sclerosis. Acute temporary ailments are usually said to be 'cured'.

Retarded ejaculation See EJACULATION, definition 3.

Retroflexed uterus A uterus that is doubled back on itself. See also RETROVERTED UTERUS.

Retrograde ejaculation See EJACULATION, definition 4.

Retrolental fibroplasia A potentially serious eye condition in PREMATURE infants who are exposed to high concentrations of oxygen during the first few days of life. The premature retina develops abnormally, the extent of abnormality depending on the oxygen concentration and time of exposure. At first the retinal blood vessels proliferate and later fibrosis may develop. In extreme cases the retina becomes detached and partial or total blindness may result.

Retroverted uterus Also *tipped uterus, tipped womb*. A condition in which the uterus, which usually tilts forward slightly at almost a right angle to the vagina, is instead tilted backward (see UTERUS). It occurs in 25 to 30 per cent of women, most of whom are not even aware of it and require no treatment. Symptoms, when they do occur, usually consist of a vague backache or, in extreme cases, pain during vaginal intercourse (because the uterus is tipped so far that it lies adjacent to the vagina). Often a tipped uterus is congenital, but sometimes it occurs after pregnancy, owing to stretching of ligaments that normally keep it tilted forward, or after multiple infections create scar tissue (adhesions) that in effect pull the uterus back. Endometriosis can also make it adhere to the back.

Rheumatoid arthritis Also *rheumatism* (pop.). A chronic, progressive, systemic disease, the principal manifestation of which is inflammation of the joints often accompanied by anaemia. It affects approximately 1.4 million people in Britain and occurs three times as often in women as in men. Although it can strike at any age, its onset typically is between the ages of twenty and forty-five or fifty. Progressive joint destruction, pain, and decreased mobility can lead to severe crippling and deformity.

Rheumatoid arthritis is the most common form of *synovitis*; that is, inflammation of the synovial membrane lining a joint. Cells in the membrane divide and grow, until the joint appears red, swollen, and feels puffy or boggy to the touch. Increased blood flow that is part of the inflammatory process makes the area feel warm. Cells release enzymes into the joint space, and these cause further irritation and pain. If the process continues for years, as it sometimes does, the enzymes may gradually digest the cartilage and bone of the joint, which becomes virtually immobile.

The earliest symptoms of rheumatoid arthritis are swelling and pain in one or more joints that persist for at least six weeks. The wrists and knuckles are the joints most often afflicted, but the knees and metatarsals (ball of the foot) are often involved as well, and indeed any joint may be affected. Diagnosis is made through a blood test that shows the presence and amount of a specific protein called the *rheumatoid factor*. X-rays are not very useful for diagnosis at the outset, although they can reveal damage to the bone and cartilage and reveal the progress of the disease over time. Other symptoms, in addition to pain in the affected joints, are general muscle aches and fatigue (similar to those of flu or another virus infection, but longer-lasting), muscle stiffness (especially first thing in the morning), and sometimes low fever.

The disease usually takes one of three courses. It may be a single brief illness, lasting a few months at the most and not leading to permanent disability; it may involve several episodes of extreme symptoms, or *flare-ups*, separated by periods of total remission, with little or no physical impairment remaining; or it may become chronic and constant, lasting several years or for life. The last is the most common course of rheumatoid arthritis.

The cause of rheumatoid arthritis is not known, but it is believed to be an auto-immune disease in which the body's immune system goes awry and it begins to make antibodies against some of its own normal tissues. Since there is no specific cure for rheumatoid arthritis, the patient must usually learn to live with it. Both overexertion and too much rest worsen joint stiffness, so a middle road between enough rest and sufficient exercise must be found. Work with a professional physiotherapist to find the right exercise programme is sometimes of great benefit. Other treatment consists of administering high doses of aspirin (under medical supervision), which helps both the pain and inflammation. Other anti-inflammatory agents may also be used. If these are not effective, anti-malarial drugs, injections of gold salts, and other more experimental medications may be tried, but they often have serious side effects. Of the drug therapies, aspirin is by far the safest. Sometimes damaged joints can be restored by orthopaedic surgery, such as hip or knee replacement, synovectomy (removal of the diseased synovial membrane) of the knee or knuckles, or resection of the metatarsis (foot). Although such surgery is a major undertaking, in severe cases it may be preferable to some of the stronger experimental drugs or a life of invalidism. Recently two preliminary studies indicated that patients who underwent X-ray therapy to suppress their immune systems showed marked improvement for up to a year and a half, but more research in this area is needed before such treatment is more broadly applied.

In women, rheumatoid arthritis affects neither the menstrual cycle nor fertility; in fact, pregnancy sometimes brings on a remission, or an exacerbation. Delivery may be complicated if the hips or spine are deformed. Oral contraceptives must be used with caution, since rheumatoid arthritis patients have circulatory problems, and intrauterine devices (IUDs) may be inadvisable if a woman is at all anaemic, since they may cause heavier menstrual flow. Though sexual response is unaffected, the sex drive may be diminished owing to both pain and fatigue, and deformities and pain may interfere with intercourse in certain positions (as well as with masturbation). See also OSTEOARTHRITIS.

Rh factor An ANTIGEN that is present in the red blood cells of most men and women, whose blood is then said to be *Rh-positive*. When it is absent, the blood is said to be *Rh-negative*. If a woman with Rh-negative blood carries an Rh-positive foetus (because the father's blood is Rh-positive), her body may become sensitized and develop antibodies to attack the Rh-positive blood cells in the foetus. This condition is called *Rh incompatibility*. In some cases it occurs when the foetal blood enters the mother's bloodstream via the placenta. More often, however, it occurs during delivery.

Rh incompatibility occurs in about 0.5 per cent of pregnancies and can result in the death of the foetus from erythroblastosis, a kind of anaemia, as early as four months along in the pregnancy. The only way to save a foetus so threatened is to give an exchange transfusion, that is, replace its blood supply with Rh-negative blood that will not react to the mother's antibodies.

All pregnant women should be tested for Rh factor, even if they plan to terminate the pregnancy. If a woman is Rh-negative and the father is also Rh-negative, no problem of incompatibility arises; if the father is Rh-positive or paternity is unknown, however, the mother's blood must be tested to see if she has developed any Rh-antibodies. Even if she has never been pregnant before, she may have been sensitized through a blood transfusion using Rh-positive blood. If no antibodies are present, the test should be repeated monthly between the twenty-eighth week of pregnancy and delivery to see if antibodies have developed. Should they be present, she must then receive special care through the remainder of the pregnancy. Antibody levels must be checked every month; if they rise significantly an intrauterine foetal transfusion may be performed. AMNIOCENTESIS is performed first to assess the extent of damage to the foetus, which can be evaluated from the level of bilirubin in the amniotic fluid. If the foetus is sufficiently well developed, premature delivery by induction may be considered.

The majority of Rh-negative women have no difficulty in a first pregnancy, but about 10 to 15 per cent become sensi-tized after one or more pregnancies. For about 90 per cent of those potentially sensitized, injection of anti-D eliminates all risk in the next pregnancy; however, it must be administered again after every pregnancy, whether ending in delivery, miscarriage, or abortion.

Rhythm method See under NATURAL FAMILY PLANNING.

Ripe cervix The softening of the cervix that occurs near term. It may be somewhat dilated (1 to 2 centimetres), show some effacement, and is usually anterior in position. This condition usually indicates that the cervix would respond favourably to INDUCTION OF LABOUR should it be necessary.

Rubella Also *German measles, three-day measles*. An infectious disease of childhood that, when contracted by a pregnant woman, can lead to miscarriage, stillbirth, or serious birth defects in the baby. The earlier in pregnancy the disease is contracted, the more serious the effects. During the first twelve weeks of gestation the foetus lacks the ability to create antibodies against the rubella virus. Therefore, if the virus is transmitted from the mother's bloodstream to the foetus, it continues to multiply at a much greater rate there. As a result, if the foetus survives early pregnancy at all, it may be born with any or all of the following defects: deafness and other ear abnormalities; cataracts and other eye disorders; brain damage; heart malformations; abnormalities of other internal organs. The danger to the foetus is greatest during the first four weeks of pregnancy, when some 60 per cent will suffer irreversible damage; 35 per cent will be affected during the second four weeks, and only about 10 per cent during the third four weeks. Because of the high risk to the unborn, a woman who contracts rubella during early pregnancy may be advised to seek an abortion, if possible. If legal, religious, or medical reasons rule out abortion, she may be given large doses of gamma globulin, though many authorities believe it to be ineffective.

The connection between rubella and birth defects was first observed in 1941, and since 1969 an effective vaccine against rubella has been available. Women who intend to bear children and have not had rubella during childhood (or think they might not have) should definitely be vaccinated at least four months before conception is planned and be sure that all of their older children (if any) have been vaccinated. Rubella vaccine is given to babies by itself, at the age of twelve months, or together with measles and mumps vaccine at fifteen months. A simple test can determine whether one has antibodies to the virus, resulting from earlier vaccination or infection. The four-month waiting period after vaccination is necessary before conceiving because the vaccine is made from attenuated (weakened) live virus; it is therefore not advisable to vaccinate a woman already pregnant. A woman already pregnant who has neither had rubella nor been vaccinated should make every effort to avoid infection.

Rubella is found everywhere and is endemic in larger cities. Typically the symptoms appear sixteen to eighteen days following exposure, though the incubation period is anywhere from two to three weeks. In children a rash consisting of pinkish raised spots, lighter than those of regular measles, is often the first sign of illness. They form on the face first and then move rapidly down the body, but since they often fade in a day or so the facial rash may be gone by the time the last of the body rash appears. Slight cold symptoms may accompany the rash. In adolescents and adults the illness is usually more severe. However, unlike measles in adults, rubella usually runs its course in a few days. Most cases are so mild that no treatment (other than aspirin, perhaps) is needed.

Newborn babies with rubella, who acquired it before delivery, may be severely ill. The worst problems are those of infants with extensive red patches caused by bleeding inside the skin, which may be symptomatic of generalized internal bleeding; more than one-third of these babies die within the first year of life. With less severe infection, there may be marked improvement after about six months, when the body finally gets rid of the virus and the child begins to gain weight and grow normally.

Rubin test Also *carbon dioxide test, tubal insufflation*. A procedure used to detect an obstruction in the Fallopian tubes that is preventing a woman from becoming pregnant. Carbon dioxide gas is blown into the cervix under pressure carefully monitored with a mercury manometer, which can indicate if the tubes are partly or wholly blocked. After the gas has passed through the tubes it escapes into the surrounding cavity, causing some shoulder pain when the woman sits up. If it cannot pass through because of blockage, it is simply expelled through the vagina. Sometimes the test itself will get rid of an obstruction, clearing the tubes of small bits of scar tissue or mucus. In many areas, however, doctors no longer perform this test, preferring the more accurate findings of HYSTEROSALPINGOGRAPHY.

S

Saddle block anaesthesia See SPINAL ANAESTHESIA.

Safe period See under NATURAL FAMILY PLANNING.

Saline abortion See under AMNIO-INFUSION.

Salpingectomy Surgical removal of one or both Fallopian tubes, a procedure usually performed in conjunction with OOPHORECTOMY and/or HYSTERECTOMY. *Unilateral salpingectomy* means removal of one tube, *bilateral salpingectomy* of both. The principal indication for unilateral salpingectomy is the removal of a foetus that has become implanted in the tube rather than the uterus (see ECTOPIC PREGNANCY).

Salpingitis Inflammation and/or infection of the Fallopian tubes, most often caused either by GONORRHOEA or as a sequel of childbirth or abortion. See PELVIC INFLAMMATORY DISEASE.

Sanitary napkin Also *sanitary towel*. An externally worn pad of absorbent material, designed to soak up menstrual flow. Such napkins were developed during World War I by Kimberly-Clark, an American manufacturer of surgical dressings that was looking for a way to use up its surplus cellucotton and marketed it as a sanitary napkin under the brand name Kotex. Prior to that – and even today, in many parts of the world – women used rags or other pieces of cloth or paper for this purpose. See also MENSTRUAL CUP; TAMPON.

Sarcoma A malignant (cancerous) TUMOUR made up of closely packed cells embedded in a homogeneous tissue. Sarcomas are often found in connective tissue, such as bone. Though in the pelvic area they are less common than other kinds of malignancy, they can affect the endometrium, ovaries, and vagina.

Scanty flow Exceptionally light bleeding during regular menstrual periods. See under MENSTRUAL FLOW.

Schiller test A diagnostic test for vaginal or cervical cancer. The cervix and vaginal walls are coated with an iodine solution (Schiller's stain or Lugol's solution), which stains normal cells brown but is not absorbed by abnormal cells, which remain pink. If abnormal tissue is revealed in this way, it is usually further examined by COLPOSCOPY, and some is removed for biopsy to determine its nature. The solution stains clothing, so one should wear a sanitary pad after this test.

Schizophrenia A group of serious emotional disorders of unknown causes that are characterized by disturbances of thought, mood, and behaviour. Typically the schizophrenic patient seems withdrawn and isolated, emotionally detached from other people. His or her fundamental perceptions of reality are fragmented and distorted. Hallucinations, especially auditory (hearing imaginary voices), are common, as are delusions of persecution. Behaviour varies. It may be torpid, silent, and apathetic, or very agitated. Moreover, symptoms vary in severity, from mild to very severe.

The onset of schizophrenia usually takes one of two forms: either it is very sudden (*reactive schizophrenia*), often triggered by some identifiable stress; or it is slow and insidious (*process schizophrenia*), with no identifiable causes. There is considerable disagreement about all aspects of schizophrenia, including its causes, classification, treatment, and outcome. Some cases seem to cure themselves spontaneously; most, however, become chronic, and may be crippling. Treatment includes a variety of drugs, principally potent TRANQUILLIZERS, as well as various forms of psychotherapy.

Sclerosing adenosis

A benign (noncancerous) lesion, often found in the breasts of relatively young women (during the childbearing years), that consists of distorted tissue of the ACINI. It is perfectly harmless but sometimes is difficult to distinguish from a malignant tumour, so to rule out cancer with certainty it is usually excised (cut out) for biopsy.

Scoliosis

A progressive lateral curvature of the spine that is four or five times more common in women than in men and most often begins at puberty, between the ages of eleven and fifteen. As the condition progresses, it contracts the ribs and compresses the lungs and heart, restricting breathing and circulation. It may also cause degenerative disease of the spine leading to osteoarthritis, disc problems, and sciatica. Eventually, without treatment, it is possible for scoliosis to cause total invalidism and death.

About 10 per cent of British adolescents have scoliosis. of these about one-quarter require medical attention of some kind, ranging from observation for future progression of the curvature to the use of a brace or surgery, depending on how advanced the curvature is at the time it is first detected. The earliest detectable symptoms are the protrusion of one shoulder blade, one hip looking higher or more prominent than the other, clothing hanging unevenly, an odd gait, and a slight thickening on one side of the neck.

There are many causes for the development of scoliosis, including various nerve and muscle disorders, diseases such as poliomyelitis, and abnormal development of the vertebrae. However, 80 to 90 per cent of the cases are idiopathic – that is, no cause can be determined. Scoliosis tends to run in families and so may be genetic, but it is not known what triggers the development of curvature or why some curves progress more than others. Scoliosis occurs in otherwise perfectly healthy individuals. Because it may appear at any time during the growing years and is painless in its early stages, it is important to check a child's spine regularly until growth is complete, especially during the rapid growth spurt of the early teen years. The easiest way to check is to have the child stand and bend forward, with the arm hanging down loosely and palms touching at

Common kinds of scoliosis

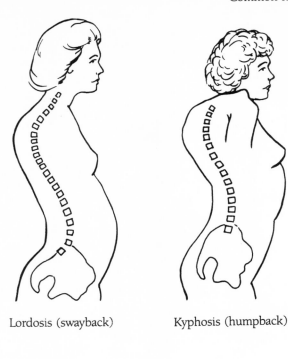

Lordosis (swayback)   Kyphosis (humpback)

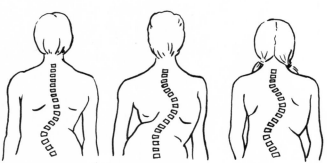

Typical scoliotic curves

almost knee level. In this position, either one shoulder higher than the other or a curve of the vertebrae, which are very prominent, is cause for suspicion. Lordosis (swayback) and kyphosis (humpback) are also indications for further checking. Some cases of scoliosis are mild enough to require no treatment. More severe cases, if caught early, may require wearing a brace twenty-three hours a day for two to three years, as well as doing daily exercises. More drastic treatment involves spinal fusion or other surgery. Because early detection is so helpful, school-based screening pro- grammes, which can be carried out by school nurses, physical education instructors, and voluteers who have some training, are highly recommended.

Scopolamine A hypnotic drug that induces amnesia and for years was given during LABOUR to make a woman forget the pain afterwards. Usually it was administered together with various narcotic drugs for their analgesic (pain-relieving) and euphoric effects, and sometimes also with barbiturates. Scopolamine induces a kind of 'twilight sleep'. However, it causes some restlessness as well, and sometimes even hallucinations and delirium. Therefore a woman given scopolamine requires constant observation by a trained attendant, and cannot co-operate in her labour or use any relaxation techniques. Its effect on babies has never been satisfactorily evaluated, and today it has been largely replaced by narcotics, especially pethidine, sometimes combined with tranquillizers to produce analgesia and sedation. A newer use of scopolamine, administered in low doses to be absorbed through the skin, is to combat severe motion sickness in adults.

Scrotum A two-chambered sac of thin, wrinkled skin that hangs between and slightly in front of a man's thighs, behind the PENIS. After puberty it is covered with pubic hair. Inside the scrotum are the TESTES. The scrotum itself it sensitive to sexual stimulation and to temperature change. In cold weather muscles in the scrotal wall contract to bring the testes closer to the body (for warmth).

Sebaceous cyst See CYST, definition 2.

Secondary sex characteristics The external physical characteristics that distinguish women from men, and are the result of increased levels of different sex hormones (oestrogen in women, androgens in men). See under PUBERTY.

Secretory phase The latter portion of the normal MENSTRUAL CYCLE where oestrogen and progesterone stimulate the uterine glands to secrete life-supporting substances in preparation for the implantation and nurture of a fertilized egg (pregnancy). If an egg is actually implanted, the secretions continue to be produced. If conception does not occur, progesterone and oestrogen levels drop sharply and the endometrium (uterine lining), unable to support the growth that took place in preparation for pregnancy, breaks down and is shed as menstrual flow. See also PROLIFERATIVE PHASE.

Semen Also *seminal fluid*. The fluid discharged when a man reaches orgasm and ejaculates. It consists of gland secretions and sperm. For semen analysis, see under SPERM. See also EJACULATION; PENIS.

Senile vaginitis See VAGINAL ATROPHY; also VAGINITIS.

Septic abortion 1 A miscarriage caused by infection in the pelvix, resulting from pelvic inflammantory disease, an intrauterine device, or some other causes. See MISCARRIAGE, definition 6.

2 An elective abortion that was improperly performed, resulting in infection, haemorrhage, or both. See under ABORTION.

Sequential pill An ORAL CONTRACEPTIVE that attempted to imitate the hormone sequence of the natural menstrual cycle, so that the pills in a four-week package consisted of oestrogen for only the first two weeks, oestrogen and progesterone for the third week, and no pills for the fourth week. However, this medication appeared to increase the risk of developing uterine cancer, and was withdrawn from use in the 1970s.

Serological test, serum See under BLOOD TEST.

Sex, determination of The establishment a baby's sex before conception, which depends on whether the particular sperm responsible for fertilization carried, after dividing, an X (girl) or Y (boy) sex CHROMOSOME. The chances for either are believed to be about equal (50 per cent). Over the years numerous theories have been developed concerning possibilities of increasing the chances of conceiving a child of the desired sex. According to one recent system that claims an 80 to 85 per cent chance of success, to conceive a boy intercourse should take place a few hours before or just at the time of OVULATION; before intercourse the woman should use an alkaline douche (2 to 3 tablespoons of baking soda per 2 pints of water); the penis should penetrate deep into the vagina at ejaculation; and the woman should experience orgasm. For a girl baby, the last intercourse should take place two to three days before ovulations, preceded by an acid douche (2 tablespoons vinegar per 2 pints of water); the penis should not penetrate too deeply at ejaculation; and the woman should not try to achieve orgasm.

Sex therapy A form of short-term therapy dealing with male and female

sexual problems that are usually solely psychological but sometimes occur in conjunction with organic disorders. The main medical problems that may contribute to SEXUAL DYSFUNCTION are diabetes, hypertension, and alcoholism.

Sex therapy is behaviourist in approach, that is, it focuses principally on changing behaviour rather than delving into its underlying causes. A therapist may treat either an individual or, more often, a couple. The treatment includes taking a detailed history of the individual's or couple's sex life, a thorough explanation of the anatomy and physiology of the sex organs and of SEXUAL RESPONSE, and, often, a series of exercises for the couple to perform at home in order to change their behaviour. These exercises help a couple to concentrate on gentle forms of touching and caressing in order to discover what they enjoy and find arousing (what William Master and Virginia Johnson called 'sensate focus exercises'; see also SEXUAL RESPONSE). Their goal is to reduce anxiety and increase pleasure, in place of feeling that one must live up to some mythical standard of 'performance'. This approach appears to work well both for women unable to achieve orgasm and for men who cannot achieve or sustain an erection (see FRIGIDITY; IMPOTENCE). For sexual problems that have deeper emotional origins, therapists tend to use a psychosexual approach, which combines behavioural tasks with psychodynamic exploration.

A couple who have difficulty with sex can seek counsel from a family doctor, gynaecologist, or psychotherapist. Sex therapy as such is still a very new field, and as the work of Masters and Johnson, Helen Singer Kaplan, and other researchers became known, numerous individuals particularly in the United States, some well qualified and others totally unqualified, set themselves up in practice. Its very nature makes sex therapy readily open to abuse by unscrupulous and/or unqualified practitioners. Reputable therapists never engage in sexual relations or exercises of any kind *with* their clients, nor do they urge clients to engage in practices that might seem morally questionable (for example, wife swapping, group sex, surrogate therapy, or indiscrimate choice of many partners).

Sexual dysfunction A disturbance or disorder that frequently or always prevents an individual from engaging in satisfactory sexual intercourse. Such dysfunctions may arise anywhere in the cycle of desire-arousal-orgasm (see also SEXUAL RESPONSE). A disorder of the desire phase is often described as a man's or woman's low LIBIDO, that is, lack of interest or desire in experiencing sexual relations. Disturbances of the arousal phase in a man result in difficulty in achieving and/or maintaining an erection (see also IMPOTENCE); in women it results in difficulty in becoming excited and achieving vaginal lubrication during sexual activity. Disorders of the orgasm phase include premature or retarded ejaculation in men (see EJACULATION) and failure to reach ORGASM in women. Another female sexual dysfunction is VAGINISMUS, making penile penetration difficult and painful, but this condition is much rarer than the other dysfunctions. The most common condition, experienced by an estimated 30 to 60 per cent of women – understandably statistics in this area are not very accurate – is failure to reach orgasm during vaginal intercourse, although they can experience orgasm with a partner by other means. The second most common problem is failure to reach orgasm with a partner although they can achieve it with masturbation. Only about 9 per cent of women are pre-orgastic, that is, have never experienced orgasm (see also FRIGIDITY). The most common dysfunction in men is premature ejaculation, experienced by about 25 per cent. See also SEX THERAPY.

Sexually transmitted disease Also *STD*. See VENEREAL DISEASE.

Sexual response A biochemical and physiological process that occurs in both men and women after puberty. Although it presumably has been experienced by countless human beings since human life began on earth, it was not clinically analyzed until the late 19th century, beginning with the work of Henry Havelock Ellis (1859–1939) and Sigmund Freud (1856–1939). Great strides were made in the 1940s and 1950s by Alfred C. Kinsey and his associates, and in the 19560s by William Masters and Virginia Johnson. It was Masters and Johnson who actually observed many of the couples they studied under laboratory conditions, and who discovered that sexual response is divided into four phases: excitement, plateau, ORGASM, and resolution. There is no real break as a person passes from one phase to another, and each phase varies in duration from occasion to occasion. The same sequence occurs in both men and women, no matter whether they are masturbating or engaging in homosexual or heterosexual relations. There is, however, a considerable difference between men and women in the time it takes to reach orgasm. The average man, proceeding without interruption, ejaculates within three minutes, whereas the average woman, proceeding at her normal pace, takes about fifteen minutes to reach orgasm.

The *excitement phase* can be activated by an enormous variety of stimuli – pictures, sounds, colours, music, smells, thoughts, daydreams – all of which can trigger sexual arousal. Direct touching of breasts, nipples, thighs, and genitals can be exciting both for the person doing it and the one being touched. The body responds in a variety of ways. Both the heart rate and breathing increase. The skin may flush. The breasts enlarge, and the nipples become erect. Both women and men experience genital vasocongestion (the dilatation of arteries in the genital area), causing an ERECTION.

In women the first physical response is usually the secretion of a lubricating fluid by the vaginal lining, which after a few minutes is felt as wetness near the vaginal entrance. The uterus moves upward into the pelvis, in effect lengthening the vagina. In men the penis becomes hard and stiff (erection);

As sexual stimulation continues, the *plateau phase* follows. Here vasocongestion gradually reaches its peak in both men and women. Heart and breathing rates increase still more. Muscle contraction and congestion in the pelvis increase. The CLITORIS becomes very sensitive and retracts (draws back) under its hood. Stimulation of the inner LABIA causes stimulation of the clitoris, by moving the hood back and forth over it. The vaginal opening swells, making the actual opening smaller; when the penis finally enters the vagina this provides a gripping sensation for it. In men the testes become engorged and draw back up to the base of the penis.

The plateau phase finally reaches a peak, resulting in *orgasm*, a sudden, almost seizure-like release of muscle tension and congestion. The muscles of the vaginal opening contract and relax in a rhythmic fashion; in men contractions of the seminal vesicles and prostrate gland push the semen into the urethra, where the muscles of the penis forcefully expel it. (See also ORGASM.)

Orgasm is followed by *resolution*. The blood flow is released and the erect tissues lose their stiffness. If there is no further stimulation the congestion subsides and the body gradually returns to its unaroused state. Men return to a low level of sexual tension rather quickly. A woman, however, can respond to continued sexual stimulation immediately and have another orgasm soon afterward, whereas a man requires a period for recovery – the refractory period – ranging from a few minutes to hours, depending on the individual and his age. Moreover, women can continue to have orgasm after orgasm. Resolution is accompanied by a sense of relaxation and satisfaction, of general well-being.

The physical changes of sexual response are controlled by the autonomic nervous system and involve involuntary muscles. However, mental processes under conscious control (thoughts, fantasies, feelings) also play a role, making a person receptive to the sexual stimulation that will set the sequence of response in motion. Moreover, this sequence, once begun, is not inevitable; it can be interrupted at almost any point (by a telephone call, a negative thought such as fear of pregnancy, etc.), so that arousal subsides. Practically the only point of no return is just before ejaculation for the man; once the seminal vesicles and prostate gland propel semen into the urethra, ejaculation cannot be delayed.

Sheehan's disease Necrosis (tissue death) of the anterior lobe of the pituitary gland following a very difficult labour or delivery, involving postpartum haemorrhage and/or shock. It is named after H. L. Sheehan, the doctor who first described it. The earliest symptoms are failure to lactate (produce breast milk) and subsequent amenorrhoea (no resumption of menstruation). Other signs are shrinking of vaginal tissue and weight gain. Progressively the patient loses her pubic and axillary hair, and then begins to lose weight markedly. Undiagnosed, the disease can end in death. The principal treatment is replacement of needed hormones. In mild cases the patient may sometimes become pregnant again, which occasionally results in considerable improvement; a pregnancy apparently stimulates the pituitary gland to grow and function better.

Shoulder presentation In childbirth, the position of the baby when one of its shoulders is the presenting part, that is, the part that leads the baby's descent into the birth canal. It occurs when the baby lies in *transverse position*, crosswise in the uterus. Shoulder presentation occurs in approximately 1 of every 200 deliveries. The diagnosis is readily made, often just by looking at the mother's abdomen, which appears very wide from side to side. In the course of labour one shoulder generally becomes tightly wedged in the pelvic canal, and often the hand and arm prolapse through the vagina.

Sickle cell disease A group of genetic disorders that affect primarily blacks, both men and women, and pose particular health problems for women. They include *sickle cell anaemia, sickle C disease*, and *sickle thalassaemia*, and they are associated with resistance to malaria, a disease long endemic in those parts of the world where sickle cell disease is most common. Sickle cell anaemia is characterized by the presence of red blood cells that are sickled (or crescent-shaped) so that they are unable to pass through small arterioles and capillaries (small blood vessels). Accumulations of sickled red blood cells lead to the formation of thrombi (blood clots) and infarcts (tissue that dies because not enough oxygen has reached it). Those sickled cells that can flow through the circulatory system are more fragile than normal red blood cells and break down easily, causing severe anaemia. The main symptoms of sickle cell anaemia are extremely painful joints, episodes of acute abdominal pain, and ulceration in the lower extremities (legs). The disease usually appears during a baby's first year and is progressive. No cure is yet known, and victims rarely survive beyond the age of forty (many die earlier).

Sickle cell anaemia is a recessive gene disease, that is, a person must have two genes for sickle cell anaemia in order to contract the disease. A couple who both have the sickle cell trait (have one gene for the disease) therefore have a 25 per cent change of producing a child with sickle cell anaemia. For this reason it is highly advisable for all blacks—men and women—to be tested for sickle cell trait (by means of a simple blood test). Furthermore, women who have sickle cell disease should never take oral contraceptives, which seem to accelerate their already existing predisposition to form blood clots. They should also never undergo a saline abortion (see under AMNIOINFUSION).

Pregnancy is a serious burden for women with sickle cell anaemia. Usually the anaemia becomes worse, and the attacks of pain more frequent. Infections and pulmonary (lung) disease are more apt to develop. One-third to one-half of babies conceived by women with the disease die in miscarriage, stillbirth, or soon after birth. The greatest danger to the mother is from blood clots, which often occur in the lungs and can be fatal. Even though extreme caution and intensive care may save both mother and baby, most authorities feel that pregnancy in most cases should be avoided, either with stringent birth control measure or sterilization. At the least, tests for sickle cell trait should be carried out, and GENETIC COUNSELLING undertaken if the trait is present. If a woman should become pregnant, AMNIOCENTESIS can reveal if her baby will have sickle cell disease. Another reliable but also more dangerous (to the foetus) procedure for detecting sickle cell disease is FOETOSCOPY.

Side effect An effect of a medication or medical procedure other than the one for which it was intended. For example, antihistamines – drugs widely used to control allergy – often have the side effect of making one drowsy or sleepy. The severity of some side effects may be such that other drugs must be substituted or all medication must be discontinued.

Sign Objective evidence of a disease or disorder, such as fever, discoloration or swelling, or the secretion of pus, which can be seen and/or measured by the doctor. See also SYMPTOM.

Silicone implant See under MAMMA-PLASTY.

Silver nitrate A metal compound that, in a very dilute solution, is used as a topical antiseptic (to destroy infection-causing organisms). Among its older uses were treating cervicitis, where it has been largely replaced by cauterization or cryo-surgery, and in treating the eyes of new-born infants to prevent a potentially blinding gonorrhoea eye infection; in the latter it must be very carefully rinsed out lest it cause conjunctivitis. Its principal other use is preventing infections resulting from severe burns.

Sims-Huhner test Also *post-coital test*. Examination of the cervical mucus to determine whether or not it is receptive to sperm. Usually this test is performed only when a couple are having trouble with conception (see INFERTILITY). The test is performed at the expected time of ovulation – some doctors say just before that time – and the woman is asked to come to the clinic within two to fifteen hours after intercourse.

Sims position Also *left lateral position*. Lying on the left side during labour, rather than on one's back. This avoids compression of a large vein (the *vena cava*) when the uterine muscles contract, thereby allowing more oxygen to reach the baby. It is also more comfortable when a woman has BACK LABOUR.

Sitz bath A bath filled to a level of six inches or so with warm water, which is used for soaking. Sitting in a sitz bath for fifteen minutes several times a day is a simple and often effective treatment for irritations affecting the genital area, among them cystitis, vaginitis, and proctitis. Warm water increases circulation to the affected parts and promotes healing. Some women use HERBAL REMEDIES in the bath water, ginger root (*Zingiber* *officinale*) to allay itching, and comfrey (*Symphytum officinale*) to promote healing.

Skene's glands Also *Skene's ducts, paraurethral ducts*. A pair of glands that run below and parallel to the female URETHRA, opening just below the outer part of the urethral opening. Their function, if any, is not known; some authorities believe they are the female counterpart of the male prostate gland. Their chief importance is the fact that they often harbour the organism causing GONORRHOEA, which may be impossible to eradicate without removing these glands. In addition, Skene's glands occasionally become infected with other organisms and develop cysts.

Skin cancer See CANCER, VULVAR; MELANOMA.

Skin changes Alterations in skin texture, pigmentation, and general health that are caused by changes in hormone balance and diet. During puberty many adolescents develop ACNE as a result of increasing androgen (male hormone) levels. For this reason acne is more common and more severe in boys than girls. During the reproductive years, either pregnancy or use of oral contraceptives, which both involve higher levels of oestrogen, can cause changes in pigmentation, such as the giant freckles of CHLOASMA or darkening of the nipples and abdominal midline in PREGNANCY. Oral contraceptives containing a considerable amount of progesterone may cause rashes and/or acne in some women.

During middle age and after menopause, women's skin becomes thinner and loses some of its flexibility and elasticity. The outermost layer of skin, the epidermis, is made up of cells that are constantly being renewed, but with age the renewal process slows down. By the time new skin cells are pushed up toward the surface they have dried and flattened out. Also, the oil and sweat glands tend to function less vigorously, which can create dry skin, sometimes causing itching and discomfort, as well as making wrinkles and lines more visible. There may also be a change in pigmentation (see LIVER SPOTS), another result of slowed-down cell renewal. Regular use of skin moisturizers and oils, avoiding very dry environments (using humidifiers or placing pans of water in heated or air-conditioned surroundings), avoiding overuse of soap, and occasionally taking a steam bath all help make drying skin look smoother and feel better. Currently researchers are experimenting with substances that speed up skin cell renewal, such as low concentration of vitamin A acid.

For skin cancer, see CANCER, VULVAR; MELANOMA.

Sleeping pills See under INSOMNIA.

Smear test See under PAP SMEAR.

Smegma A cheesy secretion of certain sebaceous (oil) glands, especially those under the PREPUCE of the penis and clitoris. Accumulated smegma needs to be washed away regularly, particularly in uncircumcised men, as it can be a source of irritation and/or harbour infection-causing bacteria.

Smoking, tobacco The habitual use of tobacco in cigars and cigarettes, an acknowledged health hazard, and especially so to women. Smokers who take ORAL CONTRACEPTIVES are at much greater risk of developing heart attacks and stroke than non-smokers, especially after the age of thirty. The rate of MIS-CARRIAGE among smokers is higher, too. Cigarette smoking during pregnancy poses dangers to the unborn child. The baby's birth weight on average will be somewhat lower than normal, and the mother has a higher risk of developing hypertension (high blood pressure). Smoking may be linked with other birth defects as well, since nicotine makes the blood vessels constrict, thereby preventing some of the blood-borne oxygen and nutrients from reaching the foetus. Nicotine is also passed on to the baby through the milk of a woman who is breast-feeding. Finally, women smokers are as much at risk as men for higher than normal incidence of emphysema, bronchitis, gum disease, and cancer of the lungs, larynx, oral cavity, and oesophagus (for these cancers smoking is considered the major cause). Also, the cancer risks are even higher if heavy smoking is associated with heavy ALCOHOL USE. Smoking is further considered a contributory factor to cancers of the bladder, kidneys, and pancreas.

Sound An instrument used to determine the length of the uterus prior to inserting an INTRAUTERINE DEVICE, performing an endometrial BIOPSY (see definition 8), or some other procedure. The uterus of a non-pregnant woman usually sounds to a depth of 6 to 8 centimetres (2 to 4 inches).

Speculum *specula* (pl.). A two-bladed metal or plastic instrument used to examine the inside of the vagina and the cervix. Inserted in the vagina with the blades closed, it is rotated to the proper position and the blades then are opened and locked in place. The blades serve to hold the walls of vagina apart (they are normally so close together they virtually touch) so that the doctor can examine both them and the cervix. For performing a PAP SMEAR a narrow spatula and then a cotton swab are inserted between the blades of the speculum to scrape surface cells from the cervix. The speculum is used for most other biopsy and vacuum curettage to vaginal hysterectomy. Specula come in a number of sizes, including a size for infants. See also under GYNAECO-LOGICAL EXAMINATION.

Sperm Also *spermatozoan* (*spermatozoa* pl.). The male reproductive cell in all animals that reproduce sexually, including human beings. *Spermatogenesis*, the production of sperm, begins at puberty. Stimulated by FSH and LH, the same pituitary hormones that cause the production of ova (eggs) in women, sperm production takes place in the testes, or male sex glands. The original sperm cells, or *spermatogonia*, take at least two months to develop before they are ejaculated as mature sperm.

A single sperm is a tiny wormlike creature, with an oval head that contains the chromosomes and a long tail whose movements enable it to move forward. From tip to tail it is about $\frac{1}{600}$ ($\frac{7}{100}$ millimetre) long, and 90 per cent of that length is the tail. The size, shape, motility, and number of sperm all affect fertility, that is, the ability to fertilize (mate with) an egg.

When a man reaches ORGASM, the pelvic muscles expel the sperm from its storage place and it is propelled, along with gland secretions (seminal fluid), through the urethra and out through the opening at the end of the penis (see PENIS for a more precise description). Each time this event, called EJACULATION, takes place, as many as 400 million sperm may be set in motion; the average *ejaculate* contains 2 to 5 millilitres of fluid, with a mean of 40 to 80 million sperm per millilitre. Most of the sperm die within a few hours; only a few reach the Fallopian tubes, where they may survive twenty-four to forty-eight hours longer. Total survival time of sperm in the female genital tract is thought to be about ninety-six hours, or four days.

For couples having trouble conceiving, one of the first tests performed in a *semen analysis* to determine if enough normal sperm are being ejaculated.

Occasionally a woman develops antibodies against her partner's sperm, in the same way the body develops antibodies against infectious organisms. Such antibodies appear in the cervical mucus, attach themselves to the sperm, and prevent them from moving up into the uterus and tubes. Since normal vaginal secretions are too acid for the alkaline-loving sperm, they soon die there. Antibody development can be a cause of infertility. For couples who want a child, one solution may be for the man to use a CONDOM for a number of months. Without the stimulation of live sperm, antibody production gradually diminishes and the levels of antibodies drop. Conception may then be possible. A blood test, called Duke's test, can determine if antibodies are being produced.

Sperm bank A storage place for frozen SPERM, to be used eventually for ARTIFICIAL INSEMINATION. For men who do not produce enough sperm at one time for successfully fertilizing an egg, one solution may be to pool numerous samples of semen and use this concentrated quantity to achieve conception. Since sperm cannot survive for more than a few hours under ordinary conditions, they are frozen. However, even in normal seminal fluid only one-quarter to one-half of the sperm may be motile (capable of moving) when they are thawed, and sperm from infertile men are even more easily damaged by freezing (sometimes no motile sperm at all can be recovered). For this reason successful artificial insemination may require a donor who can provide a fresh semen specimen. Sometimes frozen sperm from the husband are combined with fresh donor sperm to provide a mixed specimen.

Spermicide A chemical substance used to kill live sperm inside the vagina for purpose of BIRTH CONTROL. The most common forms are *spermicidal jelly* and *cream*, which are recommended for use with a DIAPHRAGM or CERVICAL CAP but sometimes are used alone, and *spermicidal foam*, *foaming tablets*, and *suppositories*, generally used alone. Each of these chemical contraceptives contains two components, a relatively inert carrier base and an active spermicidal agent (usually nonylphenoxypolyethoxyethol). They operate both mechanically, by forming a barrier (a film or coating) over the cervix to delay the movement of sperm, and biochemically, by immobilizing and destroying the sperm they have blocked. The active ingredient in them remains active for six to eight hours.

Creams and *jellies* used alone are not as effective as foam alone and have a high failure rate. Used with a diaphragm, they are more effective than foam alone. Nevertheless, creams and jellies are commonly sold with a plastic applicator to insert them into the vagina either alone or as a supplement after a diaphragm is already in place (for second intercourse, or because it was inserted more than two hours before intercourse). If the cream or jelly is used alone, it should be inserted no earlier than fifteen minutes before intercourse, with an initial application of *two* full applicators; one additional full applicator should be used for each additional act of intercourse. The stronger, more effective of the creams and jellies tend also to be more irritating, to both vaginal tissue and the penis, than weaker ones.

Foam is a white aerated cream with the consistency of shaving cream. It is generally sold in a can with a plunger-type plastic applicator. Deposited deep inside the vagina, near the cervix, no earlier than fifteen minutes before intercourse, it is more effective than either cream or jelly alone but is recommended for use only when the male partner is also using a CONDOM. (Alone it is only 70 to 90 per cent effective.) The can should be thoroughly shaken before use (a total of twenty times is recommended) and the applicator inserted into the vagina as deep as possible. The applicator should be thoroughly washed (but not boiled) after use.

Foam also comes in the form of a *vaginal suppository* or *tablet* which, after it is inserted, dissolves and releases the foam. It is approximately as effective as the aerosol foams and therefore should be used with a condom. However, it does not become effective for ten or fifteen minutes after insertion (the time it takes to melt and release foam), which may be a drawback.

All these kinds of spermicide are available in chemists without prescription. Until the late 1970s few brands bore an indication of their *shelf life* (that is, how long the ingredients remain active), which appears to be about two years. It is preferable to buy such products with a clearly marked expiration date on the package, which today is supplied by some, but not all, manufacturers. Most spermicidal jellies, creams, and foams have been found to be effective against the organisms that cause gonorrhoea, syphilis, trichomonas, and yeast infections, but the protection they give depends considerably on the care and meticulousness with which they are used.

Sphincter   A ringlike muscle that, when contracted, closes a natural opening or passage. Such muscles are particularly important in controlling the passage of urine (*urinary sphincter*) – there is one at the upper and the lower ends of the urethra – and of faeces (*anal sphincter*), as well as in the bile duct, iris of the eye, and elsewhere.

Spina bifida   Also *spina bifida operta*, *cleft spine*. A BIRTH DEFECT in which one or more individual vertebrae fail to close completely. As a result, a sac containing part of the contents of the spinal cord may protrude through the opening, which is usually at the lower end of the cord; it is called a *meningomyelocele*. Muscles and nerves in the legs and lower trunk are often affected. Symptoms are usually present at birth, although they may in some cases develop much later, during the rapid growth spurt of puberty. Among the symptoms are muscle weakness or paralysis, partial or total loss of bladder and bowel control, and, in some cases, other deformities resulting from weak muscles. Treatment for the condition depends on its severity; in some cases it is so severe, with the spine virtually completely open, that survival is impossible. In others it may be so mild that there are few obvious signs.

Spina bifida and similar open spinal defects are called *neural tube defects*. They result from a failure of development in the neural tube, which is the embryonic forerunner of the central nervous system, and they occur in nearly 2 in every 1,000 pregnancies. Since spina bifida occurs more often in children of parents with this condition, it is advisable for patients to seek GENETIC COUNSELLING before undertaking parenthood. The defect can be detected by means of AMNIOCENTESIS, but only in the case of open lesions.

Women with spina bifida face some special problems. During sexual activity, they may have increased risk of urinary and bowel incontinence during arousal. Genital sensation may be limited or totally absent, and deformities, weakness, or paralysis may interfere with intercourse in certain positions. Menstruation and fertility are not affected. Oral contraceptives are contraindicated if there are circulatory problems, and a diaphragm or intrauterine device (IUD) may be difficult to insert if there is pelvic deformity. Pregnancy not only raises the question of passing the defect on to a baby but may, during its course, aggravate back problems, incontinence, and urinary tract infections.

The results of a recent large-scale study in Great Britain indicate that the incidence of spina bifida and other neural tube defects may be greatly reduced by routinely administering vitamin supplements containing folic acid to women who are attempting to conceive.

Spinal anaesthesia Also *saddle block anaesthesia, low subarachnoid block*. A kind of REGIONAL ANAESTHESIA that is ad-ministered late in labour, as well as being used for lower abdominal surgery of various kinds. It involves injecting a local anaesthetic directly into the spinal cord through the fourth lumbar interspace, with the result that all feeling is blocked in the pelvic area (corresponding to the parts of the body in contact with a saddle, hence 'saddle block') and also the legs. In effect the woman loses all sensation from the waist down.

Spinnbarkeit See under CERVICAL MUCUS METHOD.

Split ejaculation See under OLIGO-SPERMIA.

Sponge See CONTRACEPTIVE SPONGE.

Spotting See BREAKTHROUGH BLEEDING.

Staging A procedure in which the extent of a progressive disease, usually cancer, is determined by means of diagnostic tests (X-ray, blood tests, body scans, urinalysis, etc.). In breast cancer these tests are undertaken after biopsy or mastectomy to ascertain the spread of malignancy beyond the breast.

Staining See BREAKTHROUGH BLEEDING.

STD Abbreviation for sexually transmitted disease; see VENEREAL DISEASE.

Stein-Leventhal syndrome Also *polycystic ovaries*. A condition in which both ovaries are studded with numerous small cysts, which are actually egg follicles from which the eggs cannot, for some reason, be extruded. The eggs therefore collect under the follicle capsules, making them look like small cysts. Women with this condition do not ovulate, since no eggs are released, and hence are infertile. They also menstruate irregularly or not at all, show mild or marked hirsutism (excess body and facial hair), and are often obese. The syndrome is suspected if these symptoms are present and both ovaries are enlarged. However, a conclusive diagnosis requires either CULDOSCOPY or LAPAROSCOPY.

The Stein-Leventhal syndrome, named after Irving Stein and Michael Leventhal, the doctors who first described it in 1935, is caused by a hormone imbalance, specifically an excess of male hormones produced by the adrenal glands and by the capsule that forms over the ovary. It is treated with doses of cortisone by-products given orally, or with a combination of progesterone and oestrogen. If these drugs are not effective, a surgical procedure, called *bilateral wedge resection*, can be performed, in which a wedge of the affected tissue is cut from each ovary; this procedure corrects the condition in most cases.

Sterility The condition of a man who produces very few or no SPERM, so that he cannot cause conception in a woman, or a woman who either produces no ova (eggs) or has no uterus in which a fertilized egg can grow. They are then said to be *sterile*.

See also INFERTILITY.

Sterilization Rendering a person sterile, that is, incapable of reproduction. It may result from an accident, such as over-exposure to radioactivity, be the by-product of surgery performed as treatment for some disorder, or result from a procedure performed for that very purpose, that is, a form of BIRTH CONTROL.

In women sterilization results from a HYSTERECTOMY (removal of the uterus) performed for any reason whatever (although hysterectomies commonly were, and sometimes still are, performed solely to achieve sterility).

The principal form of sterilization for birth control in women is TUBAL LIGATION, which prevents the passage of an egg through the Fallopian tubes. In men, it is VASECTOMY which prevents the passage of sperm through the vas deferens. Two other, more experimental, forms of sterilization for men are THERMATIC STERILIZATION and ULTRA-SOUND (definition 2). Vasectomy is considerably safer and simpler than any form of tubal ligation, but it does not guarantee sterility until *all* stored sperm have been ejaculated. Three negative sperm counts obtained at monthly intervals are required before one can be sure. Neither tubal ligation nor vasectomy is readily or reliably reversible, so neither procedure should be undertaken by anyone unless he or she is quite certain of not wanting any (more) children.

Steroid A hormone derived from cholesterol; see under HORMONE.

Stillbirth The delivery of a dead baby. The term is usually reserved for a foetus that is fairly close to term, that is, of twenty-eight weeks' gestation or more. See also MISCARRIAGE, definition 5; PREMATURE.

Stress incontinence Also *urinary stress incontinence* . Involuntary release of urine as a result of coughing, sneezing, laughing, or some other action that increases abdominal pressure on the bladder. It is caused by pelvic relaxation, that is, weakening of the pelvic-floor muscles, especially the pubococcygeous muscle, which often occurs after childbirth (long labour, rapid delivery, large babies, many pregnancies) or, occasionally, from strenuous physical activity. Normally the healthy pubococcygeous muscle encircles the urethra close to where it joins the bladder; it also surrounds and supports the middle third of the vagina, and encompasses the rectum just above the anal opening. When this muscle is weakened, the urethra, bladder, rectum, and uterus – any or all of these organs – may bulge into the vagina and the bladder fails to remain closed when additional pressure is placed on it, causing urine to leak. Mild stress incontinence is often relieved by KEGEL EXERCISES, which help strengthen the muscle. More severe and chronic stress incontinence may require surgery to correct it. See also URETHROCELE, CYSTO-CELE; RECTOCELE; PROLAPSED UTERUS.

Stretch marks   See STRAIE.

Striae   Also *stretch marks*. Pinkish streaks that appear on the abdomen and breasts, and sometimes also on the thighs and buttocks, in the late months of pregnancy. They are not pigment changes but result from decreased elasticity of the skin stretched over the growing uterus and enlarged breasts. At first pale pink and sometimes itchy, they later become white and look like very faint scars. Once they appear, they usually remain for life, although they become much fainter after delivery. About half of pregnant women develop striae.

Stroke   See CEREBRAL VASCULAR ACCIDENT.

Subcutaneous   Under the skin and, therefore, not very deep-lying. For sub-cutaneous mastectomy, see MASTEC-TOMY, definition 8.

Suction   See VACUUM ASPIRATION; for suction by needle, or needle aspiration, see BIOPSY, definition 3.

Suicide   Taking one's own life. In Britain it is estimated that women attempt to commit suicide two or three times more often than men, but more men than women actually succeed in killing themselves. The peak age for suicide in women is fifty-five to sixty-five. The most common cause of suicide is DEPRESSION, precipitated by marital or family strife, especially among the young, and by bereavement and physical disability, especially among the elderly. Threats to commit suicide, even if they seem to be an obvious bid for attention or an attempt to manipulate others, should never be ignored because they are often carried out. Crisis centres for potential suicides, which anyone can telephone anonymously for counselling and help, exist all over Britain; they are listed in telephone directories under 'Samaritans'.

Superfecundation   The fertilization of two eggs within a short period of time (during the same menstrual cycle) but not during the same act of sexual intercourse, resulting in the conception of fraternal twins or some other form of MULTIPLE PREGNANCY.

Superfoetation   Fertilization of two eggs during two successive ovulatory cycles, resulting in MULTIPLE PREGNANCY and birth. It is well recognized in horses and other animals, and is believed to occur in human beings as well, although it has never been verified. It requires the occurrence of ovulation during the course of (the first) pregnancy.

Suppository A medication in the form of a small, solid, bullet-shaped mass that melts readily and is administered by insertion into the vagina or rectum. Suppositories are used for administering medication for local vaginal infections. Some kinds of SPERMICIDE for birth control come in suppository form, but they are considered less reliable than jelly or foam because they do not always melt enough, or in time, for release of the active contraceptive agent. Suppositories made of glycerin and sodium stereate are commonly used to relieve temporary constipation by slightly irritating the mucous membrane of the rectum.

Surgery, unnecessary Treatment of illness, injury, or deformity by manual and/or instrumental operations that are not needed in the first place. In some countries where there is a financial incentive for the surgeon to operate consumer groups and others estimate that up to 30 per cent of surgery performed is unnecessary. Even in countries, such as Britain, with a national health service some operations may be unnecessary. Operations sometimes performed unjustifiably include HYSTERECTOMY (removal of the uterus), haemorrhoidectomy (removal of a HAEMORRHOID), tonsillectomy (removal of the tonsils) and CAESARIAN SECTION

Surgical Procedures

Classification	Examples
Emergency (immediate surgery required)	Fractured skull, certain stab or gunshot wounds, extensive burns, urinary obstruction, intestinal obstruction, ruptured appendix or Fallopian tube.
Urgent (prompt surgery required, within 24 to 48 hours)	Kidney stone, stomach obstruction, abdominal ulcer, bleeding haemorrhoid, twisted ovarian cyst, ectopic pregnancy
Required (surgery within a few weeks or months)	Cataract, spinal fusion, sinus operation, repair of heart or blood vessel defect, removal of very large fibroid
Elective (surgery should be done but no serious problem if it is not)	Simple haemorrhoids, superficial cyst, non-invasive fatty or fibrous tumour, burn scar repair
Optimal (surgery advisable but not essential)	Strabismus repair, breast reconstruction, varicose vein stripping, warm removal
Cosmetic (surgery only to improve appearance)	Removal of acne scars, nose reconstruction, breast augmentation, face lift

(surgical delivery of the baby). All operations have risks and benefits so the decision to offer surgery is made after taking these into consideration. Sometimes there are differences of opinion as to the relative risks or benefits so that surgeons may not always agree as to whether surgery is necessary. It is important that the patient is aware of the possible risks as well as the advantages of undergoing surgery. Remember that the decision to undergo surgery is yours; listen to expert opinion, get as much information as possible, but make up your own mind as to whether or not to go ahead.

Symptom Strictly speaking, subjective evidence of a disease or disorder, which is felt by the patient rather than seen by the doctor. Examples include dizziness, fatigue, and pain. However, the term is often loosely used as a synonym for SIGN. See also SYNDROME.

Syndrome A group of symptoms and/or signs that typically occur together in a particular disease or disorder. For example, numbness or paralysis on one side, dizziness, and difficulty in speaking constitute the principal symptoms of a cerebral vascular accident, or stroke, and so are sometimes called 'stroke syndrome'.

Syntocinon A brand name for synthetic OXYTOCIN, used to strengthen uterine contractions.

Syphilis Also *bad blood, lues, pox*. A VENEREAL DISEASE transmitted by sexual intercourse (vaginal, anal, oral) and caused by a microscopic organism, *Treponema pallidum*. The same organism,

a spirochete that burrows through tiny breaks in the skin and mucous membranes, also causes yaws (a skin disease), endemmic syphilis, and pinta, three disorders that occur mostly in tropical countries. Venereal syphilis, which can be fatal, is transmitted primarily by sexual contact but can also be incurred if fluid from a syphilitis sore or rash gets inside a cut on another person's skin, or by a foetus inside the womb of an infected mother. The disease has three stages: *early* (subdivided into *primary* and *secondary*), *latent*, and *late* or *tertiary*. During the primary stage a *chancre*, a painless ulcerating sore, appears at the point where the organism entered the body, in men usually on the penis and in women on the cervix or inner vaginal walls. It appears ten to ninety days (three weeks, on average) after the infectious contact and normally disappears in one to five weeks without treatment. There may also be, at the same time, painless hard swelling of the surrounding lymph nodes, especially in men. It, too, may disappear spontaneously.

The secondary stage, beginning about six weeks after the chancre appears, is characterized by a generalized non-itchy rash occurring anywhere from the scalp to the soles of the feet. There may also be flu-like symptoms such as sore throat and hoarseness, caused by rash inside the throat, occasional bone and joint pain, patchy loss of scalp hair, and eye inflammation. After some months these symptoms disappear, even without treatment, and the disease enters its latent stage, when it is detectable only by a blood test.

During the primary and secondary stages syphilis is highly infectious (catching), but during the latent stage only the foetus of an infected mother can be infected. The latent stage may last ten to fifteen years. In about one-third of cases the disease then proceeds to the tertiary or late stage, in which it attacks the heart, blood vessels, brain, spinal cord, or bone. Heart disease, blindness, loss of muscle co-ordination, deafness, paralysis, insanity, or death may result.

Congenital syphilis is acquired by an unborn baby from its mother. Pregnancy masks syphilis symptoms, making them even more dangerous. Though primary chancres in a pregnant woman may be larger than otherwise, the skin rash of secondary syphilis may be scarcely visible. The syphilis organisms travel from mother to foetus via the placenta. The placenta is not well enough developed for this transfer until sixteen to eighteen weeks into the pregnancy, so a syphilis infection detected and treated *before* the fourth month of pregnancy will not usually harm the baby. The more recent the infection in the mother, the more likely it is that the baby will be infected, and the more severe its symptoms. Almost all babies born to women with untreated primary or secondary syphilis develop the disease, and many die either before or soon after birth. However, infants born to women with latent syphilis may either escape infection or develop a case of syphilis that is not immediately life-threatening. All pregnant women in Britain must have a blood test for syphilis.

It was formerly believed that syphilis was introduced to Europe by Christopher Columbus and his crew when they returned to Spain from Haiti in 1493. In the early 1500s Europe was struck by an epidemic of syphilis, which was called the Great Pox to distinguish it from smallpox. Sceptics, however, have long questioned the fact that so few men could have started an epidemic of such size. Furthermore, there are descriptions in ancient Chinese, Hebrew, Indian, and Greek writings of a disease closely resembling syphilis, and prehistoric bones also reveal the scars of such a disorder. Further evidence suggests that other forms of syphilis, specifically yaws (which affects mainly the skin of children in moist tropical lands) and endemic syphilis, affecting the mouth, nostrils, anus, underarms, and other moist body areas in persons living in hot but some-what drier areas (in North Africa and Asia), develop in different environments. As cities grew, endemic syphilis gave way as even the very primitive sanitary facilities developed. The Treponema organism needs a perpetually moist environment to survive. In temperate climates the genital tract was the only area that continued to provide this environment, and that, along with the embarrassment, shame, and ignorance surrounding sexual relations until the most recent times, helped perpetuate the venereal form of the disease.

Systemic Bodywide, that is, not localized or limited to some particular part of the body or some particular organ. Most of the common childhood disease, such as measles and chicken pox, are systemic infections (see INFECTION), and some authorities view cancer – at least some forms of it – as a systemic disease.

Systemic lupus erythematosus Also *lupus*, *SLE*. An inflammatory disorder of the body's immune system that affects the connective tissue in numerous parts of the body and afflicts approximately 1 in every 2,000 British women (and only one-tenth as many men). It is two to three times more common in black women than in whites, and its onset occurs most often between the ages of twenty and forty. The disease is named after one of its signs, a rash in the shape of a 'butterfly' over the nose and cheeks, similar to the facial markings of a wolf (*lupus erythematosus* is Latin for 'red wolf'). However, the disease affects not only the skin but also, in different individuals and at different times, all the collagen tissues, including the joints, blood vessels, heart, lungs, brain, and, most dangerously, the kidneys. Formerly thought to be an auto-immune disease, systemic lupus is now generally described as an 'immune complex' disease, in which the patient's antibodies combine with antigens, either foreign or the patient's own, to form complexes that mediate tissue damage. There is a genetic predisposition to the development of systemic lupus, shown by the fact that if one of two identical twins gets the disorder the other twin has a 50 to 60 per cent chance of developing it, too, whereas with fraternal twins the second twin has only a 2 to 3 per cent risk.

T

Tail of Spence An extension of breast tissue toward the axilla (armpit); see BREAST.

Tampon An internally worn device of absorbent material intended to soak up menstrual flow. It comes in sizes small enough to permit insertion by most young girls, the HYMEN as a rule stretching enough to accommodate it. In efforts to improve their product and gain a larger share of the market, manufacturers have embellished tampons with various kinds of perfume to mask 'natural' odours, various kinds of applicator to make insertion easier, and various sizes and thicknesses to absorb menstrual flow ranging from light to very heavy. Occasionally their efforts have gone astray and their product has become so absorbent, for example, that it is difficult to remove because it expands so much when wet. Also, some women experience considerable vaginal irritation from some kinds of tampon.

In 1980 the use of tampons was linked to the occurrence of a rare but potentially dangerous disease called *toxic shock syndrome*, which affected primarily young women. It is characterized by very rapid onset, and symptoms include high fever, vomiting, diarrhoea, dizziness, a sunburnlike rash with peeling (especially on the hands and feet), and a rapid drop in blood pressure, frequently resulting in shock. Most cases seemed to occur in women under the age of twenty-five and to begin during a menstrual period. It is not known exactly how tampons could cause the disease, or even if they actually do – the syndrome occurs also in post-operative patients, burn victims, women who have just given birth, and men or women with boils or abscesses, who together account for 13 per cent of reported cases. However, it is believed that some or all kinds of tampons might harbour or encourage the growth of a bacterium, *Staphylococcus aureus*, in the vagina, and that this organism is responsible for the syndrome. Also, tampons might cause irritation and breakdown of vaginal tissue, thus permitting bacteria to enter the bloodstream. As a result of publicity, one brand of tampons, Rely, was withdrawn from the US market by its manufacturer, Procter and Gamble. For women who do develop symptoms of toxic shock syndrome, prompt treatment with antibiotics is essential, along with supportive measures, especially intravenous replacement of fluids and electrolytes. In addition, a woman who has had toxic shock syndrome once is at considerable risk – one study says as high as 42 per cent – of developing it again.

Tay-Sachs disease A fatal hereditary disease characterized by the absence of an enzyme, hexosaminidase-A, making it impossible for the body to assimilate certain fats. Although a child born with the disorder may seem normal at birth, symptoms appear during the first years of life, beginning with deterioration of motor ability and voluntary movement. Progressively the child becomes severely retarded and develops blindness and convulsions. Death usually occurs by the age of three or four. No cure is known. A recessive-gene disorder (see under BIRTH DEFECTS), Tay-Sachs disease is common among Ashkenazi Jews (from Central and Eastern Europe), among whom an estimated 1 of every 30 persons is a carrier (as opposed to 1 in 300 in other ethnic groups). If both parents are carriers, a fact that can be determined by a simple blood test, there is a 25 per cent risk that any child of theirs will have the disease. Its presence in a foetus can be detected by AMNIOCENTESIS. See also GAUCHER'S DISEASE.

Term See under GESTATION.

Testes See TESTIS.

Testicular feminization See ANDRO-GEN SENSITIVITY SYNDROME.

Testis Also *testicle*; *testes* (pl.). The male gonad, or sex gland, which is primarily responsible for secreting male sex hormones, or androgens, and for producing the male germ cell, or sperm. There are two testes, one hanging in each side of the SCROTUM, slightly in front of the thighs, behind the penis. Unlike the female gonads, or ovaries, which contain female germ cells at birth, the testes produce sperm only after puberty. Each testis is an oval-shaped structure about 1½ inches (3½ centimetres) long and 1

inch (2½ centimetres) thick. It is divided into some 250 compartments, each of which contains several *seminiferous tubules*. These tubules produce sperm, and cells between the tubules, called *interstitial cells*, secrete androgens. The seminiferous tubules join together into a dozen or so ducts that form the first part of the *epididymis*, a single tightly coiled duct in which sperm are stored. The cells lining the duct secrete a substance stimulating the development of sperm. Infection and the subsequent formation of scar tissue can block the epididymis, resulting in sterility. Occasionally one or both testes do not descend into the scrotum but remain in the inguinal canal or abdomen, a condition called CRYPTORCHIDISM. See also PENIS; SPERM.

Testosterone The principal male sex hormone, or androgen, produced chiefly by the male gonads, the testes. Its production is controlled in much the same way as the production of oestrogen by the ovaries in women, that is, by the pituitary hormones FSH and LH, which in turn are controlled by the hypothalamus. Before PUBERTY, which in most boys begins between the ages of ten and fifteen, the testes secrete only small amounts of testosterone. During puberty this quantity is greatly increased, and it is the substance principally responsible for the appearance of secondary sex characteristics (facial and body hair, bigger muscles, deepening voice, enlarged testes and penis) and the growth spurt characteristics of normal puberty.

In women the ovaries and adrenal glands are also capable of secreting testosterone, but, except in diseases such as the adrenogenital syndrome, they do so in very small quantity. Synthetic testosterone is used to treat disorders in which the testes do not produce sufficient amounts of the hormone.

Test-tube baby   Also *in vitro fertilization*. A procedure in which a woman's egg is removed from a ripe FOLLICLE, fertilized by sperm outside the human body, allowed to divide in a protected environment, and then is reinserted in the woman's uterus. The first pregnancy begun in this way and successfully brought to term took place in Britain in 1978.

Still considered experimental, the procedure is performed only on selected married women whose FALLOPIAN TUBES are too damaged to permit fertilization but whose other reproductive capacities are essentially normal. The procedure involves LAPAROSCOPY, whereby the doctor studies the eggs in a woman's ovary through a small incision and removes one to three mature eggs by means of a suction device. Each egg is placed in a glass dish (*in vitro* is Latin for 'in glass') with a special nutrient broth and the father's seminal fluid, containing live sperm, and after fertilization is incubated for forty-eight to seventy-two hours. If it has grown normally, it is then placed in the woman's uterus through the vagina and cervix. If all goes well, within a day or two it will implant itself in the uterine wall and develop normally for nine months, until birth. It is estimated that eventually, when the technique is perfected, about half the women undergoing this procedure will be able to bear a child.

Several newer techniques to overcome infertility are also being investigated. One, designed for women with blocked Fallopian tubes, involves removing a mature egg from the ovary and replacing it in a Fallopian tube at a point very near the

uterus where it might be fertilized (tubes tend to be blocked at the upper end, near the ovary). Another, tentatively called *artificial embryonation*, involves artificial insemination of a female donor with sperm from the husband of an infertile woman; five days following fertilization, the fertilized egg, now a tiny embryo, is removed and transferred to the uterus of the wife. This method could, when perfected, be used not only for women who are infertile but those in whom the risk of passing on an inherited birth defect is very high.

Thalidomide   A tranquillizer originally made by a West German company and commonly used in the early 1960s, especially in Europe, where it was frequently given to pregnant women. When given early in pregnancy, it was discovered to cause severe malformation in the foetus, especially interfering with the development of normal limbs (arms and legs), so that babies were born with flippers instead of limbs, or with hands attached at the shoulder, or similar structural abnormalities.

Therapy   Another word for treatment (of any kind). However, it is often used as a synonym for PSYCHOTHERAPY. See also FEMINIST THERAPY; SEX THERAPY.

Thermatic sterilization   Also *thermatic male sterilization, TMS*. A method of using heat to achieve temporary sterility in men. The fact that heat inhibits sperm has been known since ancient times, though it is still not certain whether heat kills sperm or simply slows them down (impairs their motility). In 1921 Martha Voegeli, a Swiss doctor working in India, decided to apply this principle as a means of birth control. The procedure she developed requires a man to sit in a bath with water at a temperature of 116 degrees Fahrenheit for forty-five minutes every day for three weeks; this allegedly renders him sterile for six months, whereupon his fertility is restored. Voegeli claims to have used this method successfully in India for twenty years, from 1930 to 1950. In the 1960s, several American doctors, among them John Rock, who helped develop oral contraceptives, experimented with insulated underwear, which retains body heat, for the same purpose. Apparently this method was also effective but research results are still too scanty to determine its reliability.

Thermography   A means of detecting cancer based on the fact that cancerous tissue generates more heat than surrounding healthy tissue because of its greater cellular activity (that is, its rapid growth; see CANCER). A *thermogram* is a pictorial representation of heat patterns on the surface of the skin, usually that of the breast.

Threatened miscarriage   See MISCARRIAGE, definition 2.

Thromboembolism   See   under   EMBOLISM.

Thrombophlebitis   See PHLEBITIS.

Thrombus   Also *blood clot*; (pl.) *thrombi*. A blood clot that forms within a blood vessel rather than externally. For reasons that are not understood, blood sometimes spontaneously forms such clots. A sizable clot can obstruct the blood vessel in which it formed and, if that vessel is an artery supplying oxygen and vital nutrients to an important organ, such as the heart, lungs, or brain, severe or even

fatal damage can result. Abnormal clotting within the veins or arteries is called *thrombosis*; if it occurs in one of the arteries supplying blood to the heart – the *coronary arteries* – it is called a *coronary thrombosis*, and if it affects an artery supplying blood to the brain it is a *cerebral thrombosis*. The presence of a thrombus in a vein is called *venous thrombosis*, *thrombophlebitis*, or PHLEBITIS.

Although the cause of venous clots is not known, there are certain factors that predispose to their formation, among them *stasis*, that is, sluggish blood flow through veins, which may occur with inactivity, immobilization, obstruction of the blood flow, and so on. For this reason they are more likely to form in old age, with long-term bed rest, and immediately following surgery and childbirth. Congestive heart failure and shock, oestrogen therapy, and certain infections and malignancies also increase the likelihood of thrombus formation. Thrombosis is usually treated with drugs called *anticoagulants*, which reduce the ability of the blood to form clots. One such drug is heparin, administered by injection; another is coumarin, which can be taken orally. Both interfere with the production of essential blood clotting factors and must be used with extreme caution, and never when there is danger of haemorrhage. See also EMBOLISM.

Thyroid   An ENDOCRINE gland consisting of two lobes, one on each side of the trachea (windpipe), joined by a narrow bridge. It produces two hormones, thyroxine and triiodothyronine, which help regular growth and METABOLISM and can be produced only when the body takes in adequate amounts of iodine. Like the hormones involves in the MENSTRUAL CYCLE, the secretion of thyroid hormones involves a stimulating hormone, called *thyroid-stimulating* or *thyrotrophic hormone* (TSH), which in turn requires a release factor, called *thyrotrophin-releasing hormone* (TRH) or *thyrotrophin-releasing factor* (TRF). Also as in the menstrual cycle, these hormones operate by means of a negative feedback mechanism. Increased levels of thyroid hormone suppress TSH release; when hormone levels fall, there is an increase in TRH, triggering TSH production. TRH also stimulates production of PROLACTIN and lactation.

Disorders of the thyroid gland, which occur four to five times more often in women than in men, usually involve either overproduction (*hyperthyroidism*) or underproduction (*hypothyroidism*) of these hormones. The fact that women are more prone to thyroid problems than men, especially at puberty, during pregnancy, and at menopause, suggests a possible link between thyroid and ovarian function.

Goitre, an enlargement of the thyroid gland that appears as a visible swelling on the front of the neck is estimated to be up to five times more common in women than in men. Some kinds are caused by hyperthyroidism and others by hypothyroidism. A goitre may require no treatment at all unless the enlargement causes uncomfortable pressure on adjacent organs or a tumour is suspected. Treatment is directed at restoring hormone levels to normal by means of drugs that suppress the excess, or of iodine to encourage hormone production.

The most common form of hyperthyroidism is *Graves' disease*, whose symptoms, in addition to goitre, include nervousness, heat sensitivity, weight loss despite increased appetite, tremors, muscular weakness, and bulging eyes.

Women, who are affected seven times as often as men, may also experience menstrual irregularities and impaired fertility. Treatment involves suppressing the excess hormone production by means of drugs. Sometimes partial or total surgical removal of the thyroid gland – *thyroidectomy* – is indicated; if the entire gland is removed it must be followed with life-long administration of thyroid hormones. Pregnant patients cannot be given some antithyroid drugs alone because they can affect the foetus, causing thyroid deficiency and possible permanent dwarfism and mental retardation; if they require such medication it must be given together with thyroid hormone in adequate amounts to avoid damage.

Myxoedema, caused by thyroid hormone deficiency in older children and adults, is marked by personality changes, dry and puffy skin, and oedema (fluid retention). It can delay the onset of menstruation in adolescent girls. After puberty it may cause very heavy menstrual bleeding and consequent anaemia (occasionally leading to false diagnosis of a uterine tumour), and it usually prevents a woman from becoming pregnant. This condition responds well to the administration of thyroid hormone.

TIA Abbreviation for transient ischaemic attack; see under CEREBRAL VASULAR ACCIDENT.

Tic douloureux Also *trigeminal neuralgia*. Episodes of severe sharp pain in one of the divisions of the trigeminal (fifth cranial) nerve in the upper or lower jaw, usually of brief duration (ten to fifteen seconds). Its cause is not known, but it tends to afflict women more than men, and older women more than young ones. In young people, it may be an early symptom of MULTIPLE SCLEROSIS, and it may occur in association with that disease during any of its stages. The pain of tic douloureux may be set off by touching a trigger point or by a movement of the jaws, as in chewing, shaving, or brushing the teeth. There are no objective signs of the disease, the bouts of acute pain – often many during each day – being the only symptom. Treatment is palliative, usually involving strong pain-reliever (carbamazepine is the one most commonly used).

Tipped uterus See RETROVERTED UTERUS.

Toxaemia of pregnancy See PRE-ECLAMPSIA; ECLAMPSIA.

Toxic shock syndrome Also *TSS*. See under TAMPON.

Tranquillizers
1 **Minor tranquillizers** Drugs used to treat ANXIETY. They are among the most frequently prescribed drugs in Britain, and many feel they are overprescribed, especially for women. There are two principal kinds, the benzodiazepine compounds (Librium, Valium, and others), which sedate, relax the muscles, and are anticonvulsive as well as combatting anxiety, and meprobamate (Equanil). Although very effective against anxiety, they are also potentially habit-forming and addictive, so that discontinuing the drug abruptly can lead to withdrawal symptoms. They impair alertness, often making one feel drowsy and lethargic, and in large doses can cause unsteadiness in stance and gait. They can lead to a serious adverse reaction if combined with alcohol, which therefore should be avoided by anyone taking tranquillizers. They probably should not be taken at any time during pregnancy and certainly not during the first three months, since they have been associated with birth defects. They should also be avoided by women who are breast-feeding. As with any strong medication, the risks should be carefully weighed against the benefits. On balance, the minor tranquillizers are considered useful to control distressing symptoms initially but should be used for as brief a time as possible, in conjunction with some kind of psychotherapy that is directed at determining and eliminating the causes of anxiety.
2 **Major tranquillizers** Also *neuroleptics, antipsychotics*. Drugs used to treat serious psychiatric disorders, principally schizophrenia, acute mania, and acute confusional states. They produce a state of emotional calm and virtual indifference, technically called *neurolepsy*. The principal neuroleptics are the phenothiazines, which include chlorpromazine (Largactil), thioridazine (Mellaril), and trifluoperazine (Stelazine), the butryophenones, which include halopedol (Haldol), and three other classes of drug. They usually relieve such symptoms as thought disturbances, delusions, hallucinations, and agitation, but they are very potent drugs and should not be used by pregnant women.

Transient ischaemic attack Also *TIA*. See under CEREBRAL VASCULAR ACCIDENT.

Transillumination A diagnostic technique in which a beam of strong light is passed through the breast in order to detect and differentiate between cysts and malignant (cancerous) tumours. See also CANCER, BREAST.

Transition End of the first stage of labour; see under LABOUR.

Transsexual A person who undergoes hormone treatment and/or surgery in order to changes from his or her bio-logically determined sex to the opposite sex. Although this change can be accomplished in either direction (from man to woman, or woman to man), in practice it is much easier to change from man to woman, and about 80 per cent of those seeking such a change are men who wish to become women. The penis and testes are removed, and an artificial vagina is constructed. Female sex hormones are given, and sometimes the breasts are surgically enlarged. (In changing a woman to a man, both breasts, both ovaries, and the uterus are removed, testes are constructed, and sometimes a penis is made from skin flaps; such a penis is not capable of erection but can be made to function with implants or devices of the kind sometimes used to treat impotent men. Also, male sex hormones are administered.) These operations, which are both drastic and irreversible, were devised in the mid-1960s, and by the late 1970s some surgeons were already abandoning them in the belief that they did not really change a person's life as much, or as favourably, as had been expected.

A transsexual believes he or she is really a member of the opposite sex who is trapped in the wrong body, that is, their gender identity does not match their physical identity. After surgery, trans-sexuals usually fashion new lives for themselves and, often, try to keep their old identities secret. Many marry and raise adopted children. Frequently, however, they find that their emotional adjust-ment is no better than before surgery and

hormone therapy were undertaken.

Before deciding to undergo a sex change of this kind, anyone considering it is strongly advised to seek counselling from a therapist who specializes in this specific area. At least a year of intensive counselling is recommended, and then most therapists advise the person to live in the desired role for another year before deciding on surgery. (This condition is *required* by the best of the clinics where this treatment is performed.) Many appli-cants for transsexual surgery do, in the course of these preliminary procedures, change their minds. Only 10 to 15 per cent of candidates are considered a good risk, according to some psychiatrists working in this field.

Transverse position See under SHOULDER PRESENTATION.

Trichomonas Also *trich, trichomoniasis.* A vaginal infection caused by a one-celled organism. *Trichomonas vaginalis,* that is extremely common among women but usually only if they are sexually active. Because it can be transmitted sexually, it is also considered a VENEREAL DISEASE and treatment, to be effective, must be given to both partners. Also, the organism can survive at room temperature for several hours on moist objects and so can be transmitted by a sheet, towel, wash-cloth, or toilet seat used by an infected woman.

Trichomonas causes a thin, yellow or greenish, frothy or bubbly discharge, sometimes with a foul odour, as well as itching, soreness, and inflammation of the vulva and inside the vagina. Men harbour the organism in their urinary tract and usually have no symptoms at all. In women, however, the organisms can also invade the urinary tract and cause

CYSTITIS, with symptoms of burning and urinary frequency. Unfortunately the only invariably effective drug known against trichomonas, metronidazole (Flagyl), taken orally three times a day for seven to ten days, has side effects, some of them potentially very serious. In addition, it should *never* be used during the first three months of pregnancy or while breast-feeding, and some authorities say never in pregnancy. Side effects include nausea and/or diarrhoea, headache, intolerance to alcohol – all drinking must be avoided while taking this drug and for three days Afterwards, lest it cause a severe allergic reaction – and a lowered white blood cell count. For these reasons the medication should be used with caution, and white blood cell counts should be performed before, during, and after treatment. Some authorities believe it is safer to take the drug in a single huge (2,000-milligram) oral dose or in several large doses for a few days rather than for a week or ten days. The male partner should be treated, too (a female partner needs to be treated only if she is infected). The drug is also available in vaginal suppository form.

Much safer but less effective treatments are a two-week course of a daily local application of an antibacterial agent such as Betadine, available as a vaginal gel. For a mild case, a garlic suppository (peel one clove of garlic, wrap in gauze, insert overnight, change daily) may help relieve irritation. Palliative HERBAL REMEDIES used include douching with a mixture of myrrh (*Commiphora myrrha*) and goldenseal (*Hydrastia canadensis*) twice a day for one or two weeks. Wearing tight pants of any kind should be avoided (if possible, wear no pants at all while at home), as should tampons, vaginal hygiene sprays, and sexual intercourse without a condom.

Trichomonas can be severe enough to cause an abnormal PAP SMEAR – on which, however, the organism also can be detected – and it tends to recur. Furthermore, it can encourage the development of venereal warts (see CONDYLOMA ACUMINATA) and YEAST INFECTION. Although trichomonas can cause small red lesions on the cervix, it does not invade the uterus or Fallopian tubes, nor does it affect fertility. See also VAGINITIS.

Trimester A three-month period, specifically the three such periods that make up a full-term (nine-month) pregnancy.

Tubal insufflation see RUBIN TEST.

Tubal ligation Also *tubal sterilization, tying the tubes*. A deliberate closing of the FALLOPIAN TUBES in order to prevent conception (pregnancy). Tubal ligation can be performed either through an incision in the abdomen or through the vagina, and it has been the principal form of STERILIZATION for women in the Western world since about 1880. Actually, *ligation*, meaning 'tying', is a misnomer. Formerly part of each tube was cut off and the cut ends were pinched shut and tied; newer methods use coagulation (cauterization or burning) or the placement of clips or bands around parts of each tube. All the procedures serve to block the tubes, thereby preventing the passage of sperm upward into the tubes and of eggs downward toward the uterus.

The principal form of *vaginal tubal ligation*, where a small incision is made in the vagina and the tubes are drawn through it, is CULDOSCOPY. Vaginal tubal ligation can never be performed immediately after childbirth because the vaginal tissues are still too congested. However, because the uterus is still enlarged, immediately after delivery was at one time considered the ideal time for an abdominal tubal ligation. Today it is considered preferable to wait six to eight weeks.

For traditional abdominal tubal ligation, an incision four to five inches long is made on the lower abdomen, just above the top of the pubic hair line. The incision may be horizontal (see PFANNENSTIEL) or vertical. After the abdominal cavity is entered, the tubes are closed off in one of a number of ways: 'sewn' shut with sutures; cut and sutured; cauterized (burned and sealed); or closed with metal or plastic clips or rings.

Abdominal tubal ligation is usually performed under general anaesthesia, although occasionally SPINAL or EPI-DURAL ANAESTHESIA may be used. A hospital stay of several days is required so that the incision can heal. Full recovery takes about six weeks. The principal advantage of abdominal tubal ligation is that the surgeon has adequate access to the tubes to close them off completely, even when there is scar tissue from previous surgery or infection. Also, because it is the oldest method of tubal ligation, most surgeons have considerable experience with it. However, two newer procedures, LAPAROSCOPY ('Band-aid surgery') and MINILAPAROTOMY ('minilap'), which are both simpler and less expensive for the patient, are being more widely used and are replacing the older method. Still another method of tubal ligation, used less often, is through the uterus, HYSTEROSCOPY.

The principal complication following tubal ligation is infection. Danger signs are: fever; pain not relieved by a mild analgesic such as aspirin, or pain that persists for more than twelve hours; moderate or heavy bleeding from either the incision or the vagina; faintness; chest pain; cough; shortness of breath; or pus from the incision. These symptoms should be promptly reported to the surgeon. Some women should not undergo tubal ligation at all. Among them are women who may be pregnant at the time, have an active pelvic infection, have an abnormal uterine or tubal structure (although even with scarring and adhesions an abdominal procedure may be possible), or have serious medical problems, such as asthma, heart disease, severe obesity, or others contraindicating any surgery.

Tubal ligation should be undertaken only by women who are sure they want no more children. Reconstructive surgery to re-open the tubes, called TUBERO-PLASTY, has a limited chance of success. Even when it does succeed, it carries a greatly increased risk of tubal pregnancy (ECTOPIC PREGNANCY). The effectiveness of tubal ligation, on the other hand, is quite high. When it does fail and a woman finds she is pregnant, it is due either to incomplete closing of the tubes or, in some cases, ignorance of an already existing pregnancy (one begun just before the surgery).

Tubal pregnancy See ECTOPIC PREG-NANCY.

Tuberoplasty   Also *tuboplasty*. Surgical repair of the FALLOPIAN TUBES to correct blockage resulting either from scar tissue or from TUBAL LIGATION. If previous infections have created enough scar tissue to block the tubes at the end near the fimbria (and ovaries), thereby preventing the passage of an egg into or through the tubes, a two-stage operation may be performed. First the scar tissue is removed and a small plastic hood is placed over each tube to keep it open. Then, after several months, the plastic tubes are removed. If the surgery succeeds, as it does in about one-quarter of cases, the tubes will remain open. Recently, newer techniques using laser beams rather than surgical instruments have shown great promise. In one procedure the laser is used to destroy the diseased tissue of the tube and cut a hole in the uterus, through which the surgeon then implants a healthy section of the tube.

To repair the tubes after a tubal ligation, because a woman has changed her mind and now wants a child, the two ligated ends of each tube are sewn back together, a delicate procedure best performed with the aid of a microscope (microsurgery), and a narrow plastic tube is inserted to keep each tube open until it has healed. Pregnancy following this procedure occurs in less than half of cases, and even then there is a high risk (10 to 15 per cent) of ECTOPIC PREGNANCY, with the fertilized egg becoming implanted in the tube instead of the uterus. An alternative procedure is to pull one end of each tube into the uterus and fasten it there, with the fimbria outside. This method is thought to have a higher rate of success.

To a large extent the success or failure of any repair depends on how the original ligation was accomplished. If the tubes were closed by elctrocautery (coagulation or burning) the success rate of repair is only about 10 per cent; if the fimbria were removed (fimbriectomy) it is near 0 per cent; if a plastic ring (the Falope ring) was used it may be as high as 50 to 75 per cent. Also, a great deal depends on the skill of the surgeon, so it is advisable to seek one who has had considerable experience with these procedures.

Tubes See FALLOPIAN TUBES.

Tumour Also *neoplasm*. An enlargement caused by the growth of tissue beyond its normal limits. A tumour may be benign (noncancerous), meaning it does not tend to invade other tissues or spread to other parts of the body, or it may be malignant (cancerous; see CANCER). A benign tumour may be solid or contain fluid; of the latter kinds, the most common is the CYST. Among the most common benign solid tumours that affect women is the uterine FIBROID; among the most common malignant ones are the various breast cancers (see CANCER, BREAST).

Turner's syndrome Also *ovarian dysgenesis*. A congenital condition marked by the absence of ovaries, usually owing to the absence (complete or partial) of one of the two XX sex chromosomes. Thus, instead of the normal woman's XX chromosome, there is an XO chromosome (although sometimes the configuration is somewhat different). Turner's syndrome is often not diagnosed until adolescence, when the lack of breast development and menstruation signal that something is wrong. Other signs are very short stature (usually no taller than 4½ feet), a short broad neck, and, sometimes, a webbed neck, fingers, and toes, a small receding chin, and the presence of pigmented moles. There may be associated defects in other organs as well – chiefly the heart, kidneys, and ureters, as well as hearing loss. The condition is named after Dr. H. H. Turner, who first described it in 1938. Hormone therapy can establish menstruation and secondary sex characteristics such as breast development, but it will not spur growth or make childbearing possible. Since about 1970, transplants of ovaries have been attempted, but this is still an experimental procedure. Turner's syndrome is relatively rare, occurring in about 1 of every 3,000 girls born.

Twins See under MULTIPLE PREGNANCY.

Tylectomy See MASTECTOMY, definition 7.

U

Ultrasound 1 Also *sonography, B-scan.*
A diagnostic tool in which sound echoes
provide a picture of soft-tissue structures
inside the body, among them those of the
female pelvis. It uses sound waves with
frequencies of 2.5 million to 10 million
cycles per second to scan the abdomen
and pelvic area in linear fashion and then
records their reflection (echo) on an
oscilloscope screen (the recording is
called a *sonagram*). A reflection is
recorded whenever the sound waves
meet a material of different acoustical
density. Hence ultrasound can make an
outline of soft-tissue masses in a way that
X-rays cannot. A sonogram can show the
size of the uterus, the size of a gestational
sac or foetus, the position of a foetus, the
presence of more than one foetus (twins,
triplets, etc.), and some structural defects
in the foetus. It can also detect an ectopic
pregnancy (outside the uterus), distinguish between solid tumours and cysts
of the ovaries, and between some benign
(noncancerous) and malignant (cancerous) tumours. Ultrasound has been used
to locate pelvic abscesses and wandering
intrauterine devices (IUDs), detect the
spread of cervical cancer in the pelvis,
and help diagnose breast cancer, but for
this purpose results have been less
successful, with a high margin of error.
2 A means of suppressing sperm
formation that is still considered an
experimental form of male contraception.

The man must sit with his testes resting
in a cup filled with water; the water serves
as a conductor for high-frequency sound
generated by an ultrasound transducer.
Experiments on dogs and human beings
both indicate that the ultrasound lowers
the sperm count considerably, an effect
that is believed to be reversible although
it may last for one to two years. A major
advantage of this means of contraception,
should it prove to be reliable, is that
ultrasound is quite painless and has no
harmful side effects.

Umbilical cord An organ consisting
of a semitransparent, jelly-like rope, about
55 centimetres (22 inches) long on
average (but ranging from 5 to 200 centimetres, or 2 to 80 inches, long) that
connects mother and foetus through the
PLACENTA. It contains two arteries, which
transport foetal waste products and de-
oxygenated blood to the mother, and one
vein, which transports blood containing
nutrients and oxygen from the mother
to the foetus. One of the serious complications of childbirth is a PROLAPSED
CORD, that is, delivery of the cord before
the rest of the baby, or alongside it.
Another is *cord strangulation,* in which the
cord becomes twisted around the baby's
neck. Both these risks are much greater
with abnormal presentation, especially
BREECH and SHOULDER PRESENTATION.
Another serious problem is compression

of the cord; that is, when the cord is tightly squeezed during uterine contractions, interrupting the flow of blood through it and hence periodically cutting off the baby's oxygen supply.

Almost immediately after delivery the baby, if normally developed, begins to depend on air for its oxygen supply; the foetal circulation actually changes to allow blood to pass from the right side of the heart through the lungs and from the lungs to the left side of the heart. As soon as the baby is breathing, the cord is no longer needed. The usual procedure for cutting the cord is to apply to clamps to the cord about 2 inches (5 centimetres) from the point where it joins the baby's abdomen, called the *umbilicus* or *navel*. The cord is then cut between the two clamps with sterile scissors, and a sterile tape ligature or clamp is applied about ¾ inch (2 centimetres) from the abdomen. This stump is kept clean and dry with alcohol until it drops off, a week or two later. See HERNIA, UMBILICAL.

Urea A concentrated solution of nitrogen excreted by the kidneys. It is sometimes used in second-trimester abortions, usually in conjunction with prostaglandins; see under AMNIOINFUSION.

Urethra In women, a narrow tube, about 1½ inches (3½ or 4 centimetres) long, that lies in front of the lower part of the vagina and conveys urine from the BLADDER to the outside. The upper end opens into the bladder; the lower end opens into the vestibule between the clitoris and vagina. This lower opening is called the *external urinary meatus* or *urethral orifice*. The urethra is lined with mucuous membrane similar to that of the bladder itself. A series of muscle fibres surround the urethra and neck of the bladder, which are maintained in a state of contraction by the sympathetic nervous system. The SPHINCTER muscle of the bladder neck can be relaxed voluntarily in order for urine to be passed. When the urethral or perineal muscles become less elastic, owing to repeated stretching during pregnancy and childbirth or, after menopause, to a decrease in oestrogen (which helps maintain elasticity and mucus-producing ability in the urethral as well as vaginal tissues), problems with bladder control may develop (see STRESS INCONTINENCE).

One of the most common disorders affecting women is URETHRITIS, inflammation and infection of the urethra. It often accompanies a bladder infection (see CYSTITIS) and is treated in the same way.

Urethritis Inflammation and/or infection of the URETHRA, a common disorder in women that often occurs in conjunction with bladder infection and is treated with the same medications (see also CYSTITIS). In the absence of bladder infection, it may be associated with GONORRHOEA, TRICHOMONAS, or some other infection of the vagina. For this reason it is important to find out what organism is responsible and take the appropriate medication to eliminate it (see URINE TEST). It may also be caused by irritation or injury from too vigorous intercourse, by irritation from the rim of a DIAPHRAGM or scratching, or by bacteria from the intestinal tract that enter the urethra after careless (back-to-front) wiping of bowel movements.

The symptoms of urethritis are pain, usually a burning sensation during urination, urinary frequency, and also a discharge, sometimes blood-tinged. A gonorrhoea culture is nearly always indicated for urethritis, as well as a urine culture to identify the specific bacteria involved. The organism *chlamydia trachomatis*, which may also cause some cases of nonspecific VAGINITIS, is often responsible, as is *T-strain Mycoplasma* (also called *ureaplasma*). Treatment is the same as for cystitis.

In some cases no particular organism can be found; the condition is then called *nonspecific urethritis* (NSU) or *nongonococcal urethritis* (NGU), the latter especially in men. Nonspecific urethritis is often venereal in origin (that is, sexually transmitted), although it is not caused by the same organism as gonorrhoea, and may give rise to practically no symptoms whatever in a woman, or only a thin, usually clear discharge in the urine and mild dysuria (discomfort when urinating); there may also be a slight discharge from the urethra. Symptoms occur two to three weeks after exposure. Undetected, the condition may become worse and lead to complications (see below), so a woman whose partner is diagnosed as having NGU should also be treated for the infection. Usually a broad-spectrum antibiotic such as tetracycline will clear up the condition.

In postmenopausal women the shrinking and drying of the labia often leave the urethra more exposed and more prone to infection, occasionally resulting in chronic urethritis (called *senile urethritis*). This condition may be treated with oestrogen suppositories inserted in the vagina, a treatment not without risk (see OESTROGEN REPLACEMENT THERAPY).

If neglected, urethritis can lead to serious complications, such as pelvic inflammatory disease and infertility in women, and epididymitis, a painful inflammation of the testes, in men. (However, except for NGU, urethritis is much rarer in men; see under PENIS.) Also, urethritis appears to be connected with pneumonia and eye infections in babies born of infected mothers, and has been suspected as a factor in some infections leading to stillbirth.

Urethrocele A bulging of the urethra into the vagina, owing to pelvic relaxation, that is, weakening of the muscles that normally hold the urethra in place. It usually occurs in conjunction with CYSTOCELE and is treated in the same way.

Urinalysis See under URINE TEST.

Urinary frequency See FREQUENCY, URINARY.

Urinary incontinence See STRESS INCONTINENCE.

Urine test A laboratory test performed on a urine specimen (sample) to determine the presence of blood, protein, sugar, albumin, bacteria, and/or other substances. (For urine tests performed to diagnose pregnancy, see PREGNANCY TEST.) A *dipstick urine test*, performed by many doctors in the surgery, consists of dipping a strip of chemically treated paper into a urine specimen. By changing colour, the paper reveals relative acidity, the presence of blood (haematuria), protein (albumin), bilirubin, sugar, and acetone (ketones), which in turn may indicate such disorders as diabetes, kidney or bladder infection, or, sometimes, simply contamination of the specimen by menstrual blood of vaginal discharge washed from the vulva. The presence of albumin in a pregnant woman may be a sign of PREECLAMPSIA.

A *urinalysis* is a more complex test but

still may be performed in the doctor's surgery (though more often it is done in a laboratory). It tests both the concentration and acidity of the urine. Also, the urine is spun in a centifuge for several minutes to separate solid particles from the liquid. The sediment collected at the bottom is then put on a slide and examined under the microscope for white blood cells and bacteria (present in infection) as well as red blood cells, epithelial cells, and any abnormal cell formations (which might indicate kidney disease). If bacteria are present, a *urine culture* may be performed, that is, part of the sample is put in a nutrient (usually a jelly) and incubated (heated) so that the bacteria multiply rapidly. The specific organisms can then be more readily identified, and their susceptibility to various antibiotics can be determined (called a *sensitivity test*).

Still other, more complicated urine tests include the determination of hormone levels, which may require analysis of a woman's entire urinary output over a full day (sometimes called a *24-hour test*).

Urostomy Also *urinary ostomy*. A surgical procedure in which an artificial opening is made to provide for elimination of urine because of the loss of either the bladder or bladder function. It is usually performed because of birth defects, malignancy (cancer), injury, or nerve damage. There are several kinds of urostomy. An *ileal conduit* or *ileal bladder*, the most common kind, is performed when the bladder must be removed or by-passed. The conduit is constructed by separating about a six-inch segment of the lower ileum (end of the small intestine) and implanting into it the ureters, which have been detached from the bladder. The rest of the small intestine

is then reconnected to the colon. (This procedure may be performed with a segment of the colon, in which cases it is called a *uretero-colostomy*; see also COLOSTOMY.) One end of the segment of the ileum is closed; the other end is brought through the abdominal wall to form the *stoma* (external opening), usually on the lower right abdomen. This stoma empties urine only, and an appliance (bag) must be worn at all times to collect urine and control odour. In a *vesicostomy* an opening is made directly in front of the bladder. The opening is sutured to an opening in the abdominal wall, through which urine is eliminated; a bag must be worn to collect urine. A *cutaneous ureterostomy* involves detaching one or both ureters from the bladder and bringing them through the abdominal wall, to empy outside the body; a bag must be worn at all times. A *nephrostomy* connects directly with the kidneys, from which urine drains directly (without passing through ureter or bladder) to the outside through an opening in the back or flank of the body. Either one or both kidneys may be involved. A nephrostomy is temporary usually and is drained by a tube (catheter).

In women urostomy rarely affects sexual function and, where only the bladder is affected, does not usually rule out pregnancy. In men, however, urostomy often affects potency.

Uterine polyp See POLYP, definition 3.

Uterine synechiae Also *uterine adhesions*. See ADHESION; ASHERMAN'S SYNDROME.

Uterus Also *womb*. A hollow, thick-walled muscular organ that lies in the pelvis of women, behind the bladder and in front of the rectum. It is pear-shaped, with a dome-shaped top, called the *fundus*, and a narrow neck at the bottom, called the CERVIX. The body of the uterus (that is, all but the cervix) is called the *corpus* (Latin for 'body'). In adult women who have never borne children, the corpus of the uterus is approximately 8 to 9 centimetres (3 to 3½ inches) long, and 6 centimetres (1¼ inches) at its widest point. Its walls practically touch each other. Childbearing greatly increases its size. After menopause the uterus shrinks considerably, so that cervix and corpus become about equal in length. The muscled walls of the uterus, about 1.1 centimetres (½ inch) thick, called the *myometrium*, make up almost 90 per cent of its size. On the outside they are covered with the *peritoneum*, the membrane that lines the entire pelvic and abdominal cavity. On the inside they are lined with the ENDOMETRIUM, which varies in thickness during each menstrual cycle, first being built up in preparation for pregnancy and, when no egg is fertilized during a cycle, being shed in menstrual flow, along with some blood from its blood vessels.

The uterus has three openings. At the bottom, the cervix opens into the vagina. Near the fundus, a pair of FALLOPIAN TUBES open into the corpus on either side.

The uterus is partly mobile, that is, the cervix is anchored but the corpus is free to move backward and forward. When a woman is standing her uterus is normally tilted forward at the junction of corpus and cervix, a position called *anteverted*. In about one-quarter of women, however, the uterus is tilted back (see RETROVERTED UTERUS). Anomalies of the uterus are a *septate uterus*, in which a partition of varying thickness extends

part or all of the way from fundus to cervix, dividing the corpus into two more or less separate compartments; a *bicornuate uterus*, which consists of two smaller, horn-shaped bodies, each connected to one Fallopian tube but sharing a single (although sometimes separate, or divided) cervix; and *double uterus*, in which there are two separate small bodies, each with its own cervix. These structural anomalies are all relatively rare, they are congenital (present from birth), and they can interfere with pregnancy and delivery, depending on the extent of abnormality.

The uterus is supported by three sets of strong, supple ligaments and is supplied with a rich network of blood vessels and nerves. Its principal function is to house and nourish a foetus until it is mature enough to be born, an average timespan of thirty-eight to forty-two weeks. As the foetus grows – or, in the case of multiple pregnancy, two or more foetuses grow – the muscle fibres stretch to accommodate it. Toward the end of a pregnancy the once pear-sized organ has grown to 30 centimetres (12 inches) long and increased its weight from 50 grams (2 ounces) to 900 grams (2 pounds). At some point the uterine muscles, which are involuntary, are stimulated to begin contracting, probably the the hormone OXYTOCIN, and it is their work, called LABOUR, that pushes the baby down toward the cervix and forces the cervix to widen enough to allow its passage through the vagina. This process is not without discomfort, and indeed each contraction is called a *labour pain*. Oddly, nearly all pain originating in the uterus is perceived in the same way – as a *cramp* – although differing in duration and severity, whether its cause is the contractions of childbirth, the dilatation of the cervix for a D AND C, or the shedding of endometrial tissue during a menstrual period. After delivery the uterine muscles and ligaments return to their normal size, the excess tissues being absorbed into the bloodstream and eventually excreted in urine. By the end of a week the uterus weighs 500 grams (1 pound) and, after six weeks, 50 grams (2 ounces). Occasionally the muscles and liagments weaken as a result of pregnancy and the uterus begins to sag from its normal position (see PROLAPSED UTERUS).

The body of the uterus is subject to a number of disorders and diseases (see also under CERVIX). The development of benign growths such as a FIBROID or POLYPS (definition 3) is very common. More serious conditions are infections, such as PELVIC INFLAMMATORY DISEASE, and endometrial cancer (see CANCER, ENDOMETRIAL). Two of the surgical procedures most frequently performed on women are scraping of the uterine lining for biopsy and/or treatment (see D AND C) and removal of the uterus (see HYSTERECTOMY).

V

Vacuum aspiration 1 Also *endometrial aspiration, vacuum curettage, vabra*. The removal of tissue from the uterus by means of suction for diagnostic purposes or, sometimes, to correct menstrual irregularities. It can be performed in a doctor's surgery or clinic, and is used to diagnose ENDOMETRIAL HYPERPLASIA or cancer, and to evaluate fertility. In this procedure, a SPECULUM is inserted in the vagina, the cervix is grasped and held in place with a calmp (tenaculum), and a slender plastic tube, or *vacurette*, is passed through the cervix into the uterus. The vacurette is attached either to a syringe or a special vacuum pump; when the pump is activated, shreds of tissue are removed from the uterine lining, or endometrium. The vacurette is small enough so that the cervix usually need not be dilated (widened). The procedure takes three to five minutes in all. The woman may feel mild cramping and can usually get up immediately or a few minutes later, take a short rest, and go home. See also BIOPSY, definition 8.

2 Also *suction abortion, vacuum abortion, early abortion, first-trimester abortion, early uterine evacuation*. The removal of placental and foetal tissue from the uterus by means of suction in order to terminate a pregnancy of twelve weeks or less. It is performed in a clinic, or hospital. The process is essentially the same as in definition 1 (see above) for pregnancies of four to six weeks (counting the first day of the last menstrual period as Day 1). However, some doctors prefer to wait until a patient is at least six weeks pregnant. For pregnancies of longer duration – seven to twelve weeks – a somewhat larger, nonflexible vacurette (tube) is used, and the cervix must be dilated for its insertion, usually by inserting a series of metal rods of gradually increasing diameter. To avoid the discomfort of such dilatation, most doctors use a local anaesthetic injected in the cervical area (paracervical block); unless general anaesthesia is used. Once inserted, the tip of the vacurette is rotated and moved around the walls of the uterus in order to remove the amniotic sac and also the thickened layer of endometrial tissue formed during the pregnancy. The total amount of tissue and blood removed on the average ranges (depending on the length of pregnancy) from 15 grams (1 ounce) to 150 grams (10 ounces). Some doctors follow up the suction procedure with an ordinary surgical curette (scraper) to make sure all of the foetal and placental tissue has been removed. The tissue is also carefully examined to document the pregnancy and rule out HYDATIDIFORM MOLE or some other abnormality, such as an ectopic pregnancy.

Vacuum abortion takes anywhere from six to ten minutes. For most women it is mildly to moderately uncomfortable, beginning with cramping during dilatation of the cervix, cramping and a tugging feeling in the abdomen during the suction process, and a few moderate to strong cramps near the end of the procedure, when the uterus finishes contracting. Cramps may last up to twenty minutes or so, sometimes accompanied by nausea.

Some 95 per cent of women experience little or no pain and little bleeding afterward, although light staining often continues for two weeks. Most doctors prescribe a drug to make sure the uterus contracts to normal size, and, sometimes, an antibiotic such as tetracycline for five days to eliminate risk of infection. About 5 per cent of women experience heavy bleeding temporarily and some lower abdominal tenderness, with or without fever. Following abortion douches, intercourse, and the insertion of tampons should be avoided for a week (some doctors say two weeks). In most women normal menses return within six weeks, but the first period following the procedure may be quite heavy.

Vacuum aspiration was developed in China in the late 1950s. As a method for first-trimester abortion (up to thirteen weeks from Day 1 of the last menstrual period) it has largely replaced the D AND C in the West. It is easier, cheaper, and safer than a D and C. The principal complications, which occur in only a tiny fraction of cases, are infection and incomplete abortion. Fever, severe cramps, back or rectal pain, heavy bleeding, and discharge are all symtpoms of infection, and any woman experiencing them should contact her doctor at once. Also, if signs of pregnancy persist (such as morning sickness and tender breasts) the woman should see her doctor even before the regular follow-up visit, usually scheduled for two weeks after the procedure, to make sure the curettage was complete and there is no ECTOPIC PREGNANCY (outside the uterus) or a remaining foetus (if there were twins).

Some doctors will, if the woman wishes, insert an intrauterine device (IUD) at the time of vacuum aspiration. However, many advise against it, because it increases bleeding, cramping, pain, and the risk of infection, and therefore suggest waiting until the first menstrual period. Women who use oral contraceptives may begin taking them immediately afterward, since ovulation generally will resume in two or three weeks. Women using a diaphragm should have the size checked during their follow-up visit, lest it has changed.

Vacuum extractor An instrument used in childbirth instead of FORCEPS. One or more round suctions cups fit on the baby's head, and suction is maintained by a pump linked to the extractors by a connecting tube. The instrument's great advantage is that there are no blades grasping the infant's head to add width to an already narrow passage (the mother's pelvix), and its advocates say it causes less damage to both baby and mother.

Vagina A canal lined with muscular and membranous tissue that connects a woman's external genital organs, or vulva, to the uterus. It lies between the bladder and rectum. In the average adult woman it is 9 to 10 centimetres (4 to 5 inches) long. At its far end is a cup-shaped area called the *formix*, into which the CERVIX projects; at the outer end is its external opening, called the *introitus*. In young girls the introitus is partly or completely

blocked by the HYMEN. Near the introitus is a muscular SPHINCTER that
contracts rhythmically during ORGASM.
It is this sphincter that prevents a tampon
from falling out.

The pink mucous membrane lining the
vaginal walls constantly produces small
amounts of mucus, keeping it moist.
Except near the introitus, there are
relatively few nerve endings, so the vagina
is not very sensitive to touch or to pain.
The mucous membrane is constantly
shedding old cells and replacing them
with new ones. This turnover is sometimes noticeable as a slight clear or white
discharge. Unless it is irritating or smelly,
such a discharge is normal. (See DIS-
CHARGE, VAGINAL). A healthy vagina
contains numerous micro-organisms,
among them *lacto-bacilli*, which break
down sugar stored in vaginal cells and
produce lactic acid. This acid helps
prevent infection by numerous disease-
causing organisms and also makes the
vagina inhospitable to sperm, which
cannot survive in it for more than a few
hours.

Under the mucous membrane are
layers of muscles, which make the vagina
capable of expanding enormously in size
in order to allow the passage of a baby.

The vagina has two principal functions.
It is the exit passage of the uterus, through
which its wastes (endometrial tissue and
blood) are expelled as menstrual flow and
through which babies emerge into the
world. It also is the female organ of sexual
intercourse, into which the male inserts
his penis. In rare instances a girl is born
without a vagina or with one that is
closed, a condition called *vaginal atresia*.
If the ovaries and uterus are well enough
developed for menstruation to occur at
puberty, the menstrual flow is then
retained, an accumulation that in time

becomes painful. In such cases a vaginal
passage can be surgically created.

The vagina is subject to a number of
common infections, especially YEAST
INFECTION and TRICHOMONAS, as well as
some of bacterial origin (see under
VAGINITIS). More serious are the various
VENEREAL DISEASES, transmitted by
sexual contact. Cancer originating in the
vagina is rare (except in DES daughters;
see DIETHYLSTILBOESTROL), though it
may spread there from the cervix or
vulva.

Vaginal atrophy Also *atrophic vaginitis,
senile vaginitis, vaginal dryness*. Thinning,
drying, and loss of elasticity in the tissues
lining the walls of the vagina, as well as
the urethra, vulva, and uterus, which
gradually occur in all women to some
extent in the years following menopause.
Before menopause, oestrogen stimulates
the endocervical glands to secrete a sticky,
thin, clear, alkaline mucus. After menopause, with greatly reduced oestrogen
production, much less mucus is secreted,
and the vaginal tissues become thinner,
dryer, and less elastic. The texture of the
vaginal walls changes too, becoming
smoother, and their colour changes from
a deep to a lighter pink. The pubic hair
becomes sparser and the labia majora
shrink, so that urethra, clitoris, and vagina
are all more exposed to friction. The
vagina gradually shortens and shrinks
somewhat, and sometimes the urethral
opening is pulled into and becomes part
of the outer portion of the vagina. In
severe cases these changes not only cause
burning, itching, and painful vaginal intercourse (DYSPAREUNIA) but can make
women more susceptible to urethral
inflammation and urinary infections
(principally urethritis and cystitis) as well
as vaginal infections.

Because these changes are directly related to reduced oestrogen production, oestrogen in cream or suppository form usually helps restore vaginal tone. However, oestrogen administered in this way is readily absorbed into the bloodstream and carries all the risks of oral OESTROGEN REPLACEMENT THERAPY. Consequently, it is highly advisable to try other, safer means of dealing with vaginal atrophy. To relieve painful intercourse, use of a water-soluble lubricant such as K-Y jelly often is effective. Regular sexual stimulation, either through intercourse or masturbation, helps promote secretion from the vaginal walls and offsets some of the drying. Some women have found that yoghurt inserted once a week into the vagina (with an applicator and/or diaphragm to help keep it in), used either alone or mixed with a vegetable oil such as safflower oil (1 tablespoon yogurt to 1 teaspoon oil), helps prevent drying and may also help restore the normal acid balance in the vagina (see also YEAST INFECTION for further explanation).

Vaginal hygiene Also *vaginal sprays.* See HYGIENE.

Vaginal infections See VAGINITIS.

Vaginal mycosis Also *mycotic vaginitis.* See YEAST INFECTION.

Vaginismus An involuntary spasmodic contraction of the muscles surrounding the vagina. When extreme, it can make it impossible to introduce any object (finger, tampon, penis, speculum) into the vagina. Some degree of vaginismus is not unusual in women for the first few times they engage in vaginal intercourse, especially if they are nervous or tense about coitus or fearful of possible pain caused by penetration

of the hymen. Also, if a man tries to insert his penis before a woman is fully aroused the vaginal entrance may be somewhat constricted. In true vaginismus, however, penetration becomes acutely painful or simply impossible. It is nearly always caused by an unusually strong aversion to any genital contact. Treatment consists of teaching the woman to dilate her own vaginal muscles, first with a fingertip, then a finger, then two fingers, or perhaps with dilators of graduated size, proceeding slowly and in such a way that she can relax and learn to relax those specific muscles.

Vaginitis A local inflammation that produces severe itching and burning of the vulva and is often accompanied by a vaginal discharge. The discharge may be creamy white or white (leucorrhoea; see DISCHARGE, VAGINAL) or it may be yellow, watery, or blood-tinged. In adult women such inflammation is most often the result of infection. Infections can be caused by an overabundance of the same organisms that normally reside in the vagina but have multiplied more than usual, frequently because the vaginal environment has been changed by taking oral contraceptives, hormone therapy, pregnancy, antibiotics, an illness such as diabetes, or douching.

The most common kinds of vaginitis are those caused by a yeastlike fungus called *Candida albicans* or *Monilia* and a one-celled parasite named *trichomonas vaginalis* (see YEAST INFECTION; TRICHOMONAS). Sometimes these two infections occur at the same time. Another organism frequently responsible is the bacterium HAEMOPHILUS VAGINALIS; both it and trichomonas are often transmitted through sexual intercourse and therefore are considered venereal infections. Other

Common Kinds Of Vaginitis

Disorder and/or Infectious Agent	Symptoms	How Diagnosed	Treatment
Haemophilus vaginalis	Greyish-white foul-smelling discharge	Wet smear	Antibiotic suppositories or sulpha creams
Herpes infection (*Herpes simplex* Type III)	Painful itchy blisters and open sores on vulva, sometimes inside vagina	Stained smear as for Pap smear	Local applications of sulpha creams, wet dressings, anaesthetic ointments
Trichomonas (*Trichomonas vaginalis*)	Yellow or greenish, frothy discharge, offensive odour, itching and soreness on vulva and in vagina	Wet smear	Metronidazole (Flagyl), or preferably, antibiotics suppositories and antibacterial douche
Yeast infection (*Monilia* or *Candida albicans*)	Severe vaginal and vulvar itching, white cheesy discharge with sweetish odour	Wet smear	Nystatin vaginal suppositories or propion gel or gentian violet suppositories and/or yoghurt applied locally

venereal infections responsible for vaginitis are HERPES INFECTION, which can create lesions in the cervix, vagina, and vulva, and GONORRHOEA. Both cysts and solid tumours can cause vaginitis. Cuts, abrasions, or other irritations in the vagina (from childbirth, intercourse, surgery) can become infected, and the presence of a foreign body, such as a forgotten tampon or diaphragm, also can cause infection. In children vaginitis can be induced by a variety of still other organisms, include *Escherichia coli*, normally resident in the gastrointestinal tract, and staphylococcus. Finally, some forms are known as *nonspecific vaginitis* (or *nongonococcal vaginitis*, NSV or NGV) because no particular organism can be identified, although the cause is thought to be bacterial. The organism *Chlamydia trachomatis*, which may cause nonspecific URETHRITIS, is thought to be responsible for some cases of NSV; it responds to antibiotic suppositories (tetracycline or erythromycin). Postmenopausal or *senile vaginitis* is caused by a lack of oestrogen, which leads to drying of tissues and other changes making the vaginal tissues more susceptible to the above-named infectious organisms (see VAGINAL ATROPHY).

Treatment of vaginitis depends on the cause. Specific drugs and remedies work well for many cases of yeast infection and trichomonas. For nonspecific vaginitis, local applications of antiseptic gels sometimes clear up the condition; oral antibiotics also are used. With any infection it is important to determine the cause, and with some it is necessary to treat the woman's sexual partner as well, to avoid reinfection.

In addition to specific medications, numerous preventive and palliative measures are advised for vaginitis, especially for stubborn cases with a tendency to recur. These include:

1 Keep up regular washing and gently drying of the vulva.

2 Use all-cotton underpants, which

'breathe' better than synthetic fabrics; air has a healing effect, so at home wear no underpants.

3 After bowel movements, wipe from front to back, so rectal bacteria cannot be transmitted to the vagina.

4 Avoid tight clothing in the thighs and crotch.

5 Avoid 'deodorant' soaps, tampons, and sanitary pads, which kill some of the normal organisms and make one more prone to infection by others.

6 Avoid dyed (coloured) toilet paper and all vaginal sprays.

7 In the absence of active infection, use a bland, buffered acid vaginal jelly at bedtime, such as K-Y jelly.

8 Try an acidic douche, such as 1 to 2 tablespoons white vinegar per quart of warm water, once or twice a week.

9 For yeast infections, apply yoghurt directly to the vagina, using an applicator or spoon.

10 Use a garlic suppository (one peeled clove of garlic, wrapped in thin layer of clean gauze, dipped in olive oil for easier insertion) overnight, changing daily.

11 HERBAL REMEDIES include a douche made from comfrey leaves (*Symphytum officinale*), goldenseal (*Hydrastis canadensis*), chamomile (*Matricaria chamomilla*), and sage (*Salvia officinalis*), steeped in water.

12 To relieve itching, apply cold compress of milk, yoghurt, or cottage cheese for five to ten minutes, five or six times a day; or take shallow sitz baths in plain water or in a tea made from sage, nettle (*Urtica dioica*), or chickweed (*Stellaria media*); or wash the area with sassafras bark tea.

See also DISCHARGE, VAGINAL; VULVI-TIS; WET SMEAR.

Varicocele A varicose vein in the TESTES. This condition, which is a leading cause of INFERTILITY in men, can be diagnosed simply by having the man stand and strain the muscles in the lower abdomen while the doctor probes the testes. The varicocele forms a scrotal swelling that has been described as feeling like a bag of worms. Varicocele, which inhibits sperm production (probably because of the heat generated by the swollen area), is readily corrected by surgery, which also corrects infertility in more than half of those cases where semen analysis indicates it to be the cause (see also SPERM).

Varicose vein Also *varicosity*. A permanent bulging or swelling in a vein, most commonly in one or more outer veins that run down the leg just under the skin. It can affect both men and women, but in Britain 1 in 5 women has one or more varicosities, whereas they are found in only 1 of every 15 men.

For the most part varicose veins are merely unsightly, but they can cause a feeling of heaviness, aching, and fatigue in the legs, especially near the end of the day. The ankles may swell and pain may extend down the leg, along the vein. Occasionally the overlying skin becomes scaly and itchy. Other complications are leg cramps (often at night), leg ulcers, PHLEBITIS, and blood clots.

The underlying cause of varicosities in veins lies in their structure. Veins are thin-walled blood vessels whose function is to send blood back to the heart and thence to the lungs to be reoxygenated. Since the blood travels in a steady stream in one direction, the veins are lined with one-way valves that ordinarily prevent back flow. As pressure builds behind each valve, it opens, allows blood to pass through, and then closes. (Also see

VEIN.) In the legs, however, and some other places as well – especially the rectal area (see HAEMORRHOID) – pressure may interfere with normal flow and cause the thin walls of veins to become stretched. The valves then do not close properly and blood seeps back, forming small pools that create varicose veins. When the affected part is elevated higher than the heart, the blood returns with help from the valves, and the veins empty, reducing the swelling.

It is not known why some persons develop varicose veins and others do not, but there are several predisposing factors. The disorder tends to run in families, but whether this is due to an inherited weakness in vein walls or valves or whether it reflects a familial pattern of faulty diet or some other factor is not known. High levels of oestrogen, especially in pregnancy and sometimes those resulting from oral contraceptives, appear to cause varicose veins. The varicose veins of pregnancy, which can affect the vulva as well, tend to appear in the early months and frequently disappear entirely after delivery. They are caused by the pressure of the uterus on femoral veins and the *vena cava*, causing congestion in the lower extremities that is best relieved by lying on one's side, especially the left side. Standing or sitting in one place for a long time also aggravates varicosities, while walking and other movement that activates the calf muscles helps pump blood up toward the heart and decreases the blood volume in the legs. Finally, wearing tight boots, garters, or girdles, and sitting with the legs crossed, all constrict the leg veins and contribute to varicosities. Diet may play a role, for people with high-fibre diets rarely have varicose veins; presumably a low-fibre diet results in hard stools, and the straining needed for a bowel

movement puts enormous pressure on veins of the legs and rectum. Prolonged sitting on the toilet may further aggravate the problem, since this position cuts off circulation from the rectum.

Preventive measures include a high-fibre diet (high in whole grains, raw fruits and vegetables); avoiding overweight; getting adequate leg exercise (walking, jogging, swimming); moving frequently if confined to sitting or standing positions for long period (if standing, try shifting one foot onto a low stool for a time, alternating periodically, or shift weight to toes and then back to heels alternately); wearing elastic support stockings during pregnancy, especially if either of the woman's parents had varicose veins; avoiding garments tight in the groin and leg areas; and lying on one's side whenever possible. Vulvar varicosities are also relieved by applying ice compresses and, when standing, using support from a sanitary pad.

Treatment for varicose veins other than wearing elastic support hose, which eases the discomfort, consists of either injections or surgery. The injections introduce an irritating substance directly into the affected vein, which causes a clot to form and close off that part of the vein. However, a vein so closed often opens up gain. In addition, a severe reaction can occur if any of the injected substance gets into tissues other than the vein. Surgery, called *stripping the veins*, involves threading a wire through the length of the affected vein (through several incisions made at various points on the leg) and removing the entire vein. It is usually done under general anaesthetic and involves little postoperative pain, although elastic support stockings must be worn for several weeks afterward to prevent bleeding and allow for healing. Although this procedure removes the vein or veins affected, the problem may recur in other veins, which subsequently dilate for the same·reasons as those removed did.

Vas deferens   *Vasa deferentia* (pl.). One of a pair of straight tubes, about 45 centimetres (18 inches) long, that transport sperm from each TESTIS to the male urethra (see PENIS). Without them a man is infertile (cannot ejaculate sperm). Surgical severing of both vasa deferentia, called VASECTOMY, is the principal method of male sterilization.

Vasectomy   Also *clipping the cords*. Surgically cutting each VAS DEFERENS, the pair of tubes that carry sperm from each testis, in order to render a man sterile. It is the simplest method of STERILIZATION known and has been performed for more than three centuries. The operation can be performed by a urologist or general surgeon in a hospital or a doctor's surgery, and takes about twenty minutes. Under local anaesthetic a half-inch incision is made on either side of the scrotum, over each vas deferens, though some doctors prefer to make a single incision in the centre. Each vas deferens is pulled out through the incision and a segment of it is removed. The loose ends are then closed with a suture of special metal clips, or are cauterized electrically (burned shut). The skin is closed with one or two absorbable sutures that dissolve in a week or ten days.

Following vasectomy, there is a moderate amount of pain on the day of surgery and sometimes also on the next day. Strenuous physical activity should be avoided for about one week. Wearing an athletic supporter helps prevent swelling over the area. Sexual intercourse can usually be resumed seven days after surgery. However, vasectomy is not a reliable means of contraception until the sperm stored in the upper part of the vas deferens and the seminal vesicles is emptied, which normally requires anywhere from six to fifteen ejaculations. To be absolutely safe, testing of three successive ejaculates should indicate they contain no active sperm.

After vasectomy the testes continue to produce sperm, but at a slower rate, and those that do mature simply disintegrate. The volume of seminal fluid ejaculated changes very little, however, since most of it comes from accessory glands, such as the seminal vesicles and prostate, whose secretions are not cut off. Complications from vasectomy are rare. A man who experiences fever, prolonged or heavy bleeding, or swelling and pain not relieved by applying an ice pack and taking aspirin should contact his surgeon at once, as these may be signs of postoperative infection.

Procedures other than surgery have been used in attempts to close off the vasa deferentia. Among them are the insertion of plugs, valves, and clips of various kinds into each vas deferens to serve as a mechanical barrier, and the injection of various substances into the cavity of each vas deferens in order to produce inflammation and scar tissue that will then close it off. None of these methods is considered as satisfactory as the surgical procedure.

Vasectomy should not be undertaken unless a man is quite sure he wants no more children. Reversing a vasectomy by repairing the cut ends and rejoining them, a procedure called *vasovasotomy*, is much more difficult and has at best a 50 per cent chance of success.

Vaseline   See under LUBRICANT.

Vasomotor instability See HOT FLUSHES.

VD Abbreviation for VENEREAL DISEASE.

Vein One of a system of thin-walled blood vessels that carry blood back to the heart in a steady flow. The veins are often surrounded by muscles. Unlike those of arteries (see ARTERY) their walls are not muscular enough to provide a pumping action to keep blood moving through them, and most of the blood returning to the heart must flow against the force of gravity. At least three factors play a part in maintaining blood flow through the veins. Many veins are provided with one-way valves, which permit the blood to move freely toward the heart but close to prevent movement in the opposite direction. Also, the pressure of blood behind the blood in the veins helps move it along. Finally, the usual activity of the body causes the contraction of muscles, which press against the veins and force blood toward the heart.

The most common diseases affecting the veins are VARICOSE VEINS, in which pressure causes a part of the thin wall to balloon out so that blood can pool there, and PHLEBITIS.

Venereal disease Also *VD, sexually transmitted disease, STD.* Infections that are, for the most part, transmitted by sexual contact between two persons. Despite the development of powerful new antibacterial agents during the second half of the 20th century, the incidence of certain venereal diseases—especially gonorrhoea and genital herpes infection—has been increasing in most developed countries at an alarming rate. An estimated 10 million cases of venereal disease were being diagnosed each year in the United States by 1981. Most venereal diseases attack the genital-urinary tract, with which the infecting organisms orginally come in contact, but some, notably gonorrhoea and syphilis, can attack and damage other organs, such as the heart. The principal venereal diseases are GONORRHOEA, SYPHILIS, HERPES INFECTION, CHANCROID, PUBIC LICE, LYMPHOGRANULOMA VENEREUM, GRANULOMA INGUINALE, and CONDYLOMA ACUMINATA. It is possible to be infected with more than one of them (for example, gonorrhoea and syphilis) at the same time. In addition TRICHOMONAS, nonspecific URETHRITIS, nonspecific VAGINITIS, and CYSTITIS all may be transmitted by sexual contact.

Because venereal disease is associated with sexual promiscuity (relations with many different partners), a sense of shame, embarrassment, and other feelings resulting from religious and cultural taboos often prevent its early detection and treatment. Furthermore, some of the venereal diseases, notably gonorrhoea, can be virtually without symptoms in one partner (here, the woman), who then unwittingly continues to pass on the infection. As with most infectious diseases, prevention is the best control. Measures tht may reduce the chances of infection, especially if used in combination, are:

For men: 1 Use of a condom during vaginal and anal intercourse. 2 Washing the genitals before and, even more important, right after sex, with soap and water.

For women: Use of a diaphragm with spermicidal jelly, cream, or foam, and use of these spermicides in the anus for anal intercourse. If no diaphragm is available, use of spermicides alone.

320 Veneral disease - Virginity

For both sexes, selectivity of choice in sex partners is a preventive measure; the more different partners one has, the higher the risk of infection. If one is sexually active with several partners and has any reason to suspect exposure to infection, a VD test is recommended every three to six months.

Suspicious signs on one's own body or one's partner's include sores, redness, unusual discharge, itchiness, or a foul smell in the genital area. Should these be present, either avoid sexual relations until they have been checked or at least be sure of protection with a condom and/or diaphragm and spermicides. Although spermicidal jellies, creams, and foams do kill some venereal disease organisms, oral contraceptives do not (some authorities believe they may even create a favourable environment for gonococcus growth), and use of an IUD may increase the risk of gonorrhoeal infections.

Version Turning, a term used for repositioning a foetus inside the uterus, either by manipulating the mother's abdomen from the outside, before labour has begun (*external version*), or using either the hands or instruments during labour, while the foetus still is in the uterus but the cervix is completely dilated (*internal version*).

Vertex See under CEPHALIC PRESENTATION.

Vestibule The boat-shaped female genital area surrounded by the LABIA minora (inner lips), extending from the clitoris to the point where the labia majora (outer lips) join. It contains four openings: the urethra, vagina, and the ducts of the two BARTHOLIN'S GLANDS (also called *vestibular glands*). Under the mucous membrane on each side of the vestibule are the *vestibular bulbs*, two clusters of veins about 3 to 4 centimetres (1.5 inches) long and about 1 centimetre (0.4 inch) wide. During sexual arousal these veins fill with blood, becoming congested and firm to the touch. (Also see drawing under VULVA.)

Viable Capable of surviving. The term is usually used for premature babies, those of less than twenty-four to twenty-eight weeks' gestation rarely being mature enough to survive.

Virginity The condition of a woman, called a *virgin*, who has never engaged in vaginal intercourse. In cultures where women are considered the personal property of their husbands, or in patrilineal societies, where property and authority are passed on from a father to his children, virginity is an important concept because it allegedly ensures that the husband is the first person to have vaginal intercourse with his wife and definitely establishes the paternity of her first child. Evidence of virginity traditionally was an intact HYMEN and, physically speaking, a woman is a virgin until her hymen is broken. However, the hymen can be ruptured by many means other than penile penetration, such as a tampon or physical exercise of various kinds, so virginity in this sense has largely lost its meaning. Moreover, a virgin *can* become pregnant although it does not happen often; sperm deposited on the outer genitals (the vulva) sometimes does move into the vagina and upward to fertilize an egg. In the sense of never having experienced vaginal intercourse, the old meaning of virginity persists, but since the widespread availability of birth control measures has engendered greater sexual freedom (at least in the Western world), the concept has lost much of its former significance.

Vitamin A group of nutrient chemicals that are considered essential to good health. Chemically they can be divided into two groups: the fat-soluble vitamins, A, D, E, and K, which tend to be stored in the body; and the water-soluble vitamins, the B-group and C, which except for vitamin B_{12} are not stored in the body and need frequent replenish-

ment. All of them are needed, although their mode of action is not precisely understood, and all of them are available in a wide variety of ordinary foods. Deficient vitamin intake leads to specific symptoms and diseases. Overdoses of certain vitamins, particular of the fat-soluble ones, can also make a person ill. Certain of the vitamins have a close connection to women's health. The B vitamins, especially folic acid (or folacin), are important in pregnancy, and pregnant women may need supplements of them.

Front view of vulva

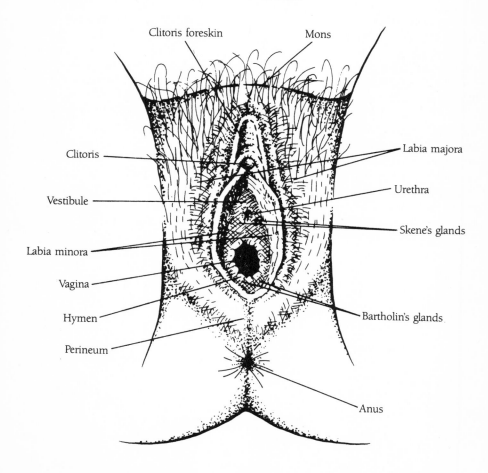

Body levels of vitamin B$_6$, folic acid, and vitamin C all seem to be decreased by taking oral contraceptives; possibly higher hormone levels decrease the body's absorption of these vitamins. Vitamin E has been found helpful by some women in relieving the HOT FLUSHES of menopause. Vitamin D, which aids calcium absorption, is thought to be particularly important for women after menopause to help prevent bone loss (see OSTEOPOROSIS). See the tables on pages 323-24, also see DIET.

Vomiting See under NAUSEA; MORNING SICKNESS.

Vulva Also *pudenda, external genitalia*. The external visible female organs of reproduction, which include the MONS VENERIS (or pubis), LABIA majora and minora (outer and inner lips), CLITORIS, VESTIBULE, opening of the URETHRA, INTROITUS (opening of the vagina), HYMEN, and BARTHOLIN'S GLANDS (also called vulvovaginal glands). See also PERINEUM. The vulva is subject to a number of disorders, the most serious of which are cancer and the various infections transmitted by sexual contact (see CANCER, VULVAR; VENEREAL DISEASE). See also VULVITIS.

Vulvectomy See under CANCER, VULVAR.

Vulvitis An inflammation or infection of the VULVA. A common cause is *contact dermatitis*, whose chief symptoms are redness, burning or itching, labial swelling, and clear blisters that eventually drain and crust over. It can be caused by soap or detergents, bubble bath, condoms, a douche, vaginal foam or other sprays, sanitary towels, or clothing. Vulvitis can result from an allergic reaction to antibiotics or other drugs taken internally. It may also be the result of an infection with PUBIC LICE ('crabs'), a HERPES INFECTION, or a vaginal infection or discharge. Treatment is chiefly palliative: sitz baths or compresses to relieve inflammation, anti-histamines and topical cortisone creams to relieve itching, and loose clothing (or better, none, since the air helps heal the condition). Meanwhile the cause should be determined and eliminated. A discharge should be checked for infectious organisms, and any suspicious lesions should be examined to make sure they are not precancerous or malignant (see CANCER, VULVA). For herbal remedies to relieve itching, see under VAGINITIS.

Principal Vitamins

Vitamin	Chief food sources	Needed for	Effects of lack / overdose	Recommended daily allowance*
A	Fish liver oils, liver, egg yolk, butter, cream, green leafy and yellow vegetables	Light reception of retina; functioning of epithelial tissue	Lack: nightblindness, drying of eye tissue, disease of cornea. Overdose: headache; skin peeling; enlargement of liver and spleen	I: 1500 i.u. C: 1000–1915 i.u. A: 2415–2500 i.u. W.O: 2500 i.u. P: 2500 i.u. L: 4000 i.u.
D	Fish liver oils, butter, egg yolk, liver; ultra-violet rays (sunlight)	Calcium and phosphorus absorption; bone calcification	Lack: rickets, softening of bone. Overdose: appetite loss; kidney failure; calcium deposits	I: 300 iu. C: 400 iu. A.W.O: 400 iu. P: 400 iu. L: 400 iu.
E	Vegetable oils, wheat germ, leafy vegetables, egg yolk, margarine, legumes	Biochemical action on cells and tissues; possible influence on various hormones	Lack: breakdown of red blood cells; muscle degeneration	I: 4–5 iu* C: 7–10 iu. A.W.O: 12 iu. P.L.: 15 iu.
K	Leafy vegetables, pork, liver, vegetable oils	Normal blood clotting	Lack: haemorrhage. Overdose: kernicterus (nerve disorder, high bilirubin levels in blood)	I: 20–20 mcg* C: 15–60 mcg A: 50–100 mcg W.O: 70–140 mcg
B₁ (thiamine)	Dried yeast, whole grains, pork, liver, other meat, enriched cereals, nuts, legumes, potatoes	Carbohydrate metabolism, nerve cell function, heart function	Lack: beriberi (disorder affecting heart and nervous system)	I: 03 mg C: 04–08 mg A: 08–09 mg W: 09–1.0 mg O: 08 mg P: 1.0 mg L: 1.1 mg
B₂ (Riboflavin)	Milk, cheese, liver, meat, eggs, enriched cereals	Protein metabolism, maintenance of nervous system, healthy skin and eyes, disease resistance	Lack: mouth, eye, skin, and genital lesions	I: 0.4 mg C: 06–1.2 mg A: 1.4–1.7 mg W.O: 1.3 mg P: 1.6 mg L: 1.8 mg
niacin (nicotinic acid, niacinamide)	Dried yeast, liver, meat, fish legumes, whole grain enriched cereals	Healthy cell metabolism; monitors cholesterol metabolism; affects metabolic rate and temperature	Lack: pellagra (disorder affecting skin, digestive tract, central nervous system)	I: 5 mg C: 7–14 mg A: 16–19 mg W.O: 15 mg P: 18 mg L: 21 mg

Principal Vitamins

Vitamin	Chief food sources	Needed for	Effects of lack / overdose	Recommended daily allowance*
B₆ (pyridoxine)	Dried yeast, liver, organ meats, whole grain cereals, fish, legumes	Healthy cell function and metabolism of amino acids and fatty acids	*Lack*: convulsions in infants; skin and nervous system disorders; mental retardation	I: 0.3–0.6 mg* C: 0.9–1.6 mg A: 1.8–2.0 mg W,O: 2.0 mg P,L: 2.5–2.6 mg
folic acid (folacin)	Fresh green leafy vegetables, fruit, organ meats, liver, dried yeast	Healthy red blood cells and synthesis of needed compounds	*Lack*: anaemia and other blood disorders; infertility; gastrointestinal disorders; may be responsible for eclampsia, miscarriage, abruptio placentae in pregnant women	I: 30–45 mcg** C: 100–300 mcg A,W,O: 400 mcg P: 800 mcg L: 500 mcg
B₁₂ (cobalamin)	Liver, beef, pork, organ meats, eggs, milk, milk products	Healthy red blood cells, nerve cell function; synthesis of DNA, enzyme synthesis	*Lack*: pernicious anaemia, other anaemias; some psychiatric disorders, dim vision	I: 0.5–1.5 mcg*** C: 2.0–3.0 mcg A,W,O: 3.0 mcg P,L: 4.0 mcg
pantothenic acid	Meat, chicken, milk, eggs, peanuts, peas, broccoli	Synthesis of several hormones, including progesterone	*Lack*: neuromotor, cardiovascular, and digestive disorders	I: 2–3 mg* C: 3–5 mg A,W,O,P,L: 4–7 mg
C (ascorbic acid)	Citrus fruits, tomatoes, potatoes, cabbage, green peppers	Healthy bone and connective tissue; circulatory function; wound healing	*Lack*: scurvy (haemorrhage, loose teeth, gum disease)	I: 20 mg C: 20–25 mg A: 25–30 mg W,O: 30 mg P: 60 mg L: 60 mg
P (C-complex, Citrus bioflavonoids, Rutin, Hesperidin)	White skin and segment part of fruit and some vegetables	Not known	*Lack*: fragile capillaries	Not known

*The allowances suggested are based on those recommended in 1980 by the Food and Nutrition Board, National Academy of Sciences—National Research Council. They are expressed in I.U. (International Units) or mg (milligrams) or mcg (micrograms). Where different amounts are recommended for different age groups, the following abbreviations mean: *I* – infants up to 12 months; *C* – children aged 1 to 10; *A* – adolescent girls aged 11 to 18; *W* – women aged 19 to 50; *O* – women over 50; *P* – pregnant women; *L* – breast-feeding women. UK RDAs are taken from Recommended Daily Amounts of Food Energy and Nutrients for Groups of People in the United Kingdom. Department of Health and Social Security Report on Health and Social Subjects 15 (1979). Those for folic acid and vitamin B₁₂ are taken from the Food Labelling Regulations S.I. No 1305, 1984.

*These figures are US RDAs. The UK authorities make no recommendations.

**These figures are US RDAs. The UK authorities suggest an overall figure of 300 mcg with no breakdown into age groups.

***These figures are US RDAs. The UK authorities suggest an overall figure of 2 mcg with no breakdown into age groups.

W

Warts, vulvo-vagina, anal See under CONDYLOMA ACUMINATA.

Wassermann test See under SYPHILIS.

Water retention See OEDEMA.

Weight, body Charts for desirable body weight, relative to height and general body frame, are widely available. In most advanced countries of the world where food is available, exceeding one's ideal weight is far more common a problem than underweight. *Weight loss*, unless it can be accounted for by increase in physical activity and decrease in food intake, may be symptomatic of numerous disorders – some of them serious ones – and warrants a thorough physical check-up. More often, however, it is increasing weight that women find troublesome. Except when it is caused by oedema (fluid retention), undesired weight gain is nearly always the result of overeating. See ANOREXIA NERVOSA; BIRTH WEIGHT; CRITICAL WEIGHT; DIET; OBESITY; WEIGHT GAIN.

Weight gain
  1 **Premenstrual** Many women regularly gain several pounds during the week preceding their menstrual period. This gain is nearly always the result of fluid retention (sometimes combined with constipation) and somewhat increased appetite, and disappears during the first few days of menstrual flow. (See also DYSMENORRHOEA, definition 5.) The same phenomenon may occur in women taking oral contraceptives, that is, the higher hormone levels seem to cause fluid retention and sometimes increased appetite, manifested in weight gain.
  2 **In pregnancy** Weight gain is both normal and necessary during pregnancy. From the 1930s to the early 1960s women frequently were advised to limit their weight gain during pregnancy to ten to fifteen pounds, in the belief that it would ease labour and delivery, prevent hypertension and preeclampsia, and help maintain an attractive figure. However, some investigators began to observe that the salt-poor, often protein-deficient diets used to restrict weight gain in pregnancy could actually be harmful, producing smaller, less healthy babies and increasing the risk to mothers. Most doctors now advise women that total weight gain of twenty-four to twenty-seven pounds during pregnancy is normal, and somewhat more than that also is not harmful. Some authorities believe that the time of weight gain also is important, recommending a gain of 1½ to 3 pounds during the first trimester, and approximately 1 pound every nine days thereafter (or 5 pounds the first trimester and 10 pounds each for the second and third). To some extent what is considered a desirable

weight gain depends on whether a woman is thin or fat before pregnancy. However, even a heavy woman should not attempt a weight-reduction diet during pregnancy, lest she deprive the foetus of needed nutrients. If she needs to lose weight, it is advisable to wait until delivery. (See also BIRTH WEIGHT; DIET).

3 **In menopause** Ideally a woman should weigh the same at menopause (average age, fifty) as her ideal weight at the age of twenty. Most women, however, tend to weigh considerably more. By the age of forty-five metabolism slows down, and only two-thirds the number of calories needed to maintain the same weight are required. After menopause another portion of the total calorie intake, which formerly supported an active reproductive system is no longer needed. Furthermore, women tend to become less physically active as they get older. Therefore, unless food intake is reduced accordingly, the unneeded calories will turn into extra body weight. Apart from being unattractive, obesity after menopause greatly increases the risk of developing serious disease, specifically arteriosclerosis and coronary heart disease, hypertension (high blood pressure), and diabetes. The moderately active menopausal woman needs approximately 14 calories per pound of body weight per day to *maintain* her weight; any calories in excess will most likely be stored as fat. See also DIET; OBESITY.

Wet smear A simple test of vaginal discharge to determine the cause of a vaginal infection, usually performed in the doctor's surgery. The doctor places a small specimen of the discharge on a slide, adds a solution of either salt or potassium hydroxide (depending on which organism is suspected), and examines the slide under a microscope. He or she can then see if the organism is *Trichomonas, Candida (Monilia) albicans,* or *Haemophilus vaginalis* (see also TRICHOMONAS; YEAST INFECTION; VAGINITIS). A wet smear cannot, however, rule out GONORRHOEA.

Withdrawal See COITUS INTERRUPTUS.

Withdrawal bleeding See under OESTROGEN; OESTROGEN REPLACEMENT THERAPY.

Womb See UTERUS.

Women's doctor See GYNAECOLOGIST.

XYZ

Xerography Also *xeroradiography, xero-mammography.* See under MAMMOGRAPHY.

Yeast infection Also *Candida albicans, Monilia albicans, moniliasis, candidiasis, fungus, vaginal thrush, vaginal mycosis, mycotic vaginitis.* One of the most common vaginal infections, caused by a yeastlike fungus called *Candida (Monilia albicans.* The main symptoms are severe vaginal and vulvar itching, and a white, cheesy discharge with a sweetish odour. The organism normally resides in the vagina of most women and gives rise to symptoms only when it multiplies more than usual. Pregnancy and oral contraceptives, which both raise oestrogen levels, may cause such an increase, as can an increase in blood sugar, antibiotic therapy, faecal contamination (by wiping from back to front after a bowel movement), or transmission from a sex partner. Some 15 to 25 per cent of women are troubled with yeast infection during pregnancy. An increase in oestrogen causes increased glycogen deposits in the walls of the vagina, making a hospitable environment for the fungus to multiply. Treatment is with local applications of a fungicidal antibiotic called nystatin, in the form of a cream or vaginal suppositories, miconazole cream, or clotrimazole vaginal tablets or cream. Alternatively, propion gel or gentian violet suppositories may also be effective, but these stain clothing. All these medications must be used for at least ten days, and sometimes longer.

A remedy found effective by some women is eating yoghrt, which suppresses the growth of fungi in the intestinal tract. It also sometimes is effective when applied locally spooned into the vagina or inserted with an applicator of the kind used for spermicides. Acidophilus capsules inserted as a vaginal suppository may have a similar effect, as may daily douches with diluted yoghurt (used for a week). Only 'natural', unpasteurized yoghurt (made at home or available in health-food shops) can be effective, because it contains live lactobacilli, which help break down the sugar of cervical discharge into lactic acid and therefore help combat the growth of organisms whose growth is encouraged by sugar. Ultrapasteurized yoghurt does not contain live lactobacilli. However, the effectiveness of yoghurt has not been documented sufficiently to recommend it with any certainty; it appears to work for some women and not for others. Also, it is not known whether it is the lactobacilli or the acidity of yoghurt that is effective; if it is the latter, vinegar douches are simpler (see below). Other home remedies include applying a poultice of natural (unpasteurized) cottage cheese on a sanitary pad, which also helps relieve itching, and douching one a day with an acidic douche (juice of half a lemon, *or* 2 tablespoons vinegar, *or* 1 teaspoon vitamin C powder, mixed in one pint of water), to make the vaginal environment more acid and less hospitable to yeast organisms. Some women find relief by using boric acid (600 milligrams in a size 0 gelatin capsule), inserting a capsule once a day for one week, and then twice a week for the next three weeks. Some doctors warn that placing unpasteurized milk products in the vagina puts a woman at risk for becoming a carrier of an organism called listeria, which in pregnancy can infect the foetus, leading to stillbirth, and cause premature labour and meningitis in the mother.

Yoghurt A dairy product that is slightly acidic and, in unpasteurized form, contains live lactobacilli, which are thought to help combat YEAST INFEC-TION. Yoghurt is also an excellent source of dietary calcium.

Zygote Also *fertilized egg*. The single cell that results from the mating of a male germ cell, or sperm, with a female germ cell, or egg (ovum), before it begins to divide (grow). It is not known exactly when the human zygote begins to divide, but it is believed to occur approximately thirty hours after FERTILIZATION, well before IMPLANTATION. Thereafter some authorities call it the EMBRYO while others use the term 'egg' (or 'ovum') for four more weeks, until organ development begins.

Subject index

This index is devised to help readers find the principal entries on a larger subject. Only the main entries are listed; where the entry consists only of a cross-reference – for example, Pill, see ORAL CONTRACEPTIVES – it is not listed in this index.

The subjects listed are:

abortion
adolescence
birth control and sterilization
breast disease
cancer
chronic disease and disability
diagnostic tests and procedures
drugs and medications
heredity and birth defects
hormones
infertility
menopause
menstruation
mental health
nutrition
pregnancy and childbirth
sexuality
venereal disease

Abortion
abortifacient 9
abortion 10
amnioinfusion 21
D and C (dilatation and curettage) 91
D and E (dilatation and evacuation) 92
hysterotomy 161
septic abortion 277
vacuum aspiration, definition 2 311

Adolescence
acne 13
adolescent nodule 15
age, childbearing 16
amenorrhoea 18
athletic ability, women's 35
critical weight 83
diet 99
growth and development 138
menarche 197
precocious puberty 250
puberty 260
scoliosis 275
secondary sex characteristics 277

Birth control and sterilization
abortion 10
barrier methods 37
basal body temperature 37
birth control 41
cervical cap 66
cervical mucus method 67
coitus interruptus 75
condom 76
contraceptive 79
culdoscopy 84
diaphragm 97

premature 254
prepared childbirth 255
primigravida 256
primipara 256
prolapsed cord 256
prolonged labour 257
psychoprophylactic childbirth 258
puerperal fever 262
puerperium 262
quickening 265
Rh factor 272
ripe cervix 272
rubella 273
scopolamine 277
sex, determination of 278
shoulder presentation 281
Sims position 282
spinal anaesthesia 287
stillbirth 288
superfecundation 289
superfoetation 289
test-tube baby 296
threatened miscarriage 297
transition 300
trimester 301
umbilical cord 305
uterus 308
vacuum extractor 312
varicose veins 316
version 320
viable 320
weight gain, definition 1 325
zygote 328

Sexuality
anus 30
apocrine gland 31
bisexual 45
chastity 70
clitoris 74
coitus 74
cunnilingus 85

defloration 93
dyspareunia 109
ejaculation 113
erection 118
fellatio 122
frigidity 130
gender identity 132
hermaphroditism 146
heterosexual 149
homosexual 151
hymen 154
impotence 163
incest 164
intercourse, sexual 168
lesbian 182
libido 183
masturbation 196
oral sex 229
orgasm 230
penis 241
sex therapy 278
sexual dysfunction 279
sexual response 279
transsexual 300
virginity 320

Venereal disease (sexually transmitted disease)
bubo 53
chancre 69
chancroid 69
condyloma acuminata 77
gonorrhoea 135
Haemophilus vaginalis 142
herpes infection 147
lymphogranuloma venereum 186
nit 219
pubic lice 261
syphilis 291
trichomonas 300
urethritis 306
vaginitis 314
venereal disease 319

Alternative health care for women

A woman's guide to self-help treatments and alternative therapies

More women than men visit the doctor, either for themselves or for their families' health care. They well know the trials of long waiting lists for operations or, for more everyday problems, the hours spent waiting for attention in the doctor's surgery. But the recent rebirth of interest in alternative medicine has at last provided a new option, and it is one in which women in particular have found both comfort and freedom.

Patsy Westcott has compiled an invaluable guide to the scope of treatment options that are attuned especially to the health and welfare of women. Individual problems and therapies are dealt with in a clear and concise manner; checklists and questionnaires provide a practical self-help method of determining what is right for *you*; and the focus throughout is the holistic view of health, which regards mental and physical well-being as part of an overall approach to wellness as a natural way of life.